DIGESTIVE DISEASES - RESEARCH AND CLINICAL DEVELOPMENTS

DISORDERS OF GASTROINTESTINAL SYSTEMS AND CLINICAL MANIFESTATIONS

DIGESTIVE DISEASES - RESEARCH AND CLINICAL DEVELOPMENTS

Additional books in this series can be found on Nova's website under the Series tab.

Additional e-books in this series can be found on Nova's website under the eBooks tab.

DIGESTIVE DISEASES - RESEARCH AND CLINICAL DEVELOPMENTS

DISORDERS OF GASTROINTESTINAL SYSTEMS AND CLINICAL MANIFESTATIONS

SENTHILKUMAR RAJAGOPAL, PHD
SENGOTTUVELAN MURUGAN, PHD
AND
SARAVANAN RAMACHANDRAN, PHD
EDITORS

NOVA BIOMEDICAL
New York

Library of Congress Cataloging-in-Publication Data

ISBN: 978-1-63485-366-8

Library of Congress Control Number: 2016940560

Published by Nova Science Publishers, Inc. † New York

CONTENTS

ACKNOWLEDGMENTS

We would like to express our gratitude to our contributors for sharing their mastery of knowledge to provide evidence-based information on *"Disorders of Gastrointestinal systems and Clinical Manifestations."*

We wish to personally thank the writers for their contributions to our inspiration and knowledge and other help in creating this book.

We are very grateful to our families for their understanding, unrelenting support and encouragement allowing us to spend extra time on completing the book in specified time.

The support provided by the Department of Biotechnology, Ministry of Science and Technology, Government of India (To Dr. Senthilkumar Rajagopal – No: BT/RLF/Re-entry/42/2012) to complete this book in a successful manner is gratefully acknowledged.

We wanted to drop a note to say thanks to the staff of Nova Publishers for their patience and assistance at various stages of the book publication.

Dr. Senthilkumar Rajagopal, PhD
Dr. Sengottuvelan Murugan, PhD
Dr. Saravanan Ramachandran, PhD

FOREWORD A

I am pleased to write a foreword for the book entitled "Disorders of Gastrointestinal Systems and Clinical Manifestations" edited by *Dr. Senthilkumar Rajagopal, Dr. Sengottuvelan Murugan and Dr. Saravanan Ramachandran* and published by Nova Publications, USA. The editors have an expertise in the gastrointestinal system and their disorders and the authors have expertise in oxidative stress, Clinical manifestations of GI tract disorders, inflammatory pathogenesis and other important fields of gastrointestinal system that is evident from their reputed publications. The book discusses comprehensively and succinctly about the gastrointestinal malabsorption, impact of alcohol in the GI tract, gall bladder diseases, role of enzymes on GI tract, flavones in gastro protection and etc.,

I am having 25 years of experience and expertise in handling multidisciplinary R&D programmes in the areas of environment and resources assessment, policy development and multilateral agreements at the National, Regional (South Asia Cooperative Environment Programme) and Global levels (Commission for Conservation of Antarctic Marine Living Resources). During April 1989, he joined as a Research Assistant in Ministry of Environment and Forests, New Delhi and was promoted to Research Officer in 1993. In 1994, I have joined as Senior Scientific Officer at Ministry of Earth Sciences (MoES), erstwhile called "Department of Ocean Development (DOD)" and associated in implementation of various nationally coordinated research programmes, *viz.*, (i) Coastal Ocean Monitoring and Prediction System (COMAPS); (ii) Integrated Coastal and Marine Area Management (ICMAM); (iii) Assessment of Marine Living Resources (MLR); and (iv) Development of potential drugs from ocean (Drugs from sea). I was the Director at the Centre for Marine Living Resources and Ecology (CMLRE), Kochi, before joining ICMAM-PD. I have provided intellectual leadership for successful implementation of R&D activities in the field of marine sciences.

This book also has contributions from eminent professors, scientists and researchers working in the field of GI tract and their complications who have provided a comprehensive and updated review of their respective topics. The elaborated description in chapters will enhance the understanding of GI biology, which will help the readers to gain an in-depth and latest development in the field of Nanotechnology in GI biology. The better understanding of regulation of oxidative stress can be utilized for devising strategies for development of novel therapeutic preparations for clinical interventions in oxidative stress and pathogenesis induced GI disorders. I am certain that the readers including faculties, researchers and students will find this book extremely informative, interesting and inspiring. Hence, I hope that you will find this book possesses sufficient disclosure and adequate utility.

Since there are not sufficient books available in this virgin area, this book may serve you to interact and improve the reader's mental horizon for better understanding among physiologists, chemists, biologist and medical practitioner.

With best wishes.

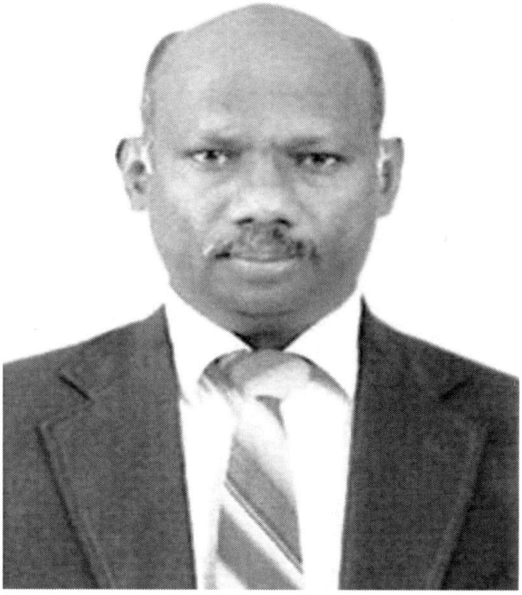

Dr. P. Madeswaran, PhD
Scientist F
Integrated Coastal and Marine Area Management - Project Directorate (ICMAM-PD)
Ministry of Earth Sciences (MoES)
Chennai, India

FOREWORD B

I am honored to write a foreword for the book entitled "*Disorders of Gastrointestinal Systems and Clinical Manifestations,*" the classic book that has lead its leadership position and enhanced its reputation in its field, edited by, *Dr. Senthilkumar Rajagopal, Dr. Sengottuvelan Murugan* and *Dr. Saravanan Ramachandran.* Knowledge and efforts in gastrointestinal physiology field are constantly changing. As new research and experience broaden our knowledge, changes in practice, treatment and drug therapy may become necessary or appropriate. A book differs in important ways from a journal. This book is an important publication and the time for it has come. The extraordinary effort required to create a book that comprehensively and authoritatively presents the state of knowledge in an arena as broad and ever expanding as gastroenterology is a taunting task.

I am currently working as an Associate Professor of Biology in National Institute of Science Education and Research (NISER), India. Before joining NISER, I was working as scientist and project leader of Bovine Enteric Disease group at the Vaccine and Infectious Disease Organization, Canada. Currently I am working on gut microbiome, probiotics and psychological stress. I am having over 12 years of experience in this area and find the current content of the book is of high value and importance for researchers and students in the field.

The continuing development of new and improved techniques of GI Physiology has to match changes in other fields. Of course, one would expect all of the "usual" chapters to be present, and the reader will not be disappointed. It is difficult to see what might be missing. I certainly could not find anything important which had been omitting. The images are well chosen and superbly produced. This book also addressed include the function, morphology, regulation, motility, secretion, digestion, absorption, transport, metabolism, immunology, and development of the gastrointestinal tract as well as the role of liver, intestinal micro flora, and dietary fiber in nutrient delivery.

Since there are not many books in these subjects, this book may also serve to start more initiatives for a closer cooperation between physiologists, chemists, biologist and medical practitioner.

With best regards,

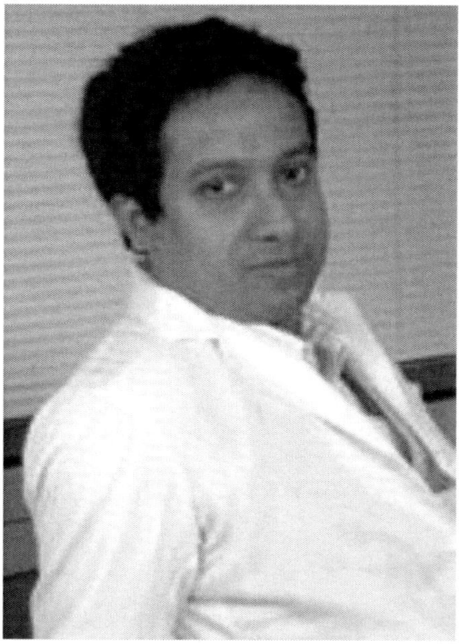

Palok Aich, PhD,
Associate Professor (G), School of Biological Sciences,
FIC/Dean, International Affairs and Resource Planning; Estate, Maintenance, Works and Library
Chairperson, Institute Works Committee and Library Advisory Committee
National Institute of Science Education and Research (NISER),
PO- Bhimpur-Padanpur, Via-Jatni,
District- Khurda, PIN- 752050, Odisha, India
e-mail: palok.aich@niser.ac.in
URL: http://www.niser.ac.in/~palok.aich/

FOREWORD C

It is great pleasure to write the foreword for a book "Disorders of Gastrointestinal Systems and Clinical Manifestations" compiled by Dr. Senthilkumar Rajagopal, Dr. Sengottuvelan Murugan and Dr. Saravanan Ramachandran and published by Nova Publications, USA. I realized that this book contained a useful solution for the dietary treatment of many gastrointestinal disorders. Thus, this comprehensive book, which is unique in that no other scientific text has devoted itself to the presentation of GI tract disorders and their treatment, is timely and highly welcome.

I obtained the doctoral degree from one of the prestigious universities of the world-Banaras Hindu University in Biochemistry. I have accumulated over 30 years of research experience in the field of cancer research, inflammation and recombinant immunology. Currently, I am privileged to lead the operations of Rx Biosciences, Ltd as its Chief Executive Officer. For last 12 years, the company has been involved in multidimensional research activities, particularly in the field of molecular biology. One of the main objectives of the company includes the discovery of new drug targets and therapeutic agents for the diseases of great public significance such as prostate cancer and Alzheimer's disease (AD). We are actively engaged in collaboration with leading pharmaceutical companies and federal government organizations within USA such as FDA, USDA and DOD. I have authored many peer reviewed scientific articles for International Journals and presented the finding in many national and international conferences. I have lead grant proposals awarded by National Cancer Institute, USA. Additionally, I have been on the reviewer's panel for National Institute of Health (NIH) along with some international scientific journals. Throughout most of my academic career, I have been ranked at the top, received prestigious honors and distinctions. I was awarded with a gold medal for ranking at the top in BS examination in the university. With all my academic achievements and professional expertise I feel very comfortable in writing about the book and would like to thank the authors for making a sincere effort to contribute in the well being of mankind.

The authors all, experts and pioneers in their field, provide both clinicians and basic scientists with an understanding of GI tract disorders, the mechanisms that govern cell and tissue responses, the methodology of treatment delivery, treatment outcomes, advantages over other treatment approaches, and potential pitfalls. It is evident that GI tract has made significant progress both in the basic understanding of mechanisms and clinical applications. The appearance of this authoritative text could not come at a more opportune time to put the spotlight on this promising gastric cancer treatment modality. It is hoped that this book will help people with GI tract disorders, especially the small intestinal and help bring it to universal approval as a treatment of choice. With the help of the chapters contributors,' drawn from India and USA, they have produced a text which is not only the first of its kind but one which I would rate as the most informed, the clearest the most up to date and indeed the best currently available in the world literature. The book is divided into 17 detailed chapters each of which is well planned, clearly written and illustrated and rounded off with comprehensive bibliography, so that more than thousands references are referred to in the text. This book will have a wide appeal to those working in many scientific and medical disciplines. The graduate and undergraduate scientific students will find sufficient breadth of knowledge and bibliography in each chapter to inform them of the basic mechanisms as they relate to GI tract deregulations.

Sincerely,

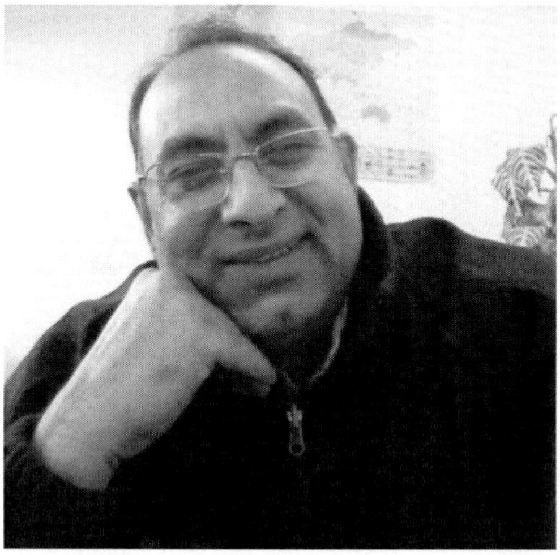

Qazi A. Hamid, Ph.D.,
Chief Executive Officer,
Rx Biosciences, Ltd.,
18908 Bonanza Way,
Gaithersburg,
Maryland 20879 USA.

ABOUT THE EDITORS

Dr. Senthilkumar Rajagopal

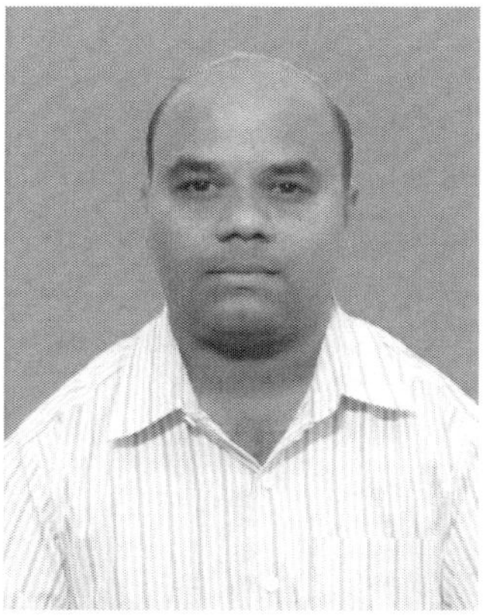

Dr. Senthilkumar Rajagopal, PhD., is a Scientist at Rayalaseema University, Kurnool, AP, India and secured his PhD in Biochemistry from Annamalai University, INDIA. He did his three Post-doctoral researches in Anesthesiology in University of Virginia, Charlottesville, Virginia, followed by Department of Cancer Immunology and AIDS, Dana Farber Cancer Institute, Harvard University, Boston, Massachusetts and, Department of Physiology and Biophysics, Virginia Commonwealth University, Richmond, Virginia, USA. Dr. Rajagopal is a recipient of Rameshwardasji Birla Smarak Kosh Endowment award from Mumbai Medical Trust, Mumbai, INDIA and Ramalingaswami Re-entry Fellowship from Department of Biotechnology, Ministry of Science and Technology, Government of India. Dr. Rajagopal has more than 10 years of research experiences in various fields such as Alcoholic hepatotoxicity, Voltage gated calcium channels, and protein kinase C phosphorylation, ADAM family, Smooth muscle physiology, G-protein coupled receptor signaling pathways, Neurotransmitters transporters to Central Nervous system.

He has published nearly 45 research articles in various peer-reviewed international journals, 14 book chapters, 7 abstracts, and 42 conferences proceedings/abstracts and attended various workshops/seminars in India, Canada and USA. He is on the editorial/reviewer board in 20 peer-reviewed international journals such as Frontiers in Cellular Neuroscience, American Journal of Biochemistry and Molecular Biology, Neuroscience, etc. He has reviewed and screened the abstracts for numerous years for National Biotechnology Conferences and Annual Biomedical Research Conference for Minority Students (ABRCMS), Reviewer for Science and Engineering Research Board (SERB), India and also served the special judge for Biophysical Society award at Virginia Piedmont Regional Science Fair-2011. He has a life member of well-known scientific associations like Indian Society for Atherosclerosis Research (ISAR), The International Science Congress Association (ISCA), Society of Biological Chemistry (SBC), Society for Free Radical Research India (SFRR), The Indian Society of Cell Biology (ISCB) and member of American Association of Pharmaceutical Scientists (AAPS) and Science Advisory Board (SAB). He conducts research in the area of G-protein coupled receptor mediated intracellular mechanisms by Alcohol-induced digestive disorders in the gastrointestinal tract. Currently, he is mentoring graduate students and having research projects from various funding agencies of Government of India.

Email: senthilanal@yahoo.com.

Dr. Sengottuvelan Murugan

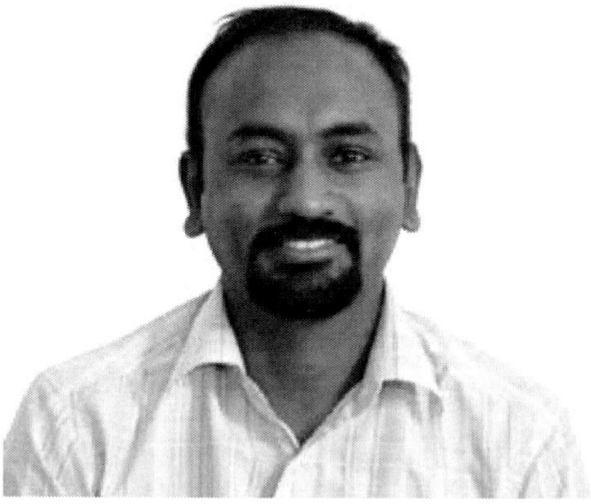

Dr. Sengottuvelan Murugan, M. Phil, Ph.D., earned his PhD in Biochemistry in November 2006 from Annamalai University, India.

Dr. Murugan began his career in cancer research, when he joined the PhD program (graduate) and he was the first recipient of a Lady Tata Memorial Trust (LTMT) Senior Research Fellowship (SRF) at Department of Biochemistry and Biotechnology, Annamalai University, for the full two years (2003-2005). After his PhD, his novel research theme was approved and he was awarded with a prestigious Japan Society for the Promotion of Science (JSPS) Postdoctoral Fellowship for foreign researchers to conduct research at Hokkaido University, Sapporo, Japan. There, Dr. Murugan was appointed as a co-investigator for one of the project funded by INSA (Indian National Science Academy – JSPS. In 2009, he moved to United Sates to do research at Rutgers University, New Jersey. In US, he received prestigious awards such as "Gallo Award" for two times (2012 and 2103) from Cancer Institute of New Jersey for outstanding cancer research.

Dr. Murugan has been elected as a member of the American Association of Cancer Research (AACR), and the American Association of Immunologists (AAI). More recently, Dr. Murugan's research is focused on elucidating the resistance mechanisms during immunotherapy at University of Pennsylvania.

Throughout Dr. Murugan's many years of cancer research, he has given countless presentations at scientific meetings, seminars, and conferences in many countries including India, Japan, and the United States. He has published more than 25 research articles in peer-reviewed journals including *Carcinogenesis*, *Cancer Research*, *Glycobiology*, *Journal of Immunology*, and *Journal of Biological Chemistry*, with more than 5 collaborators from different nations, 24 research abstracts, edited two books, an invited review and 4 book chapters, each composed with his characteristic precision. His articles have collectively been cited a total of 750 times with the h-index of 16 (Google Scholar) with a robust impact factor.

Dr. Murugan is serving on the editorial boards and as reviewer of several journals, including Pharmaceutical Biology, Scientific Reports (Nature publishing group), Tumor Biology, International Journal of Cancer Research, International Journal of Pharmacology, Cancer Research and Management, and as an editorial board member of the International Journal of Nutrition, Pharmacology, Neurological Diseases and Wyno Academic Journals. Over the past several years, Dr. Murugan has worked with and closely supervised summer trainees, undergraduate, and graduate students for their successful completion of research projects, and brought a passion for discovery to high scholarly standards.

Email: velan2009@gmail.com

Dr. Saravanan Ramachandran

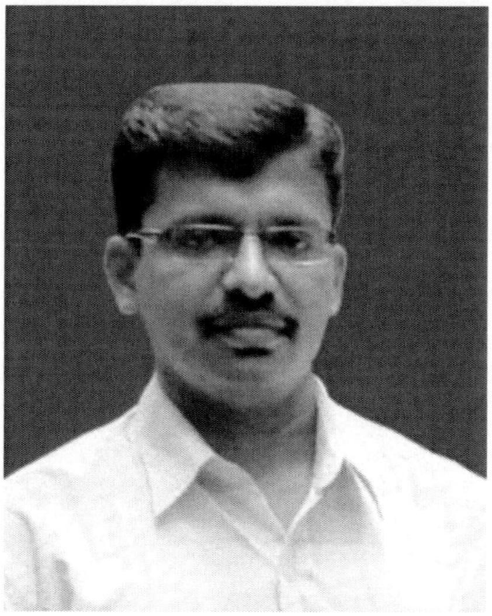

Dr. Saravanan Ramachandran, PhD., secured his doctorate in Marine Biotechnology from the Faculty of Marine Sciences, Center for Advanced Studies in Marine Biology, Annamalai University, Tamil Nadu, India in 2010. He was the recipient of the Senior Research Fellowship from Indian Council of Medical Research (ICMR), New Delhi, India and SRF from Centre for Marine Living Resource and Ecology (CMLRE), Kochi, Kerala, India. His immense interest in marine research was evident from his participation in the cruise #279 of FORV SAGAR SAMPADA expedition and covering 2560 Nautical miles along the East coast of India. His thrust research area encompasses marine glycobiology and bioactive compounds from marine sources. The highlights of his research work pertain to isolation and purification of glycaosaminoglycans, proteoglycans, glycopeptides, polyphenols, from the marine sources. From his research experience and concurrence, he has published more than 25 research publications in peer reviewed journals. He has also authored and coauthored 6 book chapters in indexed international publications such as Elsevier, Springer, Taylor and Francis, NOVA publications, etc. He is also an active reviewer for indexed journals such as Carbohydrate Polymers, International Journal of Biological Macromolecules, Applied Biochemistry and Biotechnology, etc. From his research findings, he has deposited a gene sequence in Pub Med and has also filed an Indian patent in 2013. He serves as a life time member of the International Neurotoxin Association (INA) 2015, member of Association of Pharmacy Professionals (APP), India.

Presently, he focuses on isolation of bioactive macromolecules from marine sources and screens them for their therapeutic effects on cancer, neurological and cardiovascular diseases in primates and zebra fish model.

Email: saranprp@gmail.com

SYNOPSIS

The field of Gastrointestinal Biology has been transformed by an explosion of knowledge for gastrointestinal motility, absorption, and secretion. These chapters in the book summarize the methods of molecular biology and the cell biology of gut enzymes, secreting cells and cells that respond to these enzymes.

This book is a valuable reference for students, researchers and faculties of gastrointestinal motility, absorption and secretion. No other single source covers this field so comprehensively. *The Gastrointestinal System* is more than twice the length of that textbook and contains a considerable amount of detail on subjects such as gut hormones, gut malabsorption, alcohol toxicity on the stomach and methods used in physiologic study of the digestive tract. Disease conditions are discussed only to the extent that they illustrate physiologic mechanisms. It is difficult for such a comprehensive work to remain up to date for very long, considering how rapidly our knowledge of life sciences expands. The chapters vary in the extent to which they explain the immense picture. This book, a comprehensive treatise on the causes, diagnosis, and management of gastrointestinal-motility disorders, consists of eighteen chapters with extensive references contained in slightly fewer than 300 pages. It achieves its goal through generally lucid writing and the overlap of information from chapter to chapter commonly observed in multi-authored works. Therefore, the reader is best advised to go through this book in a relaxed manner; this will allow them to finish it in a relatively short amount of time and appreciate the field of gastrointestinal motility, particularly current practice and research methods for solving its many riddles. All the chapters are clearly written, but the target audience seems to vary from medical students to practicing gastroenterologists. Despite these drawbacks, gastroenterologists, surgeons, and basic scientists wishing to bring their general knowledge of clinical motility disorders up to date will find this book useful.

Dr. Senthilkumar Rajagopal, PhD
Dr. Sengottuvelan Murugan, PhD
Dr. Saravanan Ramachandran, PhD

In: Disorders of Gastrointestinal Systems … ISBN: 978-1-63485-366-8
Editors:S. Rajagopal, S. Murugan and S. Ramachandran ©2016 Nova Science Publishers, Inc.

Chapter 1

UNDERSTANDING THE IMPACTS OF ALCOHOL: GASTRIC FUNCTIONS AND THERAPY

Senthilkumar Rajagopal[1,*], PhD, Supraj Raja Sangam[2], MTech, and Shubham Singh[3], BSc

[1]Department of Biotechnology, Rayalaseema University, Kurnool, AP, India
[2]Department of Biotechnology, JNTUH, Hyderabad, TS, India
[3]Department of Biology, IISER-Pune, Pune, MH, India

ABSTRACT

Alcohol impacts virtually on cellular and molecular functions in the body, thereby regulating the gastric acid secretion and surrounding muscles of the stomach leading to gastritis. Gastritis is known as an inflammation in the lining of the stomach. Gastric inflammation in severe cases leads to gastric cancer. Stomach is lined by a complex epithelium that forms a selective barrier between the lumen and the body. Mucosa preserves a protective balance between aggressive factors such as gastric acid, pepsin, alcohol, reactive oxygen species (ROS), non-steroidal anti-inflammatory drugs (NSAID) and infection with *Helicobacter pylori*. A neutral amino acid glycine has been studied for its ability to inhibit gastric secretion and to protect the gastric mucosa against NSAID's and stress induced ulcers. Interference in normal cellular homeostasis by redox signalling may result in cancer, cardiovascular, mitochondrial dysfunction and neurodegenerative diseases. NSAID's not only exert gastric injury, but also interrupts in the healing of ulcer lesions through a variety of local and systemic mechanisms. Alcohol hinders absorption of nutrients into small intestine and increases the transport of toxins in the intestinal walls, which may contribute to the development of alcohol-related damage to stomach and other organs in the body. Unravelling the redox signals at cellular and molecular level by free radicals is crucial for better understanding the disease pathogenesis and in designing new individual specific therapies. This book chapter focuses on the interaction between cellular and molecular aspects of alcohol and gastric functions.

---

* Corresponding author: Dr.R.Senthilkumar, PhD., DBT-Ramalingaswami Re-entry Fellow, Scientist, Dept. of Biotechnology, Rayalaseema University, Kurnool, AP, INDIA, Email:senthilanal@yahoo.com, Mo: 9566860390.

Keywords: alcohol, cancer, gastric inflammation, *H. pylori*, non-steroidal anti-inflammatory drugs, reactive oxygen species

1. Introduction

Alcoholic beverages have been socially accepted additive drug since ancient times worldwide. Addiction to alcohol is a serious medical illness and the third leading cause of preventable death (Danaei et al., 2009). The alcohol is infiltrated in the brain, liver, heart, pancreas, lungs, kidneys, and every other organ and tissue system within minutes after it passes into the blood stream (Singal and Shah, 2016). The strength of the drink will have a significant effect on absorption rates, with higher concentrations of alcohol resulting in more rapid absorption. Pure alcohol is generally absorbed faster than diluted alcohols, which are, in turn, absorbed faster than wine or beer (Rajaram et al., 2016; Iyer and Vaishnava, 2016).

Extreme alcohol consumption has drastic effect on gastric mucosa leading to acute or chronic gastritis (Singh et al., 2015). Alcohol absorption into the bloodstream takes place in gastrointestinal tract (GI) (Hiraishi et al., 1999; Bode and Bode, 1997). About 20 percent of the alcohol consumed is absorbed in the stomach, and about 80 percent is absorbed in the small intestine. The mucosa in the upper GI tract reacts with alcohol contributing to numerous metabolic and functional changes (Vassallo et al., 2015; Bode and Bode, 1997). These changes may lead to mucosal damage, resulting into acute and chronic diseases, such as acute gastrointestinal bleeding due to lesions in the stomach or small intestine. Metabolic, functional changes and mucosal damage in the intestine disturb the digestion and absorption of various nutrients into the body, thereby leading to malnutrition and weight loss (Tang et al., 2009; Siqueira et al., 2016).

The liver and other organs are severely affects by alcoholic toxic substances. Alcohol is not digested like other foods. Once alcohol is swallowed, it travels down the esophagus into the stomach and the small intestine. It avoids the normal digestive process and goes right into the bloodstream (Lieber et al., 1997). Reactive oxygen species appears to be involved in the pathogenesis of ethanol-induced gastric mucosal injury *in vivo*. Both epithelium and endothelium of the gastric cells are targeted by ethanol, because ingested ethanol diffuses into the gastric mucosa (Guth et al., 1984; Hiraishi et al., 1993). Alcohol taken in concentrated amounts can irritate the stomach lining to the extent that it produces a sticky mucous which delays absorption (Bode and Bode, 1992).

The pylorus valve which connects the stomach and small intestine may go into spasm in the presence of concentrated alcohol, trapping the alcohol in the stomach instead of passing it on to the small intestine where it would be more rapidly absorbed into the blood stream (Elshaghabee et al., 2016; Bergheim et al., 2008). The drinker who downs several straight shots in an effort to get a quick high may actually experience a delayed effect. Finally, the temperature of the beverage affects its absorption, with warm alcohol being absorbed more rapidly than cold alcohol (Bellentani et al., 1994; Baker et al., 2010).

There are two types of alcohol effect on stomach;

- *Acute alcohol:* intake show gastric erosions and peptchial hemorrhage
- *Chronic alcohol:* Chronic gastritis and acts synergistically with *H. Pylori* delays healing

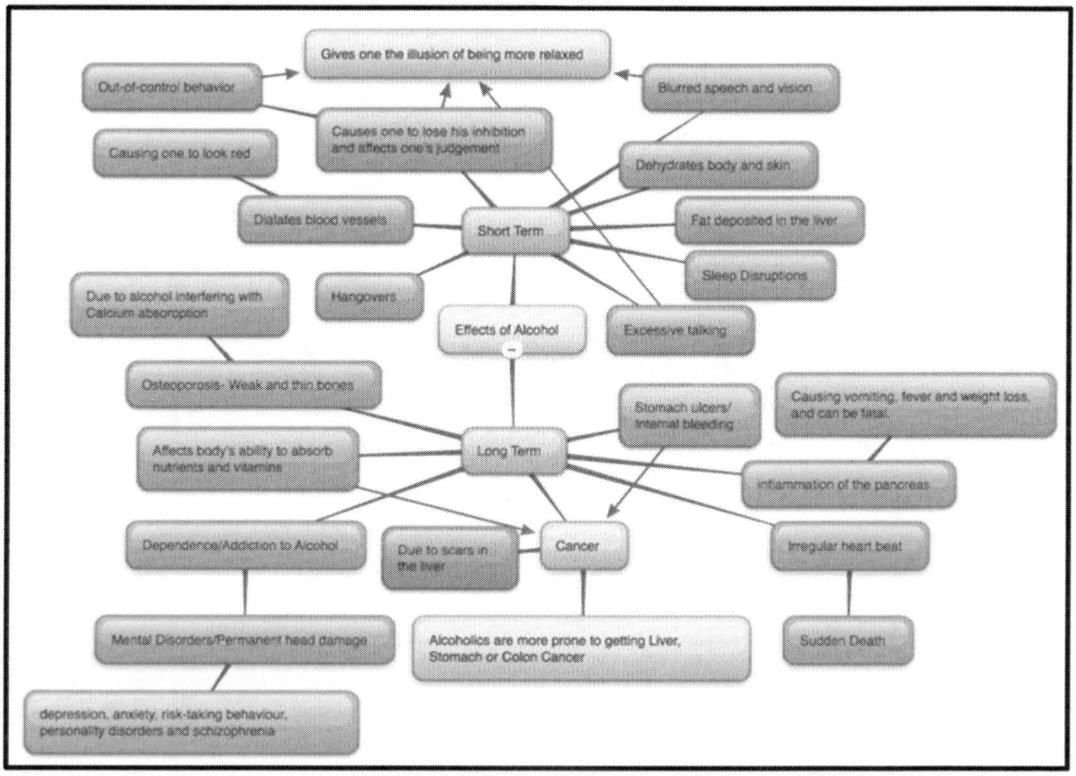

Figure 1. Short term and Long term effects of Alcohol.

2. THE GASTROINTESTINAL TRACT

Alcohol affects most of the GI organelles such as the stomach, the small and large intestines, and the pancreas. Acid secretion of stomach is increased by Alcohol. That can result in gastritis or stomach or intestinal ulcers (Hirofumi, 2011; Lindkvist, 2013). The amount of sugar in the blood is regulated by Insulin which is produced by the pancreas and the blood sugar is steep rose by drinking alcohol. Hypoglycemia or low blood sugar means that the blood sugar is dropped fast by additional secretion of insulin by pancreas (Madhavan et al., 2015; Singh et al., 2015). 70-90% of alcoholics suffer to some degree from the disorder of hypoglycemia, chronic low blood sugar, as a long term effect of their drinking (Rastrelli et al., 2015; Matsuda et al., 2009). Symptoms of hypoglycemia can include dizziness, headaches, lack of ability to concentrate, depression, anxiety, light-headedness, tremors, cold sweats, heart palpitations, loss of coordination, and upset stomach. In time, the drinker's overworked pancreas may stop producing insulin and diabetes can result. Conversely, a person with a family history of diabetes may be more vulnerable to problems with alcohol (Sagiroglu, 2008; Kartal and Kilin, 2006; Chiou et al., 2000).

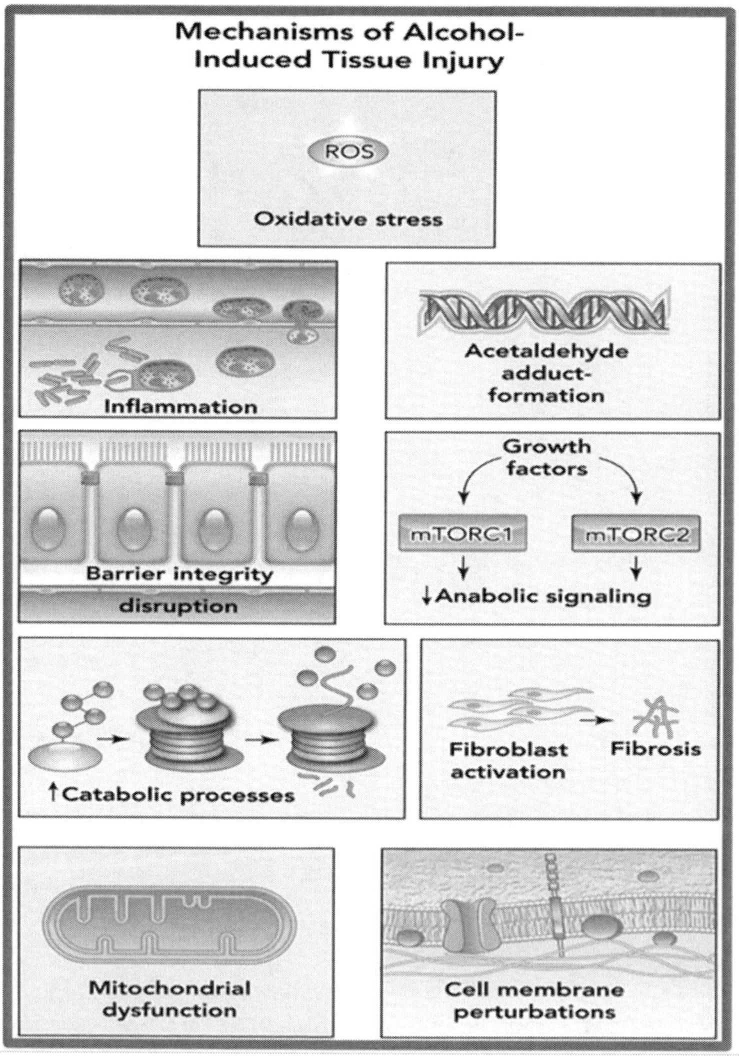

Alcohol abuse disrupts multiple cellular mechanisms, leading to altered organ function and disease. Among the most important pathophysiological mechanisms identified as causative factors in tissue and organ injury resulting from alcohol abuse include oxidative stress, inflammation, acetaldehyde generation and adduct formation, decreased barrier function, impaired anabolic signaling, up regulation of catabolic processes, fibroblast activation, mitochondrial injury, and cell membrane perturbations.

Figure 2. Principal mechanisms of alcohol-induced pathophysiology (adapted from Molina et al., 2014).

2.1. Stomach

Moderate consumption of alcohol can also alter gastric acid secretion thereby contributes to acute gastric mucosal injury and intervene in intestinal motility (Molina et al., 2014; Nassar et al., 2015; Mason et al., 2008). Hence either moderate or extreme alcohol consumption can interfere with stomach functioning. Stomach inflammation and irritation is also a known effect of prolonged alcohol use upon the body. Other systems like perforation of the stomach lining can contribute to the possible occurrence of anemia as well (Lombardo et al., 2010; Isaksen et al., 2015; McDonald et al., 1992; Li et al., 2015).

Stomach - More than 40% alcohol causes direct toxic effect on the gastric mucosa

- Back diffusion of acid from the gastric lumen into the mucosa
- Disrupts the gastric mucosal barrier
- Exacerbates acid peptide disorder (Alvarez-Suarez et al., 2011)

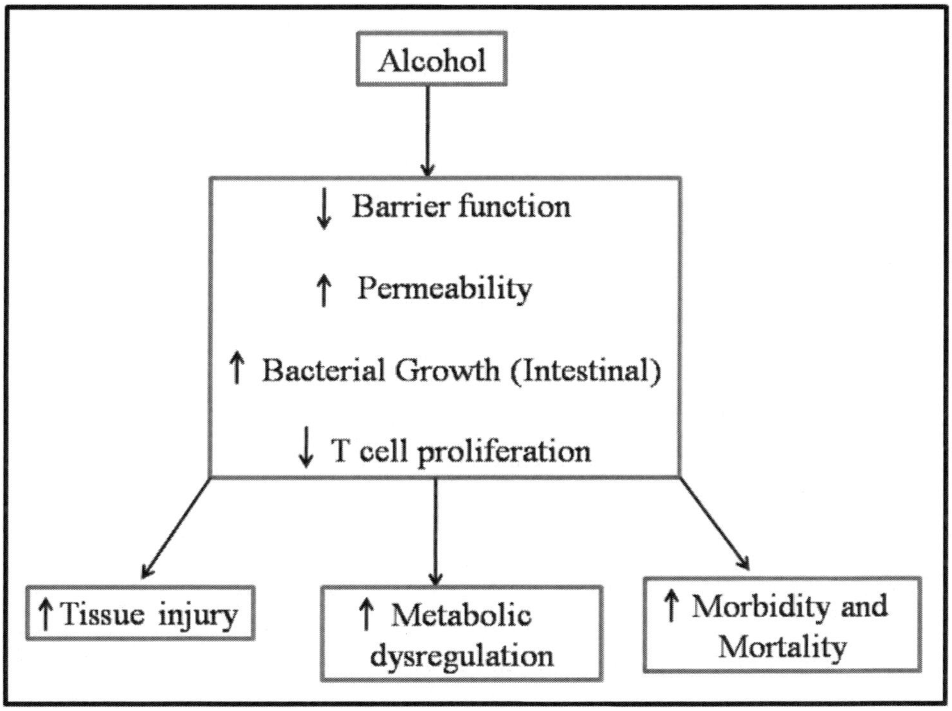

Figure 3. Pathophysiological consequences of Alcohol on stomach.

Table 1. Gastric mucosal defense mechanisms (adapted from Hirofumi et al., 2011)

1.	**Pre-epithelial mechanisms**
•	Mucous
•	Bicarbonates
•	Surface active phospho lipids
2.	**Epithelial Mechanisms**
•	Tight junction complex
•	Restitution
•	Growth factors
•	Cell profileartion
3.	**Sub-epithelial mechanisms**
•	Microcirculation of blood
•	Leukocytes

2.2. Acute Gastritis

Many decades scientists and doctors have known that alcohol consumption causes mucosal inflammation and gastric lesions. Longer administration of NSAIDs like aspirin, ibuprofen and naproxen leads to the development of alcohol induced acute gastric lesions. Scientists have proven since ages that that alcohol concentration of ten percent and more can disrupt the gastric mucosal barrier and increase the mucosa's permeability in both animals and humans (Bode et al., 1996; Salim, 1990; Mulkijanyan et al., 2013). The damages caused to the stomach and intestine, induced by moderate consumption of alcohol are reversible to certain extent. Prolonged alcohol exposure, however, disturbs the microcirculation and leads to progressive structural mucosal damage.

Several studies have suggested that the decreased formation of hormone like substances called prostaglandins might play a role in alcohol-induced mucosal injury (Ciccarelli et al., 2013; Bode et al. 1996; Webb and Starr, 2005). Prostaglandins protect the gastric mucosa from damage by agents such as aspirin that break the gastric mucosal barrier without inhibiting acid secretion. Other studies have indicated that an alcohol-dependent increase in the production of leukotrienes compounds produced by the immune system that cause allergic condition (Atkinson et al., 2004; Kim et al., 2015; Sun et al., 2015).

2.3. Chronic Gastritis

Chronic gastritis has started gaining attention since beginning of the 20th century but received more attention from 1982 after discovery of the *H. pylori* by Marshall and Warren (Forbes et al., 1996; Sgouras et al., 2015; Andrade et al., 2006). Chronic gastritis is one of the most common illnesses in human beings. The significance of chronic gastritis as a serious disease is largely underrated in clinicians, even though the role of gastritis in the pathogenesis of ordinary peptic ulcers and gastric cancers is obvious (Chamberlain, 1993; Setiawan et al., 2001; Bienia et al., 2002). It has become clear that the bacterium is the cause of gastritis in an overwhelming majority of the cases, a possible exception being gastritis of the autoimmune origin. Consequently, it has become evident that chronic gastritis can be cured with eradication of H. pylori, resulting in normalization of the gastric mucosa, at least in cases in which the gastritis is not developed to atrophic (atrophic gastritis) end stages (Vidal et al., 2016; Aasarød et al., 2016; Inagaki-Ohara, 2016).

2.4. Consequences

Consumption of alcohol leads to loss of appetite and abdominal discomfort, such as abdominal pain, fullness, gas, nausea and vomiting. The abdominal discomfort can lead to malnutrition and weight loss (Rosato et al., 2016; Garcia et al., 2015; Aguilera et al., 2001). In addition to causing abdominal complaints, alcohol plays a role in the development of cancers of the GI tract. It is likely, however, that alcohol does not cause GI-tract cancers by itself but acts in concert with other cancer inducing agents (i.e., as a co carcinogen). Alcohol abuse, like smoking, is associated with the development of cancers of the tongue, larynx (i.e., the organ of voice), and pharynx; both alcohol consumption and smoking independently increase the risk for these tumors (Bode and 1980; Han et al., 2015; Preyer et al., 2016; Sabharwal et al., 2015).

3. THERAPY

3.1. How Is Acute Gastritis Diagnosed?

The tests should be followed for acute gastritis

- A complete blood count (CBC) is used to check overall health.
- A blood, breath, or saliva test is used to check for *H. pylori*.
- A fecal test is used to check for blood in the stool.
- An esophagogastroduodenoscopy is used to look at the lining of stomach with a small camera. This is also called an endoscopy.
- A gastric tissue biopsy involves removing a small piece of stomach tissue for analysis.
- An X-ray is used to look for structural problems in the digestive system.

3.1.1. How Is Acute Gastritis Treated?

Some cases of acute gastritis go away without treatment. The treatment used will depend on what's causing the pain. Some options include:

- Medications, Antacids such as Pepto-Bismol and Milk of Magnesia can be used to neutralize stomach acid, H2 antagonists such as famotidine (Pepcid) and cimetidine (Tagamet) reduce the production of stomach acid, Proton pump inhibitors such as omeprazole (Prilosec) and esomeprazole (Nexium) inhibit the production of stomach acid, Antibiotics are only necessary if you have a bacterial infection, such as from *H. pylori*.

Lifestyle changes may also help reduce your acute gastritis symptoms. Changes that could help include:

- avoiding or limiting alcohol consumption
- avoiding spicy, fried, and acidic foods
- eating frequent, small meals
- reducing stress

Certain herbs improve digestive system health. They may also help kill *H. pylori*. Some of the herbs used to treat acute gastritis include:

- Slippery elm, myrrh, berberine, licorice, wild indigo, clove, Oregon grape.

3.2. How Is Chronic Gastritis Diagnosed?

- ➢ a test for the bacteria that causes stomach ulcers

- a stool test to look for stomach bleeding
- a blood count and an anemia test
- an endoscopy, which involves the use of a camera attached to a long tube that's inserted into your mouth and down into your digestive tract

3.2.1. The Most Common Medicines to Reduce Gastric Acid Are

antacids, such as Alka-Seltzer and Tums

- H2 antagonists, such as Zantac
- proton pump inhibitors that are available both over the counter and by prescription, such as Prilosec
- Reducing or eliminating aspirin and similar medicines is also recommended to decrease stomach irritation

3.2.2. Diet

We should avoid consuming:

- fried foods, such as french fries or other vegetables fried in oil
- citrus juices
- coffee
- alcohol

3.2.3. Recommended Foods Generally Include Foods with Small Amounts of the Following

- oil
- fat
- caffeine
- citrus

3.2.4. Recommended Foods Include

- all vegetables and fruits, except citrus fruits
- low-fat dairy products
- lean meats
- pasta and rice prepared with little or no fat (Senthilkumar et al., 2014, 2015)

SUMMARY

Alcohol consumption can interfere with the function of all parts of the gastrointestinal tract. Acute alcohol ingestion induces changes in the motility of the esophagus and stomach that favour gastroesophageal reflux and probably, the development of reflux esophagitis. Alcohol abuse may lead to damage of the gastric mucosa, including hemorrhagic lesions. Beverages with low alcohol content stimulate gastric acid secretion, whereas beverages with high alcohol content do not. In the small intestine, alcohol inhibits the absorption of numerous nutrients. The importance of these absorption disorders for the development of nutritional disturbances in alcoholics, however, is unclear. This chapter revealed the current understanding of the molecular interaction between cellular and molecular aspects of alcohol and gastric functions. We should learn, in the coming years, a great deal more about the molecular mechanisms of alcohol and intracellular cascades.

Acknowledgments

The support provided by the Department of Biotechnology, Ministry of Science and Technology, Government of India (To Dr. Senthilkumar Rajagopal – No: BT/RLF/Re-entry/42/2012) to complete this book in a successful manner is gratefully acknowledged.

References

Aasarød KM, Mosti MP, Stunes AK, Reseland JE, Basso T, Syversen U, Fossmark R. Impaired skeletal health in patients with chronic atrophic gastritis. *Scand J Gastroenterol* 2016; 8:1-8.

Aguilera A, Codoceo R, Bajo MA, Diéz JJ, del Peso G, Pavone M, Ortiz J, Valdez J, Cirugeda A, Fernández-Perpén A, Sánchez-Tomero JA, Selgas R. Helicobacter pylori infection: a new cause of anorexia in peritoneal dialysis patients. *Perit Dial Int* 2001; 21 Suppl 3:S152-6.

Alvarez-Suarez JM, Dekanski D, Ristić S, Radonjić NV. Strawberry polyphenols attenuate ethanol-induced gastric lesions in rats by activation of antioxidant enzymes and attenuation of MDA increase. *PLoS One* 2011; 6: e25878.

Andrade MC, Menezes JS, Cassali GD, Martins-Filho OA, Cara DC, Faria AM. Alcohol-induced gastritis prevents oral tolerance induction in mice. *Clin Exp Immunol* 2006; 146(2):312-22.

Atkinson W, Sheldon TA, Shaath N, Whorwell PJ. Food elimination based on IgG antibodies in irritable bowel syndrome: A randomised controlled trial. *Gut* 2004; 53 (10): 1459–1464.

Baker SS, Baker RD, Liu W, Nowak NJ, Zhu L. Role of alcohol metabolism in non-alcoholic steatohepatitis. *PLoS One* 2010; 5:e9570.

Bellentani S, Tiribelli C, Saccoccio G, Sodde M, Fratti N, De Martin, C. Prevalence of chronic liver disease in the general population of northern Italy: the Dionysos Study. *Hepatology* 1994; 20: 1442–1449.

Bergheim I, Weber S, Vos M, Krämer S, Volynets V, Kaserouni S. Antibiotics protect against fructose-induced hepatic lipid accumulation in mice: role of endotoxin. *J Hepatol* 2008; 48: 983–992.

Bhavani M, Jayabhaskar Reddy S, Vamshaj Raja S, Supraj SR. An unusual location of B-cell lymphoma involving the tongue. *Apollo Med* 2015; 12(4): 277-279.

Bienia A, Sodolski W, Luchowska E. The effect of chronic alcohol abuse on gastric and duodenal mucosa. *Ann Univ Mariae Curie Sklodowska Med* 2002;57(2):570-82.

Bode C, Bode JC. Adaptive changes in activities of enzymes of the carbohydrate metabolism in rat liver and jejunal mucosa to high fructose diets. Modifying effect of the fat content of the diet. *Z Gastroenterol,* 1980;18(1):38-44.

Bode C, Bode JC. Alcohol's role in gastrointestinal tract disorders. *Alcohol Health Res World* 1997; 21(1): 76-83.

Bode CC, Maute G, Bode JC. Prostaglandin E2 and prostaglandin F2α biosynthesis in human gastric mucosa: Effect of chronic alcohol misuse. *Gut* 1996; 39(3):348-352.

Bode JC, Bode C. Alcohol malnutrition and the gastrointestinal tract. Nutrition and Alcohol. Boca Raton, FL: CRC Press 1992; 403-28.

Chamberlain CE. Acute hemorrhagic gastritis. *Gastroenterol Clin North Am* 1993; 22(4):843-73.

Chiou A, Markidis T, Constantinou-Kokotou V, Verger R, Kokotos G. Synthesis and study of a lipophilic alpha-keto amide inhibitor of pancreatic lipase. *Org Lett* 2000 10;2(3):347-50.

Ciccarelli S, Stolfi I, Caramia G. Management strategies in the treatment of neonatal and pediatric gastroenteritis. *Infection Drug Res* 2013; 6: 133–61.

Danaei G, Ding EL, Mozaffarian D. The preventable causes of death in the United States: Comparative risk assessment of dietary, lifestyle, and metabolic risk factors. *PLoS Medicine* 2009; 6(4):1–23.

Elshaghabee FM, Bockelmann W, Meske D, de Vrese M, Walte HG, Schrezenmeir J, Heller KJ. Ethanol Production by Selected Intestinal Microorganisms and Lactic Acid Bacteria Growing under Different Nutritional Conditions. *Front Microbiol* 2016; 29:7:47.

Forbes GM, Warren JR, Glaser ME, Cullen DJ, Marshall BJ, Collins BJ. Long-term follow-up of gastric histology after Helicobacter pylori eradication. *J Gastroenterol Hepatol* 1996 Jul;11(7):670-673.

Garcia JA, Souza AL, Cruz LH, Marques PP, Camilli JA, Nakagaki WR, Esteves A, Rossi-Junior WC, Fernandes GJ, Guerra FD, Soares EA. Effects of ethanol consumption and alcohol detoxification on the biomechanics and morphology the bone in rat femurs. *Braz J Biol* 2015;75(4):983-8.

Guth PH, Paulsen G, Nagata H. Histologic and microcirculatory changes in alcohol-induced gastric lesions in the rat: Effect of prostaglandin cytoprotection. *Gastroenterol* 1984; 87:1083–1090.

Han M, Wu G, Sun P, Nie J, Zhang J, Li Y. Association of genetic polymorphisms in PTEN and additional interaction with alcohol consumption and smoking on colorectal cancer in Chinese population. *Int J Clin Exp Med* 2015; 8(11):21629-34.

Hiraishi H, Shimada T, Ivey KJ, Terano A. Role of antioxidant defenses against ethanol-induced damage in cultured rat gastric epithelial cells. *J Pharmacol Exp Ther* 1999; 289(1): 103-109.

Hiraishi H, Terano A, Ivey KJ (1993) Gastric mucosal cell culture for toxicological study. in Methods in Toxicology. 1A. In Vitro Biological Systems, eds Tyson CA, Frazier JM (Academic Press, San Diego), pp 182–191.

Hirofumi M, Osamu S, Tsuyoshi K, Yumiko N, Kanho R, Ichinosuke H. The pathophysiology of non-steroidal anti-inflammatory drug (NSAID)-induced mucosal injuries in stomach and small intestine. *J Clin Biochem Nutr* 2011; 48(2): 107–111.

Inagaki-Ohara K, Okamoto S, Takagi K, Saito K, Arita S, Tang L, Hori T, Kataoka H, Matsumoto S, Minokoshi Y. Leptin receptor signaling is required for high-fat diet-induced atrophic gastritis in mice. *Nutr Metab (Lond)* 2016; 13:7.

Isaksen AB, Østbye T, Mmbaga BT, Daltveit AK. Alcohol consumption among pregnant women in Northern Tanzania 2000-2010: a registry-based study. *BMC Pregnancy*

Childbirth 2015;15:205.

Iyer N, Vaishnava S. Alcohol Lowers Your (Intestinal) Inhibitions. *Cell Host Microbe* 2016; 10; 19(2):131-133.

Kartal F, Kilinç A. Immobilization of pancreatic lipase on polyvinyl alcohol by cyanuric chloride. Prep Biochem Biotechnol. 2006;36(2):139-51.

Kim SH, Park JG, Sung GH, Yang S, Yang WS, Kim E, Kim JH, Ha VT, Kim HG, Yi YS, Kim JH, Baek KS, Sung NY, Lee MN, Kim JH, Cho JY. Kaempferol, a dietary flavonoid, ameliorates acute inflammatory and nociceptive symptoms in gastritis, pancreatitis, and abdominal pain. *Mol Nutr Food Res* 2015;59(7):1400-5.

Li J, Tang HL, Chen Y, Fan Q, Shao YT, Jia M, Wang JC, Yang CM. Malondialdehyde and SOD-induced changes of gastric tissues in acute gastric mucosal injury under positive acceleration. *Genet Mol Res* 2015;14(2):4361-4368.

Lieber CS. Gastric ethanol metabolism and gastritis: interactions with other drugs, Helicobacter pylori, and antibiotic therapy (1957–1997) — a review. *Alcohol Clin Exp Res* 1997; 21: 1360–1366.

Lindkvist B. Diagnosis and treatment of pancreatic exocrine insufficiency. *World J Gastroenterol* 2013; 19(42):7258-66.

Lombardo L, Foti M, Ruggia O, Chiecchio A. Increased incidence of small intestinal bacterial overgrowth during proton pump inhibitor therapy. *Clin Gastroenterol Hepatol* 2010;8: 504-508.

Madhavan V, Murali A, Lalitha DS, Yoganarasimhan S. Studies on anti-hyperglycemic effect of Euphorbia antiquorum L. root in diabetic rats. *J Intercult Ethnopharmacol* 2015; 4(4):308-13.

Mason JM, Raghunath AS, Hungin AP, Jackson W. Helicobacter pylori eradication in long-term proton pump inhibitor users is highly cost-effective: economic analysis of the HELPUP trial. *Aliment Pharmacol Ther* 2008; 28:1297-1303.

Matsuda H, Asao Y, Nakamura S, Hamao M, Sugimoto S, Hongo M, Pongpiriyadacha Y, Yoshikawa M. Antidiabetogenic constituents from the Thai traditional medicine Cotylelobium melanoxylon. *Chem Pharm Bull (Tokyo)* 2009; 57(5):487-94.

McDonald AD, Armstrong BG, Sloan M. Cigarette, alcohol, and coffee consumption and prematurity. *Am J Public Health* 1992; 82:87–90.

Molina P, Jason E, Gardner D, Flavia M, Souza-Smith, Whitaker AM. Alcohol Abuse: Critical Pathophysiological Processes and Contribution to Disease Burden. *Physiol (Bethesda)* 2014; 29(3): 203–215.

Mulkijanyan K, Novikova Zh, Sulakvelidze M, Getia M, Mshvildadze V, Dekanosidze G. Ivy water extracts as gastric ulcer preventive agents. *Georgian Med News* 2013; 224:63-66.

Nasser SC, Slim M, Nassif JG, Nasser SM. Influence of proton pump inhibitors on gastritis diagnosis and pathologic gastric changes. *World J Gastroenterol* 2015; 21(15):4599-606.

Preyer O, Johansen D, Holly J, Stocks T, Pompella A, Nagel G, Concin H, Ulmer H, Concin N. γ-Glutamyltransferase and Breast Cancer Risk Beyond Alcohol Consumption and Other Life Style Factors - A Pooled Cohort Analysis. *PLoS One* 2016; 11(2):e0149122.

Rajaram P, Little B, Norvell JP, McLemore M, Veeraraghavan S. A 49-Year-Old Man With Cirrhosis and Pulmonary Fibrosis. *Chest* 2016; 149 (2): e57-e60.

Rastrelli G, Corona G, Mannucci E, Maggi M. Vascular and Chronological Age in Subjects with Erectile Dysfunction: A Cross-Sectional Study. *J Sex Med* 2015; 12(12):2303-12.

Rosato V, Abenavoli L, Federico A, Masarone M, Persico M. Pharmacotherapy of alcoholic liver disease in clinical practice. *Int J Clin Pract* 2016; 70(2):119-31.

Sabharwal R, Verma P, Syed MA, Sharma T, Subudhi SK, Mohanty S, Gupta S. Emergence of micronuclei as a genomic biomarker. *Indian J Med Paediatr Oncol* 2015; 36(4):212-8.

Sagiroglu A. Conversion of sunflower oil to biodiesel by alcoholysis using immobilized lipase. *Artif Cells Blood Substit Immobil Biotechnol* 2008;36(2):138-49.

Salim AS. Removing oxygen-derived free radicals stimulates healing of ethanol-induced erosive gastritis in the rat. *Digestion* 1990;47(1):24-8.

Senthilkumar Rajagopal, Venkateshwara Rao Joginapally, Timiri Shanmugam Prakash Srinivasan, Veerappan Ramanathan. (2014). Beneficial Effects of Dietary Amino acids on Brain Health. In: M. Mohammed Essa and Mushtaq A. Memon (Eds). Food and brain Function. Nova Publications, New York, USA, Pp: 221-24.

Senthilkumar Rajagopal, Supraj Raja sangam, Shubham Singh, Venkateshwara Rao Joginapally. (2015). Alcohol-induced Hepatotoxicity; Symptoms and Management. In: Senthilkumar Rajagopal and Sengottuvelan Murugan (Eds). Hepatotoxicity, Symptoms, Management and Health Implications. Nova Publications, New York, USA, Pp: 1-22.

Setiawan VW, Zhang ZF, Yu GP, Lu QY, Li YL, Lu ML, Wang MR, Guo CH, Yu SZ, Kurtz RC, Hsieh CC. Protective effect of green tea on the risks of chronic gastritis and stomach cancer. *Int J Cancer* 2001; 92(4):600-4.

Sgouras DN, Trang TT, Yamaoka Y. Pathogenesis of Helicobacter pylori Infection. Helicobacter, 2015; 20 Suppl 1:8-16.

Singal AK, Shah VH. Therapeutic Strategies for the Treatment of Alcoholic Hepatitis. *Semin Liver Dis* 2016; 36(1); 56-68.

Singh S, Sangam SR, Joginapalli VR, Rajagopal S. Alcohol-induced gastric inflammation. *J Pharm Biomed Sci* 2015; 5(2): 174-177.

Singh S, Sangam SR, Joginapally VR, Rajagopal S. Alcohol, Glycine and Gastritis. *International Journal of Nutrition, Pharmacology, Neurological Diseases* 2015; 5(1):1-5.

Siqueira JT, Batistela E, Pereira MP, da Silva VC, de Sousa Junior PT, Andrade CM, Kawashita NH, Bertolini GL, Baviera AM. Combretum lanceolatum flowers ethanol extract inhibits hepatic gluconeogenesis: an in vivo mechanism study. *Pharm Biol* 2016; 10:1-9.

Son DJ, Lee GR, Oh S, Lee SE, Choi WS. Gastroprotective efficacy and safety evaluation of scoparone derivatives on experimentally induced gastric lesions in rodents. *Nutrients* 2015; 7(3):1945-64.

Tang Y, Forsyth CB, Farhadi A, Rangan J, Jakate S, Shaikh M. Nitric oxide-mediated intestinal injury is required for alcohol-induced gut leakiness and liver damage. *Alcohol Clin Exp Res* 2009; 33:1220-30.

Vassallo G, Mirijello A, Ferrulli A, Antonelli M, Landolfi R, Gasbarrini A, Addolorato G. The Possible Role of Gut Microbiota Modulation in the Treatment of Alcoholic Liver Disease. *Aliment Pharmacol Ther* 2015; 41(10):917-927.

Vidal AF, Cruz AM, Magalhães L, Pereira AL, Anaissi AK, Alves NC, Albuquerque PJ, Burbano RM, Demachki S, Ribeiro-Dos-Santos Â. Hsa-miR-29c and hsa-miR-135b differential expression as potential biomarker of gastric carcinogenesis. *World J Gastroenterol* 2016; 22(6):2060-70.

Webb A, Starr M. Acute gastroenteritis in children. *Australian family physician* 2005; 34 (4): 227–31.

In: Disorders of Gastrointestinal Systems … ISBN: 978-1-63485-366-8
Editors:S. Rajagopal, S. Murugan and S. Ramachandran ©2016 Nova Science Publishers, Inc.

Chapter 2

RESVERATROL AND ITS DERIVATIVES FOR THE PREVENTION AND TREATMENT OF GASTROINTESTINAL DISORDERS: A REVIEW

Sengottuvelan Murugan[1,*], PhD,
and Deeptha Kumaraswamy, MPhil
[1]University of Pennsylvania, Perelman School of Medicine,
Division of Hematology/Oncology, Philadelphia, PA, US

ABSTRACT

Numerous studies have shown that consumption of fruits and vegetables can minimize the incidence of various diseases including gastrointestinal disorders such ulcerative colitis, colon, esophageal and stomach cancers. This chapter outlines the modulating effect of resveratrol, a polyphenolic component of various fruits and vegetables on various genes and the cell signaling pathways of gastrointestinal system.

In recent years, resveratrol and its derivatives have shown amazing biological activities including apoptosis induction, antioxidant effect in gastrointestinal diseases. However, systematic clinical trials need to be carried out to provide proof of concept. In addition, researchers worldwide should come forward to design of new resveratrol based synthetic adducts, analogs, derivatives, and conjugates that can be used as chemotherapeutic agents.

Keywords: apoptosis, cell cycle, colon cancer, gastrointestinal disorders: resveratrol, stomach cancer

INTRODUCTION

The gastrointestinal (GI) system consists of the gastrointestinal tract (mouth, pharynx, esophagus, stomach, small intestine, and large intestine) and the accessory organs (salivary

* Corresponding author: Email: velan2009@gmail.com, Phone: +1 732-688-3768.

glands, liver, gallbladder, and pancreas). Even though, gastrointestinal disorders did not received much attention worldwide as cancer, diabetes and heart disease, they results in significant human suffering and loss of economy. Extensive research in the last few years has revealed that the overall functions of the GI systems are affected by several bodies' external and internal environment including improper nutrition or a change in health practices. Maintaining a relatively healthy lifestyle and food habits such as intake of fruits and vegetables offer some health-promoting actions due to the presence of different phytochemicals (polyphenols, flavonoids, carotenoids, tannins, lignans, and phytosterols). Several molecular studies suggest that phytochemicals offer beneficial effect to GI system through the antioxidant, anti-inflammatory, anti-carcinogenic, anti-proliferative, and cellular repair properties by modulating transcription, growth factors, anti-inflammatory cytokines, protein kinases, and other enzymes.

Resveratrol is a phenol-based plant secondary metabolite (phytoalexin) present widely among plant species caught worldwide attention among researchers due to its various biological properties. In addition to resveratrol, derivatives, closely related analogs, and conjugates of resveratrol were found in nature.

Due to numerous biological, pharmacological properties and health benefits, scientists are trying to synthesize several resveratrol analogs chemically for structure–activity studies in various disease models. The potential effect of resveratrol and its derivatives *in vivo* are mainly depends on the absorption, metabolism, distribution, and excretion of these compounds within the human body.

This chapter mainly focuses on the *in vitro* and *in vivo* beneficial effect of resveratrol and its derivatives on gastrointestinal disorders, with special emphasis on ulcerative colitis, colon cancer, esophagus and stomach cancer and we discusses how resveratrol can be practically used for the benefits for human health.

Structure of Resveratrol and Its Derivatives

Resveratrol and its derivatives are basically secondary metabolites of various plant species called as "stilbene." The stilbene nucleus consists of a 14-carbon skeleton with two phenyl rings linked by an ethylene bridge.

In plants stilbenes are synthesized through phenylpropanoid pathway, starting from phenylalanine. Figure 1 shows the chemical structures of resveratrol and some of its natural monomeric derivatives.

Resveratrol and Its Derivatives in Ulcerative Colitis (UC)

Ulcerative colitis (UC) is a chronic idiopathic inflammatory disease that affects mostly the mucosa and submucosa of the colon and rectum.

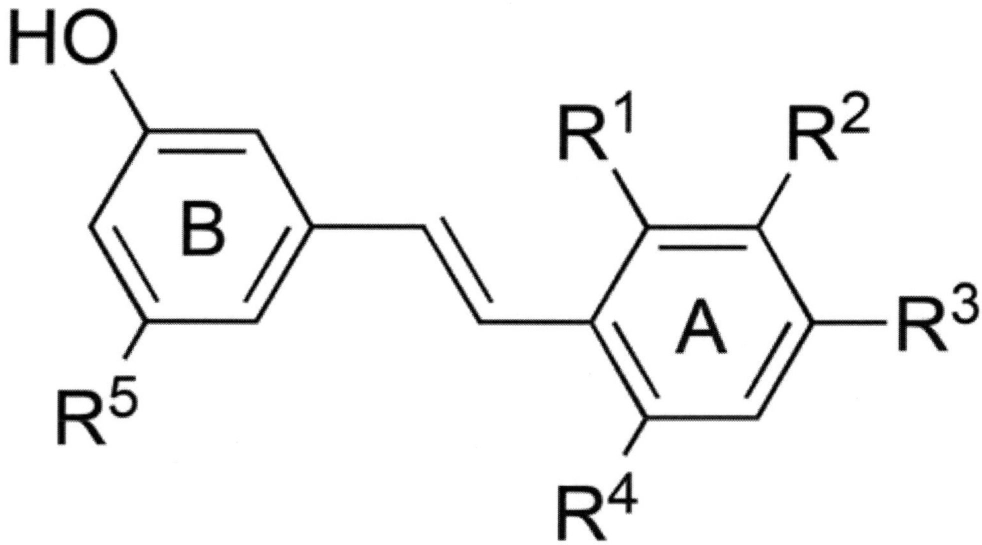

Name	R^1	R^2	R^3	R^4	R^5
Resveratrol	H	H	OH	H	OH
Oxyresveratrol	OH	H	OH	H	OH
Piceatanol	H	OH	OH	H	OH
Gnetol	OH	H	H	OH	OH
Piceid	H	H	OH	H	OGlu
Astringin	H	OH	OH	H	OGlu
Rhapontin	H	OH	OMe	H	OGlu

Figure 1. Chemical structures of resveratrol and some of its natural monomeric derivatives.

So for, the exact etiological factors for UC has not been fully elucidated, but factors such as infective agents, genetic factors and defect in the immune response to intestinal flora and life style factors such as smoking have been postulated as possible etiologic agents. The current drug therapies such as treatment with glucocorticosteroids, amino salicylates, antibiotics and anti-TNF drugs are no longer beneficial due to severe adverse effects. So, chemopreventive strategies using natural compounds, its derivatives and synthetic analogs were extensively tested as drugs to reverse or delay the progression of UC.

One among natural compounds, a number *in vivo* of studies has shown the ability of resveratrol to modulate UC (Yaoet al. 2010; Martin et al. 2006). A study shows that supplementation of dietary resveratrol to mice significantly inhibited the severity of dextran sodium sulfate (DSS)-induced colitis (Yao et al. 2010). Resveratrol exerts this effect by decreasing the colonic oxidative stress and increasing antioxidant enzymes such as superoxide dismutase (SOD) and glutathione peroxidase (GSH-Px) activities. Also, it modulated the inflammatory cytokine and factors such as tumor necrosis factors (TNF)-α, interleukin (IL)-8, Interferon gamma (IFN)-γ, p22phox, and gp91phox in the colonic tissue.

Cui et al. found that resveratrol supplementation ameliorates DSS-induced colitis in mice in a dose-dependent manner by improving inflammation score, decreasing neutrophils infiltration in the mesenteric lymph nodes and lamina propria, and modulating CD3 $^{(+)}$ T cells that express TNF-alpha and IFN-gamma (Cui et al. 2010). In addition, resveratrol downregulated the inflammation and inflammatory stress [p53 and p53-phospho-Ser(15)] markers in UC mouse model.

In the same study, they also found that resveratrol reduced the tumor incidence (80%) and tumor multiplicity in azoxymethane (AOM) + DSS induced colon cancer associated with colitis. Another study elucidates that administration of resveratrol to mice in trinitrobenzene sulfonic acid (TNBS)-induced ulcerative-colitis model significantly decreased the ulcerative area, colon mass index, colon inflammation grades, as well as histolopathological changes (Abdallah and Ismael 2011). The anti-inflammatory effects of resveratrol were mainly achieved through lowering the colonic myeloperoxidase activity, suppressing adhesive molecules such as ICAM-1 and VCAM-1 levels. In addition, resveratrol suppressed colonic nitric oxide level and lipid peroxide accumulation and restored redox balance by prevention of glutathione depletion in the colon, this effect is comparable with the standard drug sulphasalazine (Abdallah and Ismael 2011).

A study by Sánchez et al. demonstrated that resveratrol significantly attenuated the clinical signs such as loss of body weight, diarrhea and rectal bleeding in DSS induced UC model.

In addition, resveratrol substantial reduced the levels of pro-inflammatory cytokines, TNF-alpha and IL-1beta and an increase of the anti-inflammatory cytokine IL-10. The mechanisms behind the resveratrol effects is mainly due to reduction in prostaglandin E synthase-1 (PGES-1), cyclooxygenase-2 (COX-2) and inducible nitric oxide synthase (iNOS) proteins expression and downregulation of p38, a mitogen-activated protein kinases (MAPK) signal pathway (Sanchez-Fidalgo et al. 2010). In an inflammatory bowel disease (IBD) animal model, administration resveratrol to IL-10(-/-) deficient mice induces immunosuppressive CD11b (+) and Gr-1(+) myeloid derived suppressor cells (MDSCs) and decreased levels of serum amyloid A (SAA), CXCL10 and colonic TNF-α, IL-6, a chemokine called regulated on activation, normal T cell expressed and secreted (RANTES), IL-12 and IL-1β concentrations (Singh et al. 2012). Resveratrol treatment attenuated T cell proliferation, reduced IFN-γ and GM-CSF production by lamina propria (LP) derived T cells (Singh et al. 2012).

More importantly, in a randomized, double-blind, placebo-controlled study, resveratrol supplementation (500 mg) for 6 weeks improved the quality of life and clinical symptoms of colitis at least partially by reducing the inflammation and without any toxic effects to the patients (Samsami-Kor et al. 2015).

These studies in animal model and humans indicate that resveratrol is a beneficial candidate for preventing the progression of UC. In a similar fashion piceatannol (PCT), a hydroxystilbene also exerts anti-inflammatory effect in an experimental colitis mouse model through amelioration of colonic architecture, reduction in colonic myeloperoxidase (MPO) activity, and production of inflammatory mediators such as nitric oxide (NO), prostaglandin (PG) E2 (Kim et al. 2008).

Resveratrol and Its Derivatives in Colon Cancer

Colorectal cancer (CRC) is the third leading cause of cancer in males and fourth in females among western countries and the risk factors for CRC includes family history of colorectal cancer, colon polyps, and long-standing ulcerative colitis. However, several studies have shown that diet plays important role in the development of CRC in animal models and in humans. Chemopreventive effect of resveratrol against CRC has been extensively studied both in animals and in humans.

Due to high amount of resveratrol and its metabolites reaching the large intestine after metabolism, makes them a potential chemopreventive agent against CRC. Large number of *in vitro* and *in vivo* studies has shown that resveratrol possesses greater effects in prevention, suppressing and delaying development and progression of CRC. This section summarizes some interesting discoveries of resveratrol and its derivatives as chemopreventive agent for colon cancer.

Effects of Resveratrol and Its Derivatives on Colon Cancer Cells *In Vitro*

Malignant cells are defective in cell regulatory mechanisms and undergo uncontrolled division of cells; therefore blocking cell cycle would be an important target for anti-cancer effects. Numerous *in vitro* (cell culture) studies have shown that resveratrol exerts its chemopreventive effects basically through arrest of cell cycle progression and apoptotic cell death induction (Delmas et al. 2011; Ndiaye et al. 2011). Liang et al. found that resveratrol inhibited the proliferation of human colon adenocarcinoma HT29 cells by inducing cell cycle arrest at the transition S to G2/M phase by inhibition of CDK7 kinase activity (Liang et al. 2003). In another study, resveratrol was shown to inhibit cell cycle in human colonic adenocarcinoma Caco-2 cells by decreasing cyclin D1 and cyclin-dependent kinase (cdk) 4 and enhancing cyclin E and cyclin A proteins levels (Wolter et al. 2001). In 2002 Delmas et al. described that resveratrol, disrupts the cell cycle of human SW480 colorectal tumor cells through increasing cyclins A and B1 content as well as cyclin-dependent kinases Cdk1 and Cdk2. In addition, resveratrol promotes Cdk1 phosphorylation in these cells (Delmas et al. 2002).

Apoptosis is a highly organized programmed cell death process to eliminate damaged or abnormal cells. A wide range of natural compounds (phenolics, alkaloids and flavonoids etc.,) appear to exert its cytotoxic effect to cancer cells by inducing apoptosis and seems to be a reliable marker for the evaluation of cancer prevention potential. A large number of *in vitro*studies have been carried out on resveratrol to show its apoptosis inducing effect (Shankar et al. 2007; Madan et al. 2008; Mohan et al. 2006). In a study by Chen et al., reported that resveratrol induced apoptosis through MAPK MEK/ERK signaling transduction pathway in metastatic SW620 colon cancer cells(Chen et al. 2016). Resveratrol significantly increased the expression of apoptotic molecules such as Bax, Caspase 3 and Caspase 9 and decreased anti-apoptotic molecule Bcl2 in a dose-dependent manner. Also, the expression of Ras, Raf, MEK and ERK1/2 was decreased significantly by resveratrol. Crek et al. (Crek et al. 2014) have described that resveratrol induced apoptosis by altering mitochondrial membrane potential and permeability in Bax protein negative HCT- 116 colon carcinoma cell lines. Additionally, exposure of HCT-116 cells to resveratrol induced apoptosis by cleavage of PARP-1, chromatin condensation and activation of tumor suppressor gene p53 (Demoulin et al. 2015). Also, they showed that HCT-116 p53 wild type (wt) cells are more sensitive than HCT-116 p53-/- cells to resveratrol. Resveratrol induces DNA damage including double strand breaks in these cells by type II topoisomerase poisoning and activation of the Ataxia Telangiectasia Mutated (ATM) kinase. Another study compared the effect of resveratrol on Caco-2 and HCT116 human colon cancer cells and found that resveratrol had significantly higher growth inhibitory and cell cycle arresting effects on Caco-2 cells than HCT116 cells, through caspase-dependent and cyclin-CDK pathways (Liu et al. 2014).

The effects of polydatin (resveratrol-3-O-b-mono-D-glucoside, the glycoside form of resveratrol), a natural precursor of resveratrol were tested in combination with resveratrol on differentiated human adenocarcinoma colon cancer cells (Caco-2) and found that simultaneous treatment to polydatin and resveratrol induced synergistic antiproliferative effects compared with single compound treatment (De Maria et al. 2013). They also demonstrated that polydatin alone or in combination with resveratrol synergistically modulated oxidative stress, cell cycle, differentiation and apoptosis in Caco-2 cells (De Maria et al. 2013).

Molecular mechanistic studies on human colon cancer cell lines DLD-1 and LOVO shows that DMU-212, a synthetic analogue of resveratrol, showed the stronger cytotoxic activity in DLD-1 cells than that of LOVO cells, by up-regulation of pro-apoptotic Bak1, Bok, Bik, Noxa, Bad, Bax, p53 and Apaf1 and down-regulation of anti-apoptotic Bcl-2, Bcl-xL and Bag1 at transcription level (Piotrowska et al. 2013). Altogether, it seems that depending on the type of cells, resveratrol appear to activate death signals in different manner.

Effects of Resveratrol and Its Derivatives on Animal Models of Colon Cancer

Past several decades, for studying human colorectal cancer, animal models have played an important role in our understanding of carcinogenesis, tumor biology and the evaluation of novel chemopreventive agents. The ability of resveratrol and its derivatives to inhibit colon cancer development and progression has well been documented in several studies. For example Alfaras et al. demonstrated that oral administration of trans-resveratrol (60 mg/kg body weight) for 7 weeks in dimethyl hydrazine (DMH) induced colon cancer model, significantly decreased the incidence of precancerous colonic lesions such as aberrant crypt foci by 52%, and mucin depleted foci by 45% in colon (Alfaras et al. 2010).

Tessitore and colleagues reported that supplementation of resveratrol (0.2 mg/kg) for long-term (100 days) reduced number of aberrant crypt foci (ACF); a preneoplastic lesion on azoxymethane (AOM) induced colon carcinogenesis in F344 rats through modulating the cell proliferation and apoptosis molecules bax and p21 (Tessitore et al. 2000). We have also reported that supplementation of resveratrol (8 mg/kg b.w.) for 30 weeks in DMH-treated rats reduced the development of large ACF, incidence and multiplicity of tumors, which indicates that, resveratrol suppressed the progression of preneoplasia to malignant neoplasia (Sengottuvelan et al. 2006b). In addition, resveratrol attenuates the COX-2 overexpression and increased the expression of apoptotic biomarkers such as caspase 3 and heat shock protein 70 and 27 in the colonic mucosa of DMH-treated rats (Sengottuvelan et al. 2009). Supplementation of resveratrol to DMH-treated rats enhanced the activity of enzymic antioxidants such as superoxide dismutase, catalase and glutathione reductase and reduced glutathione levels; while diminished glutathione peroxidase and glutathione S-transferase overexpression in the colon (Sengottuvelan et al. 2006a).

A few authors tested the chemopreventive effects of resveratrol in genetic-based models of colorectal cancer (Schneider et al. 2001; Ziegler et al. 2004; Sale et al. 2005), for example in Apc^{Min} mice, a model where mutation of *Apc* gene makes the mouse more susceptible to develop intestinal tumors spontaneously. Resveratrol administration at 0.01% dose in drinking water for 7 weeks decreased the incidence of tumor formation in the small intestine and completely prevented the tumor formation in the colon of these animals (Schneider et al. 2001). Conversely, different doses of resveratrol (0, 4, 20, or 90 mg/kg body weight for 7 wk) were tested in Apc^{Min} mice, where higher doses of resveratrol did not affect intestinal tumor load (Ziegler et al. 2004). In addition, Sale et al. found that supplementing resveratrol at 60 mg/kg to Apc^{Min} mice did not decrease the incidence of adenomas, whereas 240 mg/kg of resveratrol reduced adenoma growth by 27% when compared with control (Sale et al. 2005).

Encouraging results from preclinical studies prompted resveratrol to clinical applications in colon cancer prevention, which results in the first clinical trial in colon cancer patients in 2009 (Nguyen et al. 2009). In this study resveratrol was given either as freeze-dried grape powder or capsules containing extracts from whole red grapes and roots of *Polygonum cuspidatum*, where the concentrations of resveratrol were 0.114 mg/d or 15.5 mg/d respectively. It appeared that in colon cancer tissue, there was no inhibition in the Wnt signaling pathway, but instead the expression of Wnt signaling target genes was reduced in normal mucosa. It suggests that low doses of resveratrol along with other bioactive compounds may have cancer chemopreventive effects in colon cancer patients (Nguyen et al. 2009). Another clinical trial conducted by Patel et al. suggests that resveratrol at 0.5 or 1.0 g doses for 8 days before the surgical resection of the colon tumor, results in 5% reduction in cell proliferation in the colonic mucosa (Patel et al. 2010).

Altogether, these findings suggest that the resveratrol and its derivatives found to be effective for chemoprevention of colon cancer in cellular systems. Further large clinical trials on testing these promising derivatives are urgently needed.

EFFECTS OF RESVERATROL AND ITS DERIVATIVES ON ESOPHAGEAL AND STOMACH CANCER

Worldwide, the incidence of esophageal and stomach cancer varies widely and undoubtedly linked with environmental and dietary factors. A number of studies have shown that resveratrol to have chemopreventive effects in esophageal cancer cells and in animal models (Zhou et al. 2003; Tang et al. 2013; Fan et al. 2014). Zhou et al. in 2003 demonstrated that resveratrol (10 mmol/L) treatment to esophageal cancer cell line EC-9706, displayed apoptotic characteristics such as morphological changes of chromatin condensation, chromatin crescent formation, nucleus fragmentation and apoptotic body formation by down-regulating the Bcl-2, an apoptosis-regulated gene and up-regulating the expression of apoptosis-regulated gene bax (Zhou et al. 2003).

In a study by Tang et al. shows that resveratrol induces apoptosis by a novel autophagy mechanism in EC109, EC9706, and K562 esophagealsquamous cell carcinoma cell lines.

Mechanistically, resveratrol-induced apoptosis by cell cycle arrest at the sub-G1 phase and autophagy by AMPK/mTORindependent pathway (Tang et al. 2013). Other investigators have examined resveratrol's effect on oesophageal adenocarcinoma cells (OAC) and showed that upon resveratrol treatment human OAC cell lines OE33 and OE19 displayed suppressed cell proliferation. This effect was due to inhibition of Skp2-mediated ubiquitylation and 26S proteasome-dependent degradation of p27Kip1 via AMPK activation to suppress OAC proliferation (Fan et al. 2014).

Few animal studies (Li et al. 2002; Woodall et al. 2009) and a study on humans (Lin et al. 2014) have shown that resveratrol is effective in the prevention of oesophageal cancer development. Li et al. evaluated the effects of resveratrol on N-nitrosomethylbenzylamine (NMBA)-induced rat esophageal tumorigenesis. Results showed that resveratrol administration at 2 mg/kg (orally, for 16 weeks), 1 and 2 mg/kg (i.p., for 16 weeks) and 1 mg/kg (i.p., for 20 weeks) significantly reduced tumor incidence to 78, 62, 54 and 48 percent, respectively when compared to NMBA alone group. Semi-quantitative RT-PCR and ELISA analysis showed that resveratrol reverted the expression of COX-1 and 2 and PGE (2) synthesis significantly in esophagealmucosa (Li et al. 2002). In an animal model, authors evaluated the effect of resveratrol on the initiation of Barrett's metaplasia and the carcinogenic progression to esophageal adenocarcinoma (Woodall et al. 2009). The study shows that intraperitoneal administration of resveratrol (7 mg/kg) decreased severity of esophagitis, incidence of intestinal metaplasia, and incidence of carcinoma as compared with both the saline and nonoperated control groups (Woodall et al. 2009).

In a Swedish nationwide population-based case-control study, it was found that three phytochemicals (lignans, quercetin and resveratrol) synergistically decrease the risk of oesophageal cancer. The study team evaluated 181 cases of oesophageal adenocarcinoma (OAC), 158 cases of oesophageal squamous-cell carcinoma (OSCC), 255 cases of gastro-oesophageal junctional adenocarcinoma (JAC) and 806 controls to come to the conclusion that these three phytochemicals may play a protective role in the development of oesophageal cancer in the Swedish population (Lin et al. 2014).

Based on many studies on stomach cancer cells and in animal models, resveratrol has been suggested as a potential cancer chemopreventive agent in stomach cancer.

Atten et al. found that when gastric adenocarcinoma SNU-1 cells were treated with resveratrol, it induces tumor suppressors p21 (cip1/WAF-1) and p53 accumulation, which is preceded by loss of membrane-associated PKC delta protein and a concomitant increase in cytosolic PKC alpha (Atten et al. 2005).

In an analysis, resveratrol treatment affected the cell cycles of human gastric SGC7901 cancer cells; for example, resveratrol increased the proportion of the G0/G1 phase and decreased S and G2/M phases. Also, resveratrol down-regulated the expression of survivin, a protein responsible for inhibitingcaspaseactivation and apoptosis (Liu and Zhang 2014). Yang et al. demonstrated that resveratrol at 25 and 50 μM concentrations inhibited the cell viability and diminished the clonogenic potential of human adenocarcinoma gastric cells (AGS), BGC-823 and SGC-7901. Resveratrol treatment arrested these cells in the G1 phase and led to senescence rather than apoptosis. Regulator proteins of the cell cycle and senescence pathways, including cyclin D1, cyclin-dependent kinase (CDK4 and 6), p21 and p16, were dysregulated by resveratrol treatment.

Their nude mice xenograft studies shows that resveratrol (40 mg/kg/d) inhibited gastric cancer development and significantly decreased the cell proliferation marker Ki67-positive cells in the tumor by Sirt1-dependent manner (Yang et al. 2013). In addition, Wang et al. demonstrated that resveratrol induced apoptosis in human gastric adenocarcinoma SGC7901 cells by via generation of reactive oxygen species (ROS), but independent of sirtuin1(Wang et al. 2012).

In a genotoxicity study, the authors found that resveratrol (20μg/mL) showed genotoxic activity (presence of micronuclei) in primary cell cultures from gastric adenocarcinoma, confirms the anticancer property (Mitrut et al. 2009).

Aquilano and colleagues found that resveratrol suppress the H_2O_2 accelerated cell growth and MEK1/2-ERK1/2 activation in AGS cells by specific inhibition of ERK1/2 phosphorylation by MEK1/2 and repression of c-Jun activation (Aquilano et al. 2009). Finally, resveratrol's chemopreventive potential against gastric cancer was tested in human gastric adenocarcinoma SNU-1 cells, where resveratrol suppressed both DNA synthesis and generation of endogenous $O2^{(-)}$ while stimulating nitric oxide (NO) synthase (NOS) activity (Holian et al. 2002).

Conclusion

Resveratrol seems to modify several cellular pathways that all may contribute to its chemopreventive effect on different cancer models. Following are some possible mechanisms that have been proposed to explain the beneficial effect of resveratrol and its analogs on gastrointestinal diseases. (1) Interactions with cell proliferation, cell-cycle delay, apoptosis, and DNA damage; (2) activation of transcription and growth factors and upregulation of genes encoding cytoprotective proteins, and enzymes involved in signaling pathways; (3) enhanced antioxidant defenses (endogenous scavengers), and detoxification enzymes; (4) selective induction of apoptosis to malignant cells compared to normal cells. Although numerous studies have revealed that resveratrol has a great potential for the treatment of a wide variety of gastrointestinal diseases, only clinical trials with large number of patients can reveal its true potential and safety of resveratrol for human consumption.

References

Abdallah D. M. and Ismael N. R. (2011) Resveratrol abrogates adhesion molecules and protects against TNBS-induced ulcerative colitis in rats. *Can. J. Physiol. Pharmacol.*, 89: 811-818.

Alfaras I., Juan M. E. and Planas J. M. (2010) trans-Resveratrol reduces precancerous colonic lesions in dimethylhydrazine-treated rats. *J. Agric. Food Chem.*, 58: 8104-8110.

Aquilano K., Baldelli S., Rotilio G., et al. (2009) trans-Resveratrol inhibits H2O2-induced adenocarcinoma gastric cells proliferation via inactivation of MEK1/2-ERK1/2-c-Jun signalling axis. *Biochem. Pharmacol.*, 77: 337-347.

Atten M. J., Godoy-Romero E., Attar B. M., et al. (2005) Resveratrol regulates cellular PKC alpha and delta to inhibit growth and induce apoptosis in gastric cancer cells. *Invest. New Drugs,* 23: 111-119.

Chen H., Jin Z. L. and Xu H. (2016) MEK/ERK signaling pathway in apoptosis of SW620 cell line and inhibition effect of resveratrol. *Asian Pac. J. Trop. Med.,* 9: 49-53.

Crek C., Mutlu Altundag E., Karademir B., et al. (2014) The effect of resveratrol on signal transduction pathways and the role of pro-apoptotic Bax protein on apoptosis in HCT-116 colon carcinoma cell lines. *Free Radic. Biol. Med.,* 75 Suppl. 1: S27.

Cui X., Jin Y., Hofseth A. B., et al. (2010) Resveratrol suppresses colitis and colon cancer associated with colitis. *Cancer Prev. Res. (Phila),* 3: 549-559.

De Maria S., Scognamiglio I., Lombardi A., et al. (2013) Polydatin, a natural precursor of resveratrol, induces cell cycle arrest and differentiation of human colorectal Caco-2 cell. *J. Transl. Med.,* 11: 264.

Delmas D., Passilly-Degrace P., Jannin B., et al. (2002) Resveratrol, a chemopreventive agent, disrupts the cell cycle control of human SW480 colorectal tumor cells. *Int. J. Mol. Med.,* 10: 193-199.

Delmas D., Solary E. and Latruffe N. (2011) Resveratrol, a phytochemical inducer of multiple cell death pathways: apoptosis, autophagy and mitotic catastrophe. *Curr. Med. Chem.,* 18: 1100-1121.

Demoulin B., Hermant M., Castrogiovanni C., et al. (2015) Resveratrol induces DNA damage in colon cancer cells by poisoning topoisomerase II and activates the ATM kinase to trigger p53-dependent apoptosis. *Toxicol. In Vitro,* 29: 1156-1165.

Fan G. H., Wang Z. M., Yang X., et al. (2014) Resveratrol inhibits oesophageal adenocarcinoma cell proliferation via AMP-activated protein kinase signaling. *Asian Pac. J. Cancer Prev.,* 15: 677-682.

Holian O., Wahid S., Atten M. J., et al. (2002) Inhibition of gastric cancer cell proliferation by resveratrol: role of nitric oxide. *Am. J. Physiol. Gastrointest. Liver Physiol.,* 282: G809-816.

Kim Y. H., Kwon H. S., Kim D. H., et al. (2008) Piceatannol, a stilbene present in grapes, attenuates dextran sulfate sodium-induced colitis. *Int. Immunopharmacol.,* 8: 1695-1702.

Li Z. G., Hong T., Shimada Y., et al. (2002) Suppression of N-nitrosomethylbenzylamine (NMBA)-induced esophageal tumorigenesis in F344 rats by resveratrol. *Carcinogenesis,* 23: 1531-1536.

Liang Y. C., Tsai S. H., Chen L., et al. (2003) Resveratrol-induced G2 arrest through the inhibition of CDK7 and p34CDC2 kinases in colon carcinoma HT29 cells. *Biochem. Pharmacol.,* 65: 1053-1060.

Lin Y., Yngve A., Lagergren J., et al. (2014) A dietary pattern rich in lignans, quercetin and resveratrol decreases the risk of oesophageal cancer. *Br. J. Nutr.,* 112: 2002-2009.

Liu B., Zhou Z., Zhou W., et al. (2014) Resveratrol inhibits proliferation in human colorectal carcinoma cells by inducing G1/Sphase cell cycle arrest and apoptosis through caspase/cyclinCDK pathways. *Mol. Med. Rep.,* 10: 1697-1702.

Liu M. L. and Zhang S. J. (2014) Effects of resveratrol on the protein expression of survivin and cell apoptosis in human gastric cancer cells. *J. buon.,* 19: 713-717.

Madan E., Prasad S., Roy P., et al. (2008) Regulation of apoptosis by resveratrol through JAK/STAT and mitochondria mediated pathway in human epidermoid carcinoma A431 cells. *Biochem. Biophys. Res. Commun.,* 377: 1232-1237.

Martin A. R., Villegas I., Sanchez-Hidalgo M., et al. (2006) The effects of resveratrol, a phytoalexin derived from red wines, on chronic inflammation induced in an experimentally induced colitis model. *Br. J. Pharmacol.,* 147: 873-885.

Mitrut P., Burada F., Enescu A., et al. (2009) The genotoxicity study of resveratrol in primary gastric adenocarcinoma cell cultures. *Rom. J. Morphol. Embryol.,* 50: 429-433.

Mohan J., Gandhi A. A., Bhavya B. C., et al. (2006) Caspase-2 triggers Bax-Bak-dependent and -independent cell death in colon cancer cells treated with resveratrol. *J. Biol. Chem.,* 281: 17599-17611.

Ndiaye M., Kumar R. and Ahmad N. (2011) Resveratrol in cancer management: where are we and where we go from here? *Ann. N Y Acad. Sci.,* 1215: 144-149.

Nguyen A. V., Martinez M., Stamos M. J., et al. (2009) Results of a phase I pilot clinical trial examining the effect of plant-derived resveratrol and grape powder on Wnt pathway target gene expression in colonic mucosa and colon cancer. *Cancer Manag. Res.,* 1: 25-37.

Patel K. R., Brown V. A., Jones D. J., et al. (2010) Clinical pharmacology of resveratrol and its metabolites in colorectal cancer patients. *Cancer Res.,* 70: 7392-7399.

Piotrowska H., Myszkowski K., Amarowicz R., et al. (2013) Different susceptibility of colon cancer DLD-1 and LOVO cell lines to apoptosis induced by DMU-212, a synthetic resveratrol analogue. *Toxicol. In Vitro,* 27: 2127-2134.

Sale S., Tunstall R. G., Ruparelia K. C., et al. (2005) Comparison of the effects of the chemopreventive agent resveratrol and its synthetic analog trans 3,4,5,4'-tetramethoxystilbene (DMU-212) on adenoma development in the Apc(Min+) mouse and cyclooxygenase-2 in human-derived colon cancer cells. *Int. J. Cancer,* 115: 194-201.

Samsami-Kor M., Daryani N. E., Asl P. R., et al. (2015) Anti-Inflammatory Effects of Resveratrol in Patients with Ulcerative Colitis: A Randomized, Double-Blind, Placebo-controlled Pilot Study. *Arch. Med. Res.,* 46: 280-285.

Sanchez-Fidalgo S., Cardeno A., Villegas I., et al. (2010) Dietary supplementation of resveratrol attenuates chronic colonic inflammation in mice. *Eur. J. Pharmacol.,* 633: 78-84.

Schneider Y., Duranton B., Gosse F., et al. (2001) Resveratrol inhibits intestinal tumorigenesis and modulates host-defense-related gene expression in an animal model of human familial adenomatous polyposis. *Nutr. Cancer,* 39: 102-107.

Sengottuvelan M., Deeptha K. and Nalini N. (2009) Influence of dietary resveratrol on early and late molecular markers of 1,2-dimethylhydrazine-induced colon carcinogenesis. *Nutrition,* 25: 1169-1176.

Sengottuvelan M., Senthilkumar R. and Nalini N. (2006a) Modulatory influence of dietary resveratrol during different phases of 1,2-dimethylhydrazine induced mucosal lipid-peroxidation, antioxidant status and aberrant crypt foci development in rat colon carcinogenesis. *Biochim. Biophys. Acta,* 1760: 1175-1183.

Sengottuvelan M., Viswanathan P. and Nalini N. (2006b) Chemopreventive effect of trans-resveratrol--a phytoalexin against colonic aberrant crypt foci and cell proliferation in 1,2-dimethylhydrazine induced colon carcinogenesis. *Carcinogenesis,* 27: 1038-1046.

Shankar S., Siddiqui I. and Srivastava R. K. (2007) Molecular mechanisms of resveratrol (3,4,5-trihydroxy-trans-stilbene) and its interaction with TNF-related apoptosis inducing ligand (TRAIL) in androgen-insensitive prostate cancer cells. *Mol. Cell Biochem.,* 304: 273-285.

Singh U. P., Singh N. P., Singh B., et al. (2012) Role of resveratrol-induced CD11b(+) Gr-1(+) myeloid derived suppressor cells (MDSCs) in the reduction of CXCR3(+) T cells and amelioration of chronic colitis in IL-10(-/-) mice. *Brain Behav. Immun.,* 26: 72-82.

Tang Q., Li G., Wei X., et al. (2013) Resveratrol-induced apoptosis is enhanced by inhibition of autophagy in esophageal squamous cell carcinoma. *Cancer Lett.,* 336: 325-337.

Tessitore L., Davit A., Sarotto I., et al. (2000) Resveratrol depresses the growth of colorectal aberrant crypt foci by affecting bax and p21(CIP) expression. *Carcinogenesis,* 21: 1619-1622.

Wang Z., Li W., Meng X., et al. (2012) Resveratrol induces gastric cancer cell apoptosis via reactive oxygen species, but independent of sirtuin1. *Clin. Exp. Pharmacol. Physiol.,* 39: 227-232.

Wolter F., Akoglu B., Clausnitzer A., et al. (2001) Downregulation of the cyclin D1/Cdk4 complex occurs during resveratrol-induced cell cycle arrest in colon cancer cell lines. *J. Nutr.,* 131: 2197-2203.

Woodall C. E., Li Y., Liu Q. H., et al. (2009) Chemoprevention of metaplasia initiation and carcinogenic progression to esophageal adenocarcinoma by resveratrol supplementation. *Anticancer Drugs,* 20: 437-443.

Yang Q., Wang B., Zang W., et al. (2013) Resveratrol inhibits the growth of gastric cancer by inducing G1 phase arrest and senescence in a Sirt1-dependent manner. *PLoS One,* 8: e70627.

Yao J., Wang J. Y., Liu L., et al. (2010) Anti-oxidant effects of resveratrol on mice with DSS-induced ulcerative colitis. *Arch. Med. Res.,* 41: 288-294.

Zhou H. B., Yan Y., Sun Y. N., et al. (2003) Resveratrol induces apoptosis in human esophageal carcinoma cells. *World J. Gastroenterol.,* 9: 408-411.

Ziegler C. C., Rainwater L., Whelan J., et al. (2004) Dietary resveratrol does not affect intestinal tumorigenesis in Apc(Min/+) mice. *J. Nutr.,* 134: 5-10.

In: Disorders of Gastrointestinal Systems ... ISBN: 978-1-63485-366-8
Editors:S. Rajagopal, S. Murugan and S. Ramachandran ©2016 Nova Science Publishers, Inc.

Chapter 3

ANTI-INFLAMMATORY EFFECT OF POLYMER FROM CEPHALOPOD AGAINST EXPERIMENTALLY INDUCED INTESTINAL BOWEL DISEASE IN ZEBRA FISH MODEL

V. Manigandan[1,*], R. Karthik[1,*] and S. Ramachandran[2,†], PhD

[1]Department of Medical Biotechnology,
Chettinad Academy of Research and Education,
Kelambakkam, Tamil Nadu, India
[2]Faculty of Allied Health Sciences,
Chettinad Academy of Research and Education,
Kelambakkam, Tamil Nadu, India

ABSTRACT

Despite advances in the progress of substitutes in the biomedical field to using animals in research, scientists still frequently quote necessitate to use live animals in trials. Human anti-inflammation has commonly been replicated using animal models, such as zebra fish has added terrific interest as a model system. The root cause of the regular form of inflammatory bowel diseases (IBD) remains blurred. The remedies (Nonsteroidal anti-inflammatory drugs - NSAID) currently used to treat IBD produce major limitations such as stimulation of apoptosis, inhibition of angiogenesis etc. The concept of cephalopod biopolymers has been raised to be future of medicine for IBD. Glycosaminoglycans (GAG) and its derivative oligosaccharides are isolated from various natural marine resources, which have widely been used drug candidate for IBD on the benefit of humankind. IBD are experimentally induced in zebra fish model, various concentration of biopolymer from cephalopods is added to the zebra fish experimental set up. The zebra fish are anesthetized, sectioned, stained and observed. The changes in colon length, colon length: weight ratio were determined. The histology of the intestine is studied using hematoxylin-eosin, alcian blue and Sudan black staining. Mean survival

---

* Equally contributed.

† Corresponding author: Dr. Saravanan Ramachandran, PhD., Department of Marine Pharmacology, Faculty of Allied Health Sciences, Chettinad Academy of Research & Education, Kelambakkam, Chennai-603 103, Tamil Nadu, India, E mail: saran_prp@yahoo.com, Phone: +91 044 4741 9038, Fax: +9147413300.

time of the treated and control group was also determined. The results of the present study establish the ameliorative abilities of the fractionated GAG (f-GAG) from cuttlefish against IBD in zebra fish model.

Keywords: anti-inflammation, f-GAG, inflammatory bowel diseases, nonsteroidal anti-inflammatory drugs, zebra fish

1. Introduction

The inflammatory bowel diseases (IBD) are caused by a decreased lenience to intestinal bacteria and a strange activation of intestinal cellular immunity, which consists of Ulcerative Colitis (UC), Crohn's Disease (CD) and Indeterminate Colitis (IC).

1.1. Types of IBD

1.1.1. Crohn's Disease (CD)

CD has an effect on any part of the GI tract, from the mouth to the anus. It most usually affects the end of the small intestine especially in the ileum where it joins the beginning of the colon. CD may appear in "patches," affecting a few parts of the GI tract while leaving other segments completely untouched. In CD, the inflammation may extend through the entire thickness of the bowel wall.

1.1.2. Ulcerative Colitis (UC)

Ulcerative colitis is limited to the large intestine (colon) and the rectum. The inflammation occurs only in the innermost layer of the lining of the intestine. It usually begins in the rectum and lower colon, but may also spread continuously to involve the entire colon.

1.1.3. Indeterminate Colitis (IC)

In some individuals, it is difficult to determine whether their IBD is Crohn's disease or ulcerative colitis. In these rare cases, people are given the diagnosis of indeterminate colitis (IC).

1.2. Historical Perspective and Research Advances

CD was first described in 1932 by three doctors - Burrill Crohn, Leon Ginzberg, and Gordon D. Oppenheimer. At the time, any disease in the small intestine was thought to be intestinal tuberculosis. These medical practitioners pooled data from 14 patients with symptoms of abdominal cramps, diarrhea, fever, and weight loss, which showed that the symptoms were not the result of tuberculosis or any other known disease. They described a new disease entity, which was first called regional ileitis, and later, CD. In the years since inflammatory bowel diseases were identified, major scientific advances, specifically in the fields of genetics, immunology, and microbiology, have led to greater understanding of the underlying mechanisms involved in IBD, resulting in the development of increasingly effective treatments.

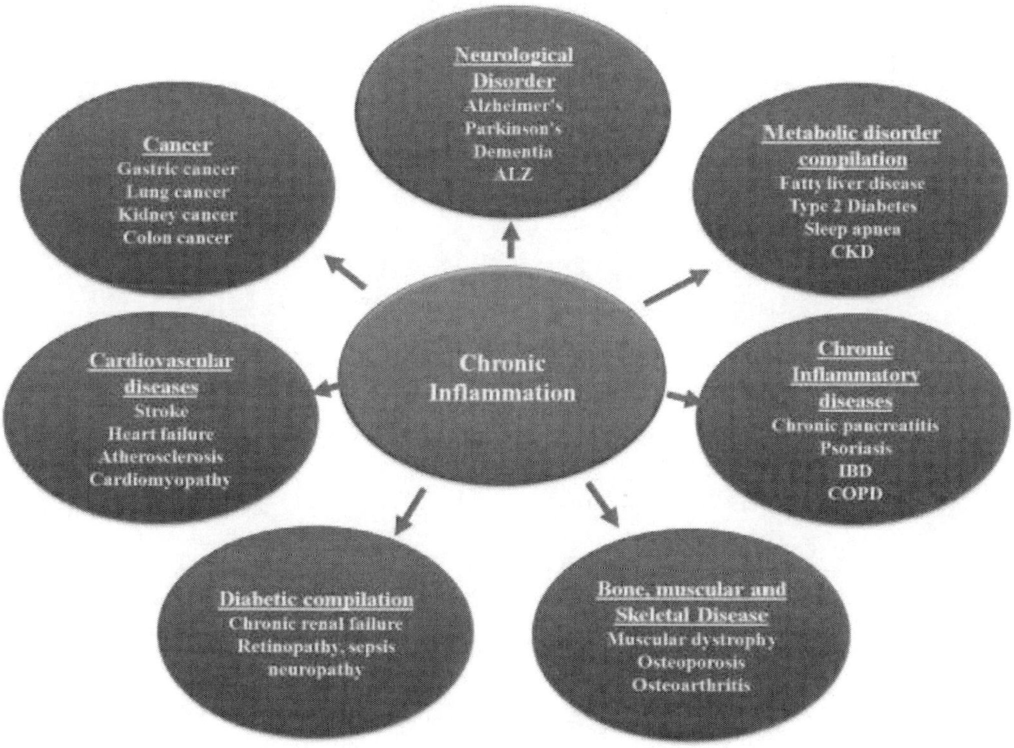

Figure 1. Chronic Inflammation and associated disease complications.

UC was first described in 1875 by two English physicians, Wilks and Moxon, who distinguished it from diarrheal diseases caused by infectious agents. Reports of a disease with similar symptoms to ulcerative colitis date back to before the Civil War and even many years before that, although it was not named as a distinct disease until 1875. IBDs are characterized by unrelieved inflammation of the gastrointestinal tract (GIT) which can influence any portion of the GIT. The incidence of IBD has increased dramatically over the past half century, which is in genetically predisposed individuals of IBD are pictured to environmental risk factors (Mikhailov, and Furner, 2009; Danese and Fiocchi, 2004; Podolsky, 2002). This tale effort shacks glow on the environmental factors of IBD (Figure 2) that are equally divided diagonally the world and that are discrete in Asia. In addition, many of the risk factors are amendable and thus suggest the opening for main hindrance to avoid the frequency of IBD in Asia from resembling that in Australia, North America and Europe (Kaplan, 2014). Although development has been made in understanding these diseases of IBD, but their etiology is unidentified hitherto. Their incidence is increasing worldwide, and the diseases remain incurable.

IBD places a heavy burden on populations because it decreases quality of life and capacity for work and increases disability.

The predominance of IBD is surplus 200 cases per 100,000 citizens in the West Asia, and IBD has a foremost impact on health care resources. Most IBD data is based on epidemiology and the IBD history have been taken from residents-based researches performed in Scandinavia and in Olmsted County, Minnesota, between the duration of 1950–1970; Disease evolution and prediction significantly revolutionized radically with the discoveries of steroid based therapies in the 1950s, latter immunosuppressant are introduced in the year of 1970s. Although these treatments do not have severe complications and improve quality of life, it is not clear whether they are able to modify the long-term course of the diseases (Cosnes et al., 2011).

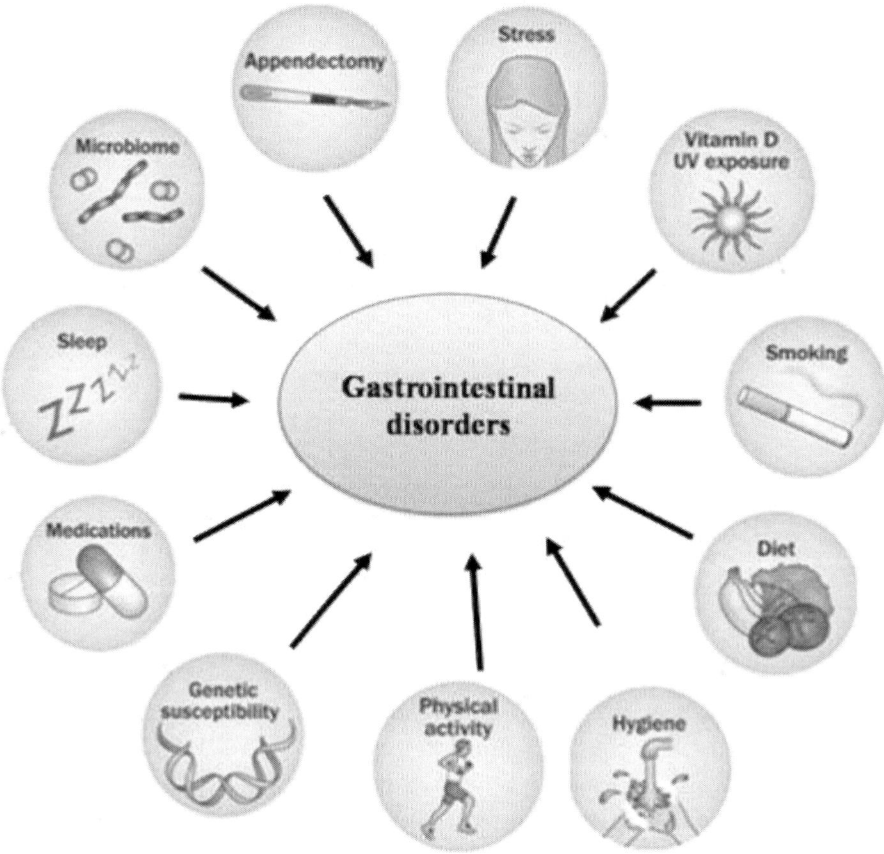

Figure 2. Environmental factors associated with IBD.

Few decades back the etiology of IBD has been extensively studied (Podolsky, 2002); still, the disease pathogenesis is not completely understood (Mikhailov, and Furner, 2009; Cosnes et al., 2011). Substantial disparity in the epidemiology of IBD has been reported around the globe, with an ample array of approximations both within and connecting the geographic regions. The prevalence of IBD in North America and Europe are believed to be associated with industrialization of nations (Bernstein et al., 1999) and the incidence of IBD may be increasing in developing countries as they have turned into industrialized (Zheng et al., 2005; Desai and Gupte, 2005). However, the epidemiology of IBD are population-based data collected in an identical trend in developing nations are meager. Several invention have been reported that the incidence of IBD has risen distinctly over the latter period of the 20th century, while other research have proposed a plateau or even refuse in frequency in certain geographic areas (Logan, 1998, Loftus, 2004). The highest incidence rates of IBD are habitually reported in Northern and Western Europe over and above North America, whereas lower rates are recorded in Africa, South America and Asia. It is more common in developed, more industrialized nations, pointing at urbanization as a latent risk factor of IBD (Russel, 2000, Xia et al., 1997).

1.3. Does an Environmental Factor Play a Role in IBD?

In the past half century the incidence of IBD has increased spectacularly. Though surplus 160 genetic risk loci have been recognized that lie beneath disease predilection, these loci have not fully elucidated the disease etiology. Outstanding epidemiological surveillance counting the increasing incidence in developing countries and the raised risk of disease in immigrant residents incriminate the magnitude of environmental persuades on genetic predisposition (Ng et al., 2013). In 2013, the study of Ng et al., explained that the occurrence of IBD varies transversely in Asia but is still poorer than in the Western counties. However, the appearance of IBD in Asia specifies a vital role for environmental factors in the pathogenesis and suggests a single prospect to study etiological factors, mostly factors connected with 'Westernisation' including amends in diet, global industrial exposure, frequent childhood exposure to antibiotics, vaccination and developed hygiene. Numerous of these environmental risk factors have not been survived in populations of increasing incidence.

1.4. "Westernization"

The developed countries such as United States, United Kingdom and Scandinavia are facing the most prevalent disease of IBD (Andres and Friedman, 1999; Loftus and Sandborn, 2003). The raised episode of IBD observed in industrialized countries and the remarkable raise in cases throughout the 20th century hold the theory that environmental factors lead to disease development (Krishnan and Korzenik, 2002; Sandler and Loftus, 2004). This may possibly in addition description for the north-to-south deviation and higher occurrence in metropolitan communities compared with rural areas. Fascinatingly, augments in incidence have newly been lesser in southern countries and Asia and among emigrants to first-world countries (Andres and Friedman, 1999; Loftus and Sandborn, 2003). It is suggested that this is the effect of "westernization" of way of life, for instance modifications in diet, smoking, and differences in experience to sunlight, pollution, and industrial chemicals (Loftus and Sandborn, 2003).

1.5. Sanitation and Exposure to Infection

IBD is a disease of spotlessness. In widespread with diseases for example asthma, multiple sclerosis and rheumatoid arthritis, it exhibits a contrary association with the degree of sanitation: poor sanitation emerges to shield against IBD. The propensity for infection associated with overcrowding may also be a factor. For example, children increased in more spacious circumstances (i.e., diminished sharing of sleeping lodging and rest rooms) have a greater risk of developing CD. It is claimed that advanced sanitation modifies the intestinal flora by decreasing contact to certain dangerous microorganisms. There is also an increased incidence of UC and CD in higher socioeconomic groups (Krishnan and Korzenik, 2002; Farrell and LaMont, 2002).

1.6. Occupation

Both UC and CD are the most prevalent in white-collar compared with blue-collar professions (Krishnan and Korzenik, 2002; Loftus et al., 1996; Sonnenberg, 1990). Higher death rate of IBD has been pointed in managerial, clerical and sales spots, which typically occupy deskbound, interior work. Not in any way, transience consequence from IBD is low down in among cultivators and civil employees (Sonnenberg, 1990; Sandler and Loftus, 2004) Sonnenberg (1990) suggests that revamp occupying outside air and corporal exploit is defensive against IBD, but exertion in artificial locations presents an boosted hazard. This theory could simplify the advanced risk for IBD in northern atmospheres (e.g., more indoor exposure) and in colonizers to expanded countries, as well to the unstable times among ethnic groups in dissimilar regions (Andres and Friedman, 1999).

1.7. Diet

Researches seeking to link diet and IBD are generally indecisive. There are several confirmations that an excess intake of fatty acids increases the risk for IBD (Krishnan and Korzenik, 2002). Similarly, Persson et al., 1992 proposes that frequent fast-food intake presents a 3- to 4-fold greater risk for IBD.

1.8. Tobacco Smoking

The physically powerful environmental risk factor for IBD is tobacco smoking, predominantly amid customers of cigarettes. The correlation involving IBD and smoking is intricate, signifying exclusive pathophysiological factors for jointly UC and CD. Several case-control reports have demonstrated that existing smoking is defending against UC, with effects that are constant across different geographic regions. The decreased risk for UC in smokers appears to be dose dependent. In distinguish to UC; cigarette smoking is an important risk factor for the improvement of CD (Lindberg et al., 1988; Erpecum et al., 1996; Merrett et al., 1996).

1.9. Genetic Factors

Epidemiological and family histories reveal that genetic factors play a vital role in the propensity to IBD. The infection is, conversely, genetically complex and cannot be clarified by a particular gene model alone. It is consideration that UC and CD may be coupled polygenic disorders splitting numerous but not all susceptibility loci. Primarily, the disease phenotype is caused by several risk factors; containing relation between allelic variants at a number of loci, in addition to genetic and environmental influences. As a result, the occurrence of a mutated gene does not agree that IBD will form, nor does it envisage who will develop it, underlining the significance of cofactors in precipitating the disease (Boyko et al., 1988; Reif et al., 1995; Satsangi et al., 2003).

1.10. Familial and Ethnic Syndromes

The present prevalence of IBD is increased in first- and second-degree comparatives and a higher relative risk among siblings. The ancestral occurrence of IBD ranges from 20% to 30% in referral-based reports and between 5% and 10% in population reviews (Binder, 1998). Yang et al., (1993) observed the higher risk for IBD found in Jewish population and they suggest that genetic factors may play a major role in some subpopulations (Satsangi et al., 2003). In families with a high frequency of IBD between the first degree relatives, 75% of those influenced are concordant for both UC and CD, while 25% are not concordant, with some groups having UC and others having CD (Binder, 1998). This invention highlights that multiple, overlapping genetic factors may donate to disease pathogenesis. Additional support for a genetic vulnerability comes from the finding of a connection between IBD and other syndromes with a genetic predisposition (Satsangi et al., 2003).

2. Current Limitations of IBD Treatment

Accelerated research over the last five years has led to immense move forwards in scientific invention and has enlarged our accepting of the IBD and their original pathophysiologic systems. Researchers have afforded confirmation for the hypothesis that IBD are consequence of a genetic predisposition that guides to a mucosal immune regulatory cell deficiency and weakness to environmental activates, mostly luminal bacteria, covering specific antigens and pathogen-connected molecular patterns. Foremost currently it has become obvious that this dysfunction happens from an uncharacteristic association between innate immune reactions to bacterial cells mediated via toll and other inventors and the adaptive immune reaction. A disproportion between several effectors cell types, counting T cells and NK-T cells, and an immense group of T regulatory cells is the possible root of inflammation. As well as these findings, there have been numerous new pathways and definite targets upon which to hub new remedies. The "holy grail" of IBD management is to evade chronic steroid practice in an attempt to avoid disease sequence.

The utilization of azathioprine (AZA) signifies an important remedial advance in the cure of IBD as an entrenched second-line treatment for refractory and steroid-dependent patients and for reduction maintenance. Nevertheless, at the innovative proposed standard dosage of up to 2.5 mg/kg/day, AZA has to be discontinued in about 15% of both adult and pediatric patients due to cruel hematotoxicity (e.g., pancytopenia) and gastrointestinal adverse effects such as hepatotoxicity, pancreatitis, and gastrointestinal disturbances. The most common sudden adverse effects include nausea, pancreatitis, fever, allergic reactions, hepatitis, infections and probably malignancy and bone marrow inhibition (Present et al., 1989; Connell et al., 1993; Kirschner, 1998).

It has now been certified that the collection of agents known as nonsteroidal anti-inflammatory drugs (NSAIDs) can have deadly effects on small bowel and colonic mucosa as well as the upper GI tract. NSAIDs have been demonstrated to particularly cause ulceration and constraints of the jejunum, ileum, and colon. The clinical symptoms of NSAID-associated small and large bowel tract toxicity are wide and include abdominal pain, diarrhea, colitis and perforation, blood and protein loss (Felder et al., 2000).

3. Drug Discovery and Zebra Fish Research

Drug discovery involves a multiple repetitious technique on cellular and biochemical assays, followed by validation in animal models, and ultimately in human's trials. There is also steep pressure to reduce animal use to situations in which they are absolutely necessary, especially in safety assessment and preclinical toxicity. Zebra fish are beginning to be used at various platforms of the drug discovery process and can be a cost-effective and useful alternative to some mammalian models - rodents, dogs and pigs (Zon and Peterson, 2005). Zebra fish is a small tropical indigenous fish to India and south Asia, it belongs to the subphylum (Vertebrata) and the subclass (Teleostei). These fish raise and breed easily in the laboratory conditions, Females are capable of laying 100–200 eggs in a day, on a weekly basis, which are externally fertilized by the males. For optimum breeding and collection of eggs, males and females (2:1) ratio are maintained in a tank with shallow water overnight and eggs are separated. It's possible to induced breed the entire year around in laboratory conditions.

Zebra fish serves as popular model for exploring in bio-medical research against various diseases and disorders - cardiovascular disorder, cancer, hemophilia, angiogenesis, central nervous disorders, osteoporosis, kidney and liver diseases (Schloz et al., 2008, Kabashi et al., 2010, Ben-Moshe et al., 2014). Advantage that include rapid embryonic development, larval transparency and high genetic and physiological to humans (81%) compared to rodents or non-human primates. Zebrafish particularly open to high - throughput drug testing given their simple handling, reduced size and low cost with an economy that is not feasible in other vertebrates (Pinho et al., 2015). The transparency of zebra fish embryos allow to study the scoring of toxic effects, developmental toxicity and teratological effects easily with ecological end points. Various studies have been documented and proved that zebra fish assay has studied of the teratogenic potential of different chemicals showing a good concordance with *in vivo* results in humans. (Teixido et al., 2013)

3.1. Zebra Fish - Inflammation Research

The immune system of all the vertebrates from fish to mammals is similar in nature. Zebra fish are transparent during their embryo and larval stages, which allows them optimally matched for non-invasive imaging of the behavior of immune cells during development and disease. The inflammatory response of zebra fish has been well characterized most relied on physical damage and genetically induced chronic inflammatory condition (Renshaw SA et al., 2007). The major pathological features studying in zebra fish are comparable to those of human, due to clear visualization of disease progression, availability of transgenic fluorescent reporter lines and the conservation of the integral components of the innate immune system of larval or adult model in *in-vivo* screening are the greater advantage of inflammation research compare to other animal models. The availability of both forms as larvae and adult has greater advantage of examine molecules by directly dissolving them in small volumes of fish water; usually a solvent to allow diffuse of the compounds to all tissues (Alencon et al., 2010).

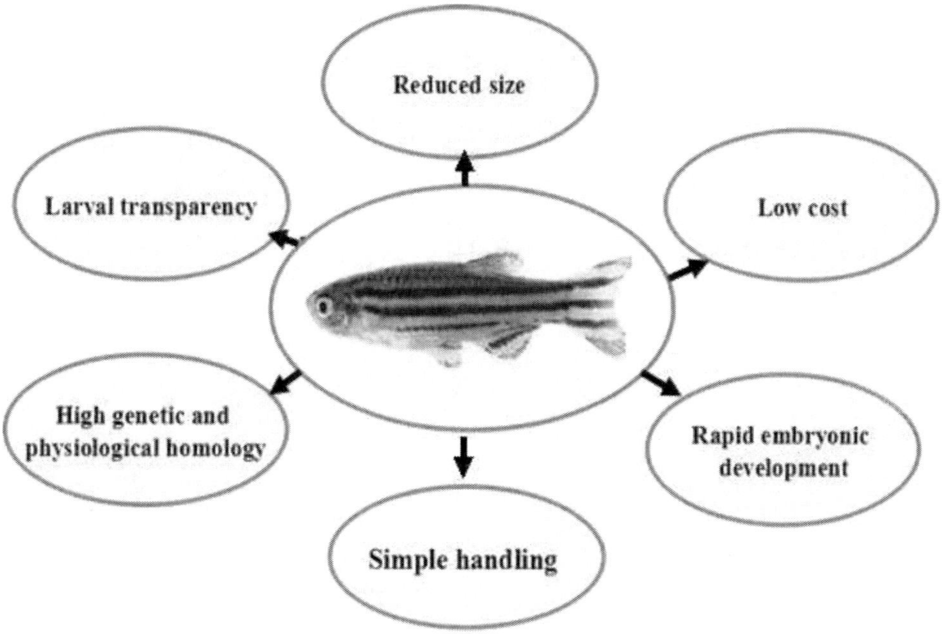

Figure 3. Zebrafish as an ideal model for Inflammatory diseases.

4. Microbes Causing Inflammation

Bacteria are present several millions in the digestive tract and intestine helps us to digest the food, protects against pathogenic bacteria and producing a variety of substances that have an important nutritional value. Gut bacteria have an intricate relationship with our immune system. Various factors may disturb the mutually beneficial relationship between the microbial flora and the body. When this happens, bacteria that can cause disease may take hold. Some specific bacteria that can cause infection of the stomach leads to the development of diseases, such as dyspepsia, gastritis), and ulcers in the stomach, duodenum and other serious complications. (Sartor et al., 2012) Inflammatory bowel disease (IBD) is a condition that involves chronic inflammation in all or part of the digestive tract. Often painful and debilitating, IBD can lead to life-threatening complications as well as increase the risk for colon cancer.

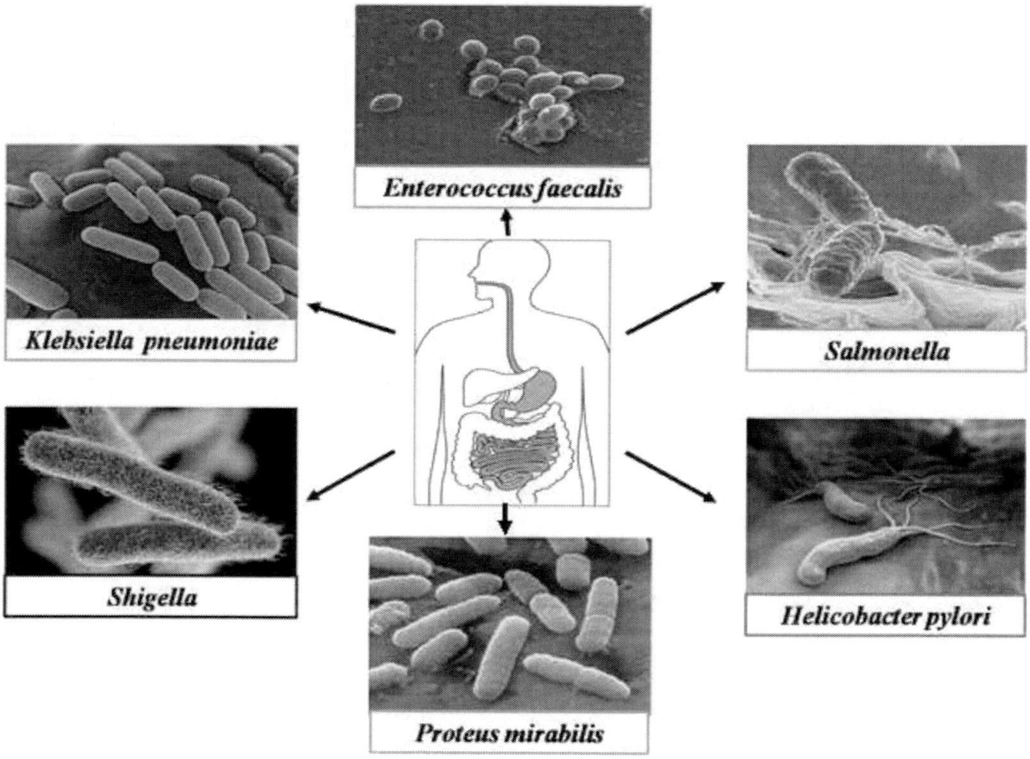

Figure 4. Intestinal microbiota associated with IBD.

5. Experimental Setup

5.1. Extraction and Isolation of Fractionated Glycosaminoglycans (f-GAG)

The cuttlefishes *S. pharaonis* were collected from the catchment areas of the Kasimedu landing Center, Chennai, Tamil Nadu, India. The crude GAG was isolated following the extraction procedure of Saravanan and Shanmugam, 2010. The crude GAG was fractionated in amberlite IRA 900 Cl^- anion exchange resin and the active fractions were pooled (Vidhyanandhini et al. 2014). The fractionated GAG (f-GAG) characterized using FT-IR (data not shown) was further studied for its protective role in ameliorating the inflammatory processes caused by IBD.

5.2. Maintenance of Stocks and Collection of Embryos

Wild type zebra fishes were reared following standard conditions in a circulating system attached with filters and aerators at a temperature of 26°C-28°C, optimal pH and under 14:10 light dark cycle (Avdesh et al., 2012). Male and female adult fishes were partnered to allow natural spawning following standard breeding protocol in a male: female ratio 2:1. Embryos were collected and the viable ones observed under a microscope (Nikon Eclipse Ni-U, USA) were reared in embryo medium (5 mM NaCl, 0.33 mM $CaCl_2$, 0.33 mM Mg_2SO_4, 0.17 mM KCl and 1% methylene blue) which was changed daily and maintained at 27°C-28°C (Dhillon et al., 2013).

5.3. Induction of IBD

2, 4, 6-Trinitrobenzenesulfonic acid or Picryl sulfonic acid was a nitroaryl oxidizing acid. IBD was induced using a stock solution of 1 mg/mL 2, 4; 6-trinitrobenzenesulfonic acid (TNBS; Sigma) in embryo medium was used for the induction of IBD. The zebra fish larvae (2/well in 250 µl) were introduced into "U" bottom micro titer plates (Greiner Cellstar, USA) 3 days post fertilization (d.p.f.) in embryo medium. The larva were divided into 4 groups of control, IBD induced, f-GAG treated for a total of 20 larvas per group. The larva's were pretreated with the f-GAG from *S. pharaonis* in serial dilutions. The zebra fish were then subjected to freshly prepared TNBS (75 µg/ml) for the concomitant induction of IBD. The experimental conditions were reinstated daily for 3 days (8 d.p.f.). The zebra fish larvae were constantly monitored for intestinal inflammation and treatment effects in a microscope (Nikon Eclipse Ni-U, USA) (Oehlers et al., 2013).

5.4. Optical Observation

The control and treated groups of zebra fish larva (8 d.p.f.) were observed under an Opticam optical microscope (Nikon Eclipse Ni-U, USA) for the infiltration of neutrophils. Owing to their transparent anatomy, the larvas were observed for localized accumulation of neutrophils in the gastrointestinal tract.

5.5. Histology and Staining

On termination of the study, the zebrafish larva were anaesthetized using tricaine (120 µg/ml) solution and the larva are processed for histopathology. The larvas are fixed in 10% neutral buffered formalin and were subjected dry heat at 70°C. The dehydrated larvae are fixed with molten paraffin wax. The zebra fish larvas fixed in paraffin were embedded transverse axes in paraffin blocks. The paraffin blocks were trimmed and sections of 3 µ thickness were taken using a microtome (brand, make). The sections were kept at 70°C for 10 minutes, deparaffinized in multiple washes of xylene, rehydrated using absolute alcohol and 70% alcohol. The rehydrated sections were stained using hematoxylin and exosin, alcian blue (1%) and Sudan black (0.7%). The stained sections were washed in running distilled water, rehydrated using alcohols, cleared using xylene and mounted using DPX mountant and visualized under the dissection microscope (Nikon Eclipse Ni-U, USA) for cytological changes associated with induction of inflammation by IBD.

5.6. Alcian Blue Staining

Alcian blue is a water soluble polyvalent basic dye, blue in colour due to the presence of copper. Alcian blue stains carboxylated and sulfated acid mucopolysaccharides sialomucins by forming salt linkages with the acid groups. Acidic mucosubstances were observed in excessive amounts during inflammation and early lesions of atherosclerosis. The zebra fish larva were subjected to 1% alcian blue solution and incubated at 28.5°C for 30 minutes. The stained larvas were visualized for the uptake of the alcian blue dye by the mucopolysaccharides lining the gastrointestinal tract.

5.7. Sudan Black Staining

Sudan Black (SB) is an azo dye that specifically stains the lipids with dark staining of the cytolymph. SB shows preferential staining to neutrophils than other cell types and is an excellent indicator of the inflammatory processes associated with IBD. The zebra fish larval sections after hydration are stained with 0.7% SB, dehydrated, mounted and observed in microscope.

5.8. Antibacterial Activity

The intestinal micro biota was highly associated with the development and prognosis of IBD. The presence of the micro biota such as *E. coli, Salmonella* and *Pseudomonas* sp. have been reported to be highly implicated in the development of IBD (Sartor et al., 2012). The potentials of the f-GAG to inhibit the growth of the micro biota could be established as a protective measure against the inflammation caused by IBD. The inhibitory activity of the f-GAG from *S. pharaonis* was determined by the antibacterial susceptibility testing assay. Initially the isolated colonies of the selected gram positive and gram negative bacteria were inoculated into sterile Luria Beltane (LB) broth and incubated at 37°C for 1 h. The bacterial concentration in the broth was estimated in a UV-visible spectrophotometric using the McFarland's standard 0.5. All the media (LB and MHA) and the fluoroquinolone antibiotic ciprofloxacin were purchased from Himedia laboratories.

5.9. Antibacterial Susceptibility Testing

The gram negative bacterial strains *Escherichia coli* 25922, *Pseudomonas aeroginosa, Salmonella typhimurium* ATCC 51812, were obtained from the archives of the Department of Microbiology, Chettinad Hospital and Research Institute, Kelambakkam, Tamil Nadu, India. The standard Kirby-Bauer antibiotics susceptibility test was performed to determine the inhibitory effect of the tested compounds against the selected strains of gram positive and gram negative bacteria. Sterile MHA medium was poured into petridishes to obtain an agar of 3-4 mm thickness. Sterile cotton swabs were dipped into broth cultures of the bacteria grown to a McFarland's standard of 0.5 containing approximately 1.2 – 1.5 X 10^8 CFU/ml. The cotton swabs with bacterial culture were swabbed onto the MHA plates evenly on the surface and incubated briefly for 5 min. Wells of 8 mm diameter were punched in the agar at equal distances allowing space for zone formation. The wells were filled with the f-GAG of concentrations 100 μg, 200 μg and 500 μg in DMSO. A well containing Ciprofloxacin (10 μg) served as the positive control and a well with DMSO was used as the negative control. After few minutes, the plates are incubated at 37°C for 24 h and 48 h. Finally the plates are observed for the formation of zones of inhibition and measured (Karthik et al., 2015).

5.10. Statistics

All experiments were performed in triplicates and were statistically analyzed using SPSS software version 21.0.

6. Results and Discussion

Increased infiltration of leucocytes caused due to leucocytosis was an important pharmacological process associated with the infection of IBD. Migration of macrophages and neutrophils to the intestinal sites are primary mediatory processes of immune responses to IBD. TNBS has been shown to induce robust inflammation and has been exemplified using zebra fish larva. The marine f-GAG from *S. pharaonis* has been found to show commendable protective activity from TNBS induced IBD in zebra fish model.

6.1. Optical Observation

The zebra fish larva showed evidences of IBD pathogenesis by prominent inflammation and variation in intestinal morphology compared to non-induced control group. The induced larva showed reduction in intestine length, breadth ratio, which was observed to be restored in the larva treated with f-GAG. The length breadth ratio was considerably reduced in zebra fish in TNBS induced IBD, which was restored in larva treated with f-GAG. The length/breadth ratio in the control zebra fish larva was 3.2 whereas it was 1.6 in larva induced with TNBS and 2.8 in larvas treated with f-GAG. The infiltration of neutrophils to the site of inflammation was observed in larva induced with TNBS (Figure 5 (a-c).

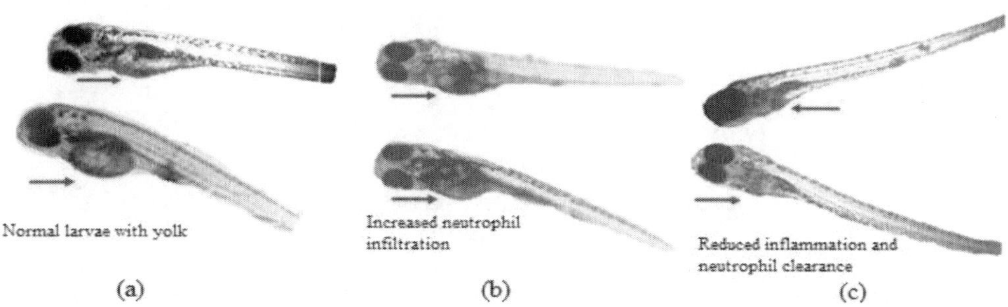

Figure 5. Optical imaging of (a) control (b) IBD induced and (c) f-GAG treated zebrafish larva 8 dpf (as indicated by arrows).

6.2. Histology

The histology of the sections revealed the inflammatory processes in the control, TNBS treated and f-GAG pretreated zebra fish larva. The larval sections stained with hematoxylin and eosin established the inflammation in TNBS induced IBD in zebra fish larva, which was restored in a dose-dependant manner in f-GAG-pretreated TNBS induced IBD. The IBD pathogenesis was illustrated with decreased intestinal vasculature, increased leukocyte recruitment, increased cellular proliferation and skin damage (Figure 4). H & E staining of the sections revealed pronounced inflammation by increase in intestine size, while increased goblet cell population (stained dark blue) was observed by AB staining in TNBS induced zebra fish larva. However, the histological sections of larva treated with f-GAG showed significant reduction in AB staining, demonstrating potential preventive effects of inflammation in TNBS induced IBD.

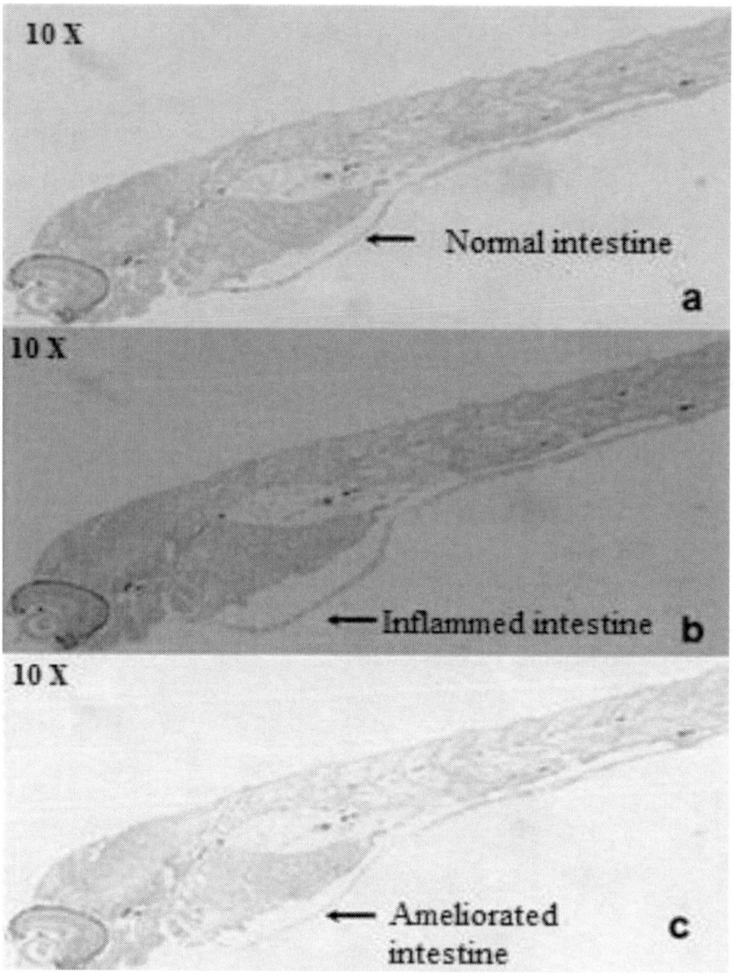

Figure 6. Hematoxylin and Eosin staining of (a) control; (b) IBD induced and (c) f-GAG treated zebrafish larva 8 d.p.f.

6.3. Alcian Blue Staining

Goblet cells were glandular cells distributed in the intestinal epithelium. Alcian blue staining of the acidic mucus producing Goblet cells showed the inflammatory process of TNBS induced IBD in the zebra fish larva 8 dpf. Increased staining of the goblet cells (Figure 3(a-c)) showed the mucus production of the goblet cells due to the induction of IBD. The larva pre-treated with f-GAG from *S. pharaonis* resulted in dose-dependent reduction in the uptake of alcian blue; thereby protecting the intestine against TNBS induced IBD.

6.4. Antibacterial Activity of f-GAG

The f-GAG exhibited significant inhibitions against IBD associated micro biota, *E. coli, Salmonella* sp. and *Pseudomonas* sp. (Figure 6). The f-GAG exhibited maximum inhibition at 200 ug concentrations with a zone of inhibition of 1.8 cm against *E. coli*, 2.4 cm against *Salmonella* sp. and 2.0 cm against *Pseudomonas* sp. The positive control ciprofloxacin demonstrated inhibition zones of 2, 3.2 and 3.0 cm against *E. coli, Salmonella* and *Pseudomonas* sp. respectively. The f-GAG thus demonstrated significant inhibitions against the bacteria associated with IBD, thereby serving as a potential protective anti-inflammatory agent.

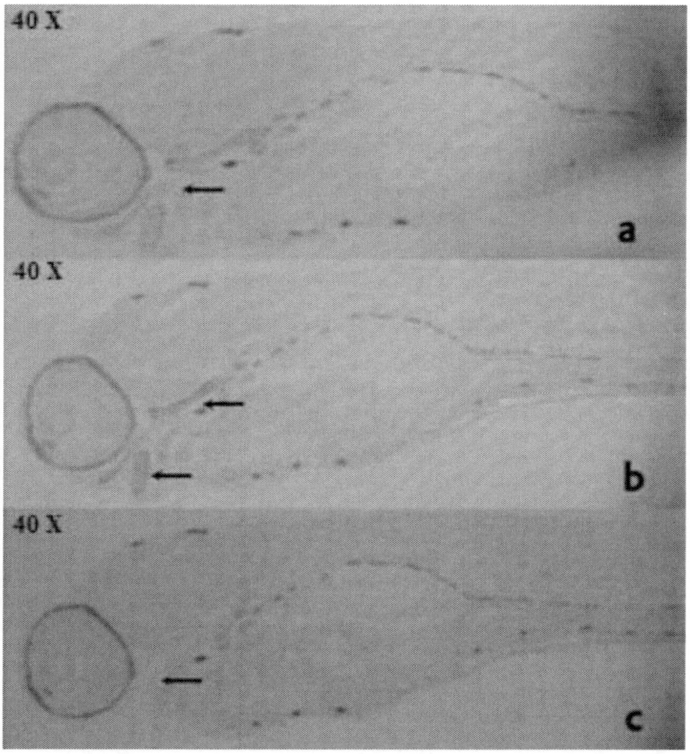

Figure 7. Alcian Blue staining of goblet cells in (a) control; (b) IBD induced; (c) f-GAG treated zebrafish larva 8 d.p.f. (as indicated by arrows).

7. Hypothetical Mechanism of Action

Zebra fish display similar immune mechanisms to humans showing migratory and phagocytic responses and release of inflammatory factors. Neutrophils are the chief patrollers of immune defense which destroy and en route; eliminate invading foreign pathogens through phagocytosis, and ROS formation by degranulation. These powerful effector functions must be limited to avoid persistent inflammation; this can be achieved by either the well-characterized process of neutrophil apoptosis or by neutrophil reverse migration. An essential step toward achieving successful inflammation resolution is the clearance of tissue neutrophils.

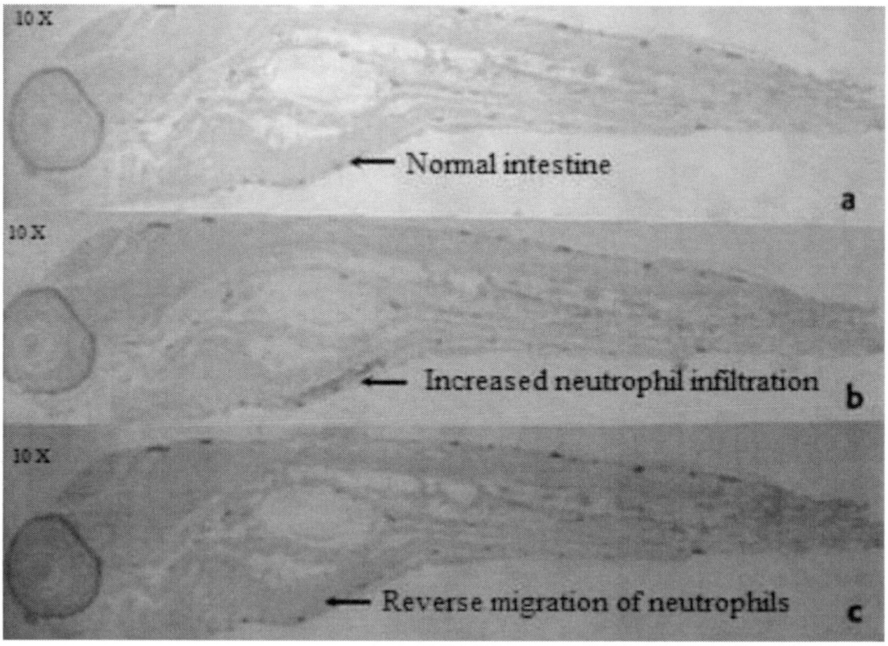

Figure 8. Sudan Black staining of (a) control; (b) IBD induced and (c) f-GAG treated zebrafish larva 8 d.p.f.

In the present study, the f-GAG significantly reduced the infiltration of neutrophils to the site of inflammation viz. the intestine, thereby reducing the resolution of inflammation in the zebra fish larva. The ameliorative effect of the f-GAG could have occurred by the retrograde chemotaxis of the neutrophils. Oehlers' et al., in 2011 reported the use of pharmacological agents such as acetyl salicylic acid and prednisolone as possible therapeutic agents for TNBS induced enterocolitis in zebrafish larvae. McCarty in 1998 reported the role of extrinsic heparin in managing IBD by inhibiting neutrophil activation, adhesion and chemotaxis. He studied the implication of vascular glucosamine in limiting the ability of leukocytes to penetrate the endothelial barrier by degradation of intrinsic heparan sulfates and its potential to be used as a pharmaceutical adjunct with conventional modalities for management of IBD. The curbing of effector functions of the neutrophils has been studied as a potential mechanism to prevent inflammation caused in IBD (Ishiwata et al., 2003; Robertson et al., 2014). Day et al., in 1999 reported the hypothetical therapeutic role of heparin in IBD by restoration of response to fibroblast growth factor, thereby increasing syndecan-1 expression. Matzner et al., In 1984 also reported the inhibitory effect of heparin and related GAG on neutrophil chemotaxis, functioning as a negative regulator of inflammation.

From these results, it could be hypothesized that the f-GAG acts on the pro-inflammatory pathway of immune response bringing about ameliorative action on the inflammatory response in experimentally induced IBD in zebra fish model. Further, the validation is required through molecular techniques and IBD associated genetic and protein markers.

The f-GAG by virtue of its inhibitory potentials against the micro biota associated with IBD also holds potentials of preventing incumbent infection leading to IBD and related complications. However, the mechanism of bacterial inhibition of the f-GAG has to be studied in detail in future.

Conclusion

The chapter deals with the causes and complications associated with the gastrointestinal tract infection IBD. It encompasses the pathogenicity and etiology of the IBD and its related complications, CD and EC. It also describes in detail the potential usage of zebra fish as an animal model for the study of IBD and the ameliorative effect of the marine derived polymer f-GAG from *S. pharaonis* as a potential anti-inflammatory agent in future.

Acknowledgments

The authors gratefully acknowledge Dr. R. Vijayashree, Head, Department of Pathology, CHRI for permission to utilize the histopatholgical services. The authors (V. M and R. K) are gratefully acknowledged to CARE for providing the JRFs.

References

Andres, P.G, Friedman, L. S 1999. Epidemiology and the natural course of inflammatory bowel disease. *Gastroenterol. Clin. North. Am.* 28,255–281.

Ben-Moshe, Z, Foulkes, N.S, Gothilf, Y, 2014. Functional Development of the Circadian Clock in the Zebrafish Pineal Gland. *Biomed. Res. Int.* 235781.

Bernstein, C.N, Blanchard, J.F, Rawsthorne, P, Wajda, A, 1999. Epidemiology of Crohn's disease and ulcerative colitis in a central Canadian province: a population-based study. *Am J Epidemiol.* 149(10),916-924.

Binder, V, 1998. Genetic epidemiology of inflammatory bowel disease. *Dig Dis.*16,351–355.

Boyko E.J, Perera D.R, Koepsell T.D, et al., 1988. Effects of cigarette smoking on the clinical course of ulcerative colitis. *Scand J Gastroenterol.* 23, 1147–1152.

Brown, R.A, Lever, R, Jones, N.A, Page, C.P, 2003. Effects of heparin and related molecules upon neutrophil aggregation and elastase release in vitro. British. *J. of pharmacol.* 139(4), 845-853.

Carr, I, Mayberry, J.F, 1999. The effects of migration on ulcerative colitis: a three year prospective study among Europeans and first- and second-generation South Asians in Leicester (1991–1994). *Am. J. Gastroenterol.* 94,2918–2922.

Connell, W.R, Kamm, M.A, Ritchie, J.K, Lennard-Jones, J.E, 1993. Bone marrow toxicity caused by azathioprine in inflammatory bowel disease: 27 years of experience. *Gut.* 34,1081–1085.

Cosnes, J, Gower-Rousseau, C, Seksik, P, Cortot, A, 2011. Epidemiology and natural history of inflammatory bowel diseases. *Gastroenterology.* 140(6),1785-1794.

Crohn's and Colitis Foundation of America. Living with Crohn's Disease (educational brochure). Available at: http://www.ccfa.org. Accessed August 19, 2005.

D'Alencon CA, Pena OA, Wittmann C, Gallardo VE, Jones RA, Loosli F, et al., 2010. A high-throughput chemically induced inflammation assay in zebrafish. *BMC Biology.* 8(1),1-16.

Danese S, Sans, M, Fiocchi, C, 2004. Inflammatory bowel disease: the role of environmental factors. *Autoimmun Rev.* 3(5), 394-400.

Day, R, Ilyas, M, Daszak, P, Talbot, I, Forbes, A, 1999. Expression of syndecan-1 in inflammatory bowel disease and a possible mechanism of heparin therapy. *Digestive diseases and sciences.* 44(12), 2508-15.

Desai, H.G, Gupte, P.A, 2005. Increasing incidence of Crohn's disease in India: is it related to improved sanitation? *Indian J Gastroenterol.* 24(1), 23-24.

Farrell, R.J, LaMont, J. T, 2002. Microbial factors in inflammatory bowel disease. *Gastroenterol. clin. of North Am.* 31(1), 41-62.

Felder, J.B, Korelitz, B.I, Rajapakse, R, Schwarz, S, Horatagis, A.P, Gleim, G, 2000. Effects of nonsteroidal antiinflammatory drugs on inflammatory bowel disease: a case-control study. *The American journal of gastroenterology.* 95(8), 1949-1954.

Fleming, A, Jankowski, J, Goldsmith P 2010. In vivo analysis of gut function and disease changes in a zebrafish larvae model of inflammatory bowel disease: a feasibility study. *Inflammatory bowel diseases.* 16(7), 1162-1172.

Ishiwata, Y, Okamoto, M, Yokochi, S, Hashimoto, H, Nakamura, T, Miyachi, A, et al., 2003. Non-steroidal anti-inflammatory drug, nabumetone, prevents indometacin-induced gastric damage via inhibition of neutrophil functions. *The Journal of pharmacy and pharmacology.* 55(2), 229-237.

Kabashi, E, Lin, L, Tradewell, M.L, Dion, P.A, Bercier, V, Bourgouin, P, et al., 2010. Gain and loss of function of ALS-related mutations of TARDBP (TDP-43) cause motor deficits in vivo. *Human Molecular Genetics.* 19(15), 3102.

Kaplan, G.G, 2014. IBD: Global variations in environmental risk factors for IBD. Nat Rev Gastroenterol. Hepatol. 11(12), 708-709.

Karthik, R, Saravanan, R, Ebenezar, K.K, Sivamalai, T, (2015). Isolation, purification, and characterization of avian antimicrobial glycopeptide from the posterior salivary gland of *Sepia pharaonis. App. Biochem. Biotechnol.* 175(3), 1507-18.

Kirschner, B.S, 1998. Safety of azathioprine and 6-mercaptopurine in pediatric patients with inflammatory bowel disease. *Gastroenterol.* 115,813–821.

Krishnan, A, Korzenik, J.R, 2002. Inflammatory bowel disease and environmental influences. *Gastroenterology clinics of North America.* 31(1), 21-39.

Kwon, O.K, Kim, S.J, Lee, Y.M, Lee, Y.H, Bae, Y.S, Kim, J.Y, et al., 2016. Global analysis of phosphoproteome dynamics in embryonic development of zebrafish (Danio rerio). *Proteomics*. 16(1), 136-49.

Langholz, E, Munkholm, P, Davidsen, M, Binder, V, 1994. Course of ulcerative colitis: analysis of changes in disease activity over years. *Gastroenterol.* 107(1), 3-11.

Lapidus, A, Bernell, O, Hellers, G, Lofberg, R, 1998. Clinical course of colorectal Crohn's disease: a 35-year follow-up study of 507 patients. *Gastroenterol.* 114(6),1151-1160.

Lindberg, E, Tysk, C, Andersson, K, et al., 1988. Smoking and inflammatory bowel disease: a case control study. Gut.29, 352–357.

Loftus, E.V, Jr, Sandborn W.J. 2003. Epidemiology of inflammatory bowel disease. *Gastroenterol. Clin. North. Am.* 31,1–20.

Loftus, E.V, Jr, 2004. Clinical epidemiology of inflammatory bowel disease: Incidence, prevalence, and environmental influences. *Gastroenterol.* 126(6),1504-1517.

Loftus, E.V, Jr., Sandborn, W.J, Tremaine, W.J, Mahoney, D.W, Zinsmeister, A.R, Offord, K.P, et al., 1996. Primary sclerosing cholangitis is associated with nonsmoking: a case-control study. *Gastroenterol.* 110(5), 1496-502.

Logan, R, 1998. Inflammatory bowel disease incidence: up, down or unchanged? *Gut*.42(3), 309-311.

Matzner, Y, Marx, G, Drexler, R, Eldor, A, 1984. The inhibitory effect of heparin and related glycosaminoglycans on neutrophil chemotaxis. *Thrombosis and haemostasis*. 52(2), 134-137.

McCarty, M.F, 1998. Vascular heparan sulfates may limit the ability of leukocytes to penetrate the endothelial barrier--implications for use of glucosamine in inflammatory disorders. *Medical hypotheses*. 51(1), 11-15.

Merrett, M.N, Mortensen, N, Kettlewell, M, et al., 1996. Smoking may prevent pouchitis in patients with restorative proctocolectomy for ulcerative colitis. *Gut*.38, 362–364.

Mikhailov, T.A, Furner, S.E, 2009. Breastfeeding and genetic factors in the etiology of inflammatory bowel disease in children. *World J Gastroenterol*. 15(3), 270–279.

National Institute of Diabetes and Digestive and Kidney Diseases. Digestive Diseases in the United States: Epidemiology and Impact. Washington, DC: US Government Printing Office; 1994. NIH publication 94-1447.

Ng, S.C, Tang, W, Ching J.Y, Wong, M, Chow, C.M, Hui, A.J, et al., 2013. Incidence and phenotype of inflammatory bowel disease based on results from the Asia-pacific Crohn's and colitis epidemiology study. Gastroenterol. 145(1),158-65.

Oehlers, S.H, Flores, M.V, Okuda, K.S, Hall, C.J, Crosier, K.E, Crosier, P.S, 2011. A chemical enterocolitis model in zebrafish larvae that is dependent on microbiota and responsive to pharmacological agents. Developmental dynamics: *an official publication of the American Association of Anatomists*. 240(1),288-298.

Persson PG, Ahlbom A, Hellers G, 1992. Diet and inflammatory bowel disease: a case-control study. Epidemiology (Cambridge, Mass3(1),47-52.

Pinho, B.R, Reis, S.D, Guedes-Dias, P, Leitao-Rocha, A, Quintas, C, Valentao, P, et al., 2016. Pharmacological modulation of HDAC1 and HDAC6 in vivo in a zebrafish model: Therapeutic implications for Parkinson's disease. *Pharmacol. Res.* 03:328-39.

Podolsky D.K, 2002. Inflammatory bowel disease. *N. Engl. J. Med.* 347, 417– 429.

Present, D.H, Meltzer, S.J, Krumholz, M.P, Wolke, A, Korelitz, B.I, 1989. 6-Mercaptopurine in the management of inflammatory bowel disease: short- and long-term toxicity. *Annals of internal medicine*. 111(8),641-649.

Reif, S, Klein, I, Arber, N, et al., 1995. Lack of association between smoking and inflammatory bowel disease in Jewish patients in Israel. *Gastroenterology*.108,1683–1687.

Renshaw, S.A, Loynes, C.A, Elworthy, S, Ingham, P.W, Whyte, M.K. 2007. Modeling inflammation in the zebrafish: how a fish can help us understand lung disease. *Exp Lung Res*. 33(10): 549-54.

Robertson, A.L, Holmes, G.R, Bojarczuk, A.N, Burgon, J, Loynes, C.A, Chimen, M, et al., 2014. A zebrafish compound screen reveals modulation of neutrophil reverse migration as an anti-inflammatory mechanism. *Science translational medicine*.6, (225).

Roth, M.P, Petersen, G.M, McElree C, Feldman E, Rotter, J.I, 1989. Geographic origins of Jewish patients with inflammatory bowel disease. *Gastroenterology*. 97(4), 900-904.

Russel, M.G, 2000. Changes in the incidence of inflammatory bowel disease: what does it mean? *Eur. J. Intern. Med*. 11(4),191-196.

Sandler, R.S, Loftus, E.V, Jr, 2004. Epidemiology of inflammatory bowel disease. In: Sartor RB, Sandborn WJ, eds. Kirsner's Inflammatory Bowel Diseases, 6th ed. Philadelphia, PA: WB Saunders:245–262.

Saravanan, R, and Shanmugam, A. 2010. Isolation and characterization of low molecular weight glycosaminoglycans from marine mollusc Amussium plueronectus (Linne) using chromatography. *Appl. Biochem. Biotechnol*. 160, 791-799.

Sartor, R.B, Mazmanian, S.K, 2012. Intestinal Microbes in Inflammatory Bowel Diseases. *Am. J. Gastroenterol Suppl*. 1(1),15-21.

Satsangi, J, Morecroft, J, Shah N.B, Nimmo, E, 2003. Genetics of inflammatory bowel disease: scientific and clinical implications. *Best practice and research Clinical gastroenterology*. 17(1), 3-18.

Scholz, S, Fischer, S, Gundel, U, Kuster, E, Luckenbach, T, Voelker, D, 2008. The zebrafish embryo model in environmental risk assessment--applications beyond acute toxicity testing. *Environ. Sci. Pollut. Res. Int*. 15(5), 394-404.

Shivananda, S, Lennard-Jones, J, Logan, R, Fear, N, Price, A, Carpenter, L, et al.,1996. Incidence of inflammatory bowel disease across Europe: is there a difference between north and south? Results of the European Collaborative Study on Inflammatory Bowel Disease (EC-IBD). *Gut*. 39(5),690-697.

Sonnenberg, A, 1990. Occupational distribution of inflammatory bowel disease among German employees. *Gut*. 31(9),1037-1040.

Teixido, E, Pique, E, Gomez-Catalan, J, Llobet, J.M. 2013. Assessment of developmental delay in the zebrafish embryo teratogenicity assay. Toxicol. In Vitro.; 27(1): 469-78.

Van Erpecum, K.J, Smits, S.J, van de Meeberg, P.C, et al., 1996. Risk of primary sclerosing cholangitis is associated with nonsmoking behavior. *Gastroenterology*. 110,1503–1506.

Vidhyanandhini, R, Saravanan, R, Vairamani, S, and Shanmugam, A. 2014. The anticoagulant activity and structural characterization of fractionated and purified glycosaminoglycans from venerid clam Meretrix costa (Chemnitz). *J. Liquid. Chrom. Related. Tech*., 37: 917-929.

Xia B, Shivananda S, Zhang GS, Yi JY, Crusius, J.B.A, Peka, A.S, 1997. Inflammatory bowel disease in Hubei province of China. *China Natl J New Gastroenterol*. 3, 119-120.

Yang, H, McElree, C, Roth M.P, et al., 1993. Familial empirical risks for inflammatory bowel diseases: differences between Jews and non-Jews. *Gut*.34, 517–524.

Yang, L.L, Wang, G.Q, Yang, L.M, Huang, Z.B, Zhang, W.Q, Yu, L.Z, 2014. Endotoxin molecule lipopolysaccharide-induced zebrafish inflammation model: a novel screening method for anti-inflammatory drugs. *Molecules*.19(2), 2390-2409.

Zheng, J.J, Zhu, X.S, Huangfu, Z, Gao Z.X, Guo, Z.R, Wang, Z, 2005. Crohn's disease in mainland China: a systematic analysis of 50 years of research. *Chin J Dig Dis*.6(4),175-181.

Zon, L.I, Peterson, R.T,2005. In vivo drug discovery in the zebrafish. Nature reviews *Drug discovery*. 4(1), 35-44.

In: Disorders of Gastrointestinal Systems … ISBN: 978-1-63485-366-8
Editors:S. Rajagopal, S. Murugan and S. Ramachandran ©2016 Nova Science Publishers, Inc.

Chapter 4

THE INFLUENCE OF GUT MICROBIOME ON GASTROINTESTINAL DISEASE

Ali Al-Yasari*[*1,2], MS, Kamil Sochacki[1] and Miguel Cabrera[1]

[1]Endocrine Research Facility, Department of Animal Sciences, Rutgers University, New Brunswick, NJ, US
[2]College of Veterinary Medicine, Al-Muthanna University, Al-Samawa City, Al-Muthanna Province, Iraq

ABSTRACT

The influence of gut microbiome is one of the most important manifestations in gastrointestinal diseases. The microbiome is the full complement of microorganisms that inhabit the lining of the gastrointestinal tract, skin, and mucosal surfaces of mammalian hosts. Mammalian-microbe interactions described in the gastrointestinal mucosa are critical in priming the immune system and if dysregulated can contribute to metabolic disorders and autoimmune disease. Variability in genetics, environmental exposures, and diet between individuals can influence the composition of microbiota and host responses to commensally and pathogenic microbes. The alteration of microbial populations associated with disease is highlighted in studies on Crohn's disease which has shown changes in bacterial colonies in the terminal ileum. Similarly, diet-induced obesity studies in rodents have demonstrated multi-factorial associations between obesity, glucose/lipid metabolism, diet, and microbiota composition. Phenotypes observed in metabolic disorders may arise from the action of bacterial secretions, surface polysaccharides, or metabolic by-products on host cell structure (cellular permeability) and function. In this chapter, we will describe the role host microbiota play in the onset of diabetes mellitus, Crohn's disease, and ulcerative colitis, by modulating the host immune response.

[*] Corresponding author: Dr. Ali Mosa Rashid Al-Yasari, MS., Endocrine Research Facility, Dept. of Animal Sciences, Rutgers University, 67 Poultry Farm Lane, New Brunswick, NJ-08901. College of Vet. Medicine, Al-Muthanna University, Al-Samawa City, Al-Muthanna Province, Iraq. Email: ali.alyasari@rutgers.edu, alialyasari81@gmail.com Phone number: +1 (732) 640-4245.

Keywords: commensal microbes, crohn's disease, diabetes mellitus, gastrointestinal tract, microbiota

INTRODUCTION

The microbiome is the vast and complete assembly of microbes that make their niches throughout the human body. Microbial cells outnumber human somatic cells by a ratio of 10:1 and although bacteria comprise a large percentage of organisms that make up the microbiome, archaeans, protozoans, fungi as well as viruses and parasites also make their home in human hosts. Recent findings in the literature indicate that the human gut alone contains between 400-1,000 different species and strains of bacteria (Mazmanian, Round and Kasper, 2008), while approximately 10^{11} bacterial cells can be found per gram of colon contents (Guarner and Malagelada, 2003). Technological advances in the last decade in genomic sequencing have tremendously aided the characterization of microorganisms that colonize the skin, mouth, gastrointestinal tract as well as the vagina in humans. Phylogenetic classification of bacteria is based on differences in nucleotide sequence from the variable region of bacterial ribosomal RNA subunit (16S rRNA) in addition to other unique sequences. Metagenomic data collected by the Human Microbiome Project (HMP) revealed the heterogeneity and distribution of bacterial species in different environments and between different individuals which demonstrated that in almost every subject specific body sites were colonized by a single or by a few signature taxa which dominated the community (National Institutes of Health, 2013). Two dominant phyla in particular are the gram-positive Firmicutes and gram negative Bacteroidetes. These phyla, in addition to members of Actinobacteria, Verrucomicrobia, Proteobacteria, Fusobacteria and Cyanobacteria phyla (Sommer and Backhed, 2013) colonize the gut, are present in most individuals, and are specifically adapted to certain body sites. Genetic studies from the HMP also examined metabolic pathways and cellular processes to characterize the function and activity of host-microbe and microbe-microbe interactions. Unlike the high level of taxonomic diversity described above, genetic studies show that many metabolic pathways are ubiquitous in most subjects examined; thus suggesting that host-microbe interactions may be critical to proper health in human subjects.

The existence of commensal bacteria in the gut is necessary for a balanced microbiome and optimal gastrointestinal and immune function. This balance is achieved by commensal organisms which can break down macromolecules and aid in host nutrient absorption in addition to secreting a menagerie of metabolites, short chain fatty acids, and amino acids that support bacterial survival and may improve the mucosal barrier and recruit immune effectors (Sekirov et al., 2010). Additionally, these beneficial bacteria have been shown to limit the ability for enteropathogens to produce toxins by uptaking metabolites required by pathogenic biosynthetic pathways in the intestinal lumen (Cordonnier et al., 2016). Commensals also reinforce the mechanical integrity of the mucosal-intestinal barrier by binding to the intestinal mucous to competitively inhibit the colonization of pathogenic organisms as a mechanism to prevent septicemia and infection (Salzman et al., 2007). This phenomenon is known as colonization resistance (CR) and disruption of CR can lead to an opportunity for pathogen growth. Successful pathogenic overgrowth and colonization of the gut does occur and results in subsequent dysbiosis, a state in which the populations of microbes have deviated from the norm. Several factors influence the ability for enteropathogens to successfully compete with commensal species including, colonization resistance, psychological and physical stress, chronic inflammation, in addition to host diet and genetics, antibiotic use and drug use (Dethlefsen et al., 2011; Hillet al., 2010; Wu et al., 2011; Walker et al., 2011). Collectively, these findings may suggest that although there is incredible microbial diversity within individuals, some taxa may play more important roles than others in maintaining balance between host and microbe and that these taxa can influence neuroendocrine and neuroimmune effects throughout the host.

Host-Microbe Interactions Are Mediated by the Enteric Nervous System

Selective pressures have resulted in the evolution of microbes specialized to exist throughout the gastrointestinal tract and to maintain the integrity of the mucosal barrier, provide nutrients, and aid indigestion. This has led to the notion that the microbiome is a *supraorganism* made up of human and microbial cells which are in constant cross-talk to regulate organ function and maintain homeostasis (Rogers, 2015). The enteric nervous system, embedded in the walls of the gastrointestinal tract, is comprised of the myenteric plexus and the submucosal plexus: networks of intrinsic primary afferent neurons, motor neurons, and interneurons (Sharkey and Savidge, 2014; Lomax et al., 2010; Furness, 2012) which are innervated by extrinsic primary afferents, parasympathetic and sympathetic fibers. Neuronal control of gut function is mediated by muscarinic cholinergic, vasoactive intestinal peptide, and nitric oxide signaling pathways which are controlled locally by the myenteric plexus or communicate with signals emanating from postganglionic sympathetic and parasympathetic branches. Studies on the influence of the microbiome on homeostasis revealed that germ-free animals exhibited physiological and metabolic abnormalities as well as impaired gut motility and increased visceral nociception; abnormalities not seen in animals with an existent microbiome (Caenepeel et al., 1989; Slack et al., 2009; Hapfelmeier et al. 2010; Geuking et al., 2011; Kunii et al., 2011; Hansen et al., 2012; Macpherson et al., 2012; Olszak et al., 2012). Given that differences in homeostatic function arise between germ free and control animals, it has been presumed this a result of cross-talk between the peripheral tissues (i.e., stomach, intestine, pancreas, spleen, liver, etc.) and the branches of the autonomic nervous system. The first instances of microbe-host communication arise from the colonization of the early gut which occurs during parturition as the offspring exits the birth canal. Thus, microbial colonization during the early postnatal period is especially crucial to establishing proper structure and function of the enteric nervous system. Collins et al. 2014 demonstrated that the myenteric plexi of germ free P3 mice exhibited decreased contractility and nerve density in the ileum and jejunum not observed in specific pathogen-free mice. This is consistent with seminal findings that show germ free animals exhibit atypical gut afferent-efferent functions, consisting in delayed gastric emptying and intestinal transit (Abrams and Bishop, 1967; Iwai et al., 1973). In order to better characterize the primary afferent neurons of the enteric nervous system, which terminate near the intestinal epithelium, McVey Neufeld et al., 2012 used segments of the myenteric plexus from the jejunum of 8-12 week old germ free and pathogen free mice to study their electrophysiology? Findings revealed sensory-enteric neurons of germ free animals exhibited decreased excitability and lower resting membrane potentials suggest that bacterial colonization of the intestine can regulate neuronal firing patterns for proper function.

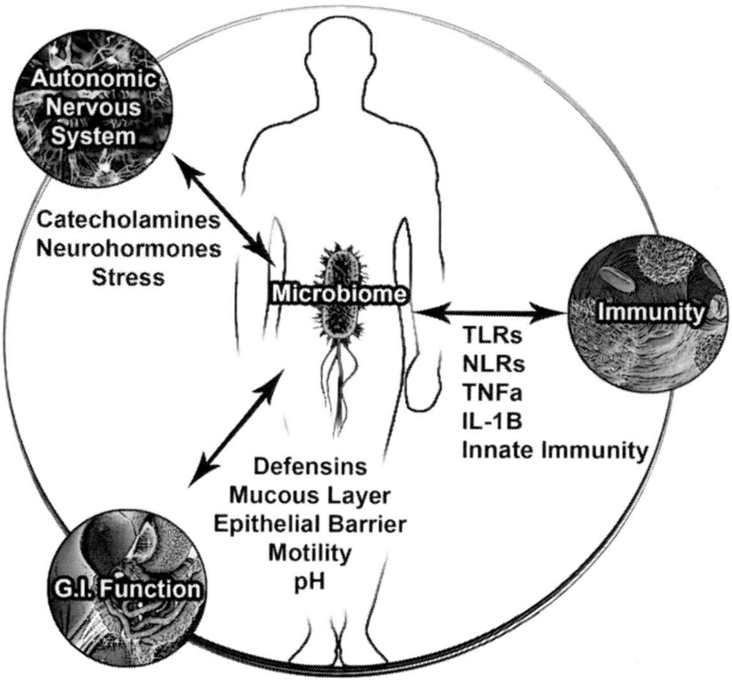

Figure 1. The microbial communities are in constant cross-talk with the enteric nervous system, the gastrointestinal system and immune systems. Bacteria are known to affect the complexity and electrophysiology of myenteric plexus neurons. The enteric nervous system also surveys the gut environment and digestive function. Gut motility and mucous production are under the control of metabolic hormones in addition to the gut bacteria known to secrete factors and metabolites which can alter gut function and trigger immune responses. The immune system is partly controlled by autonomic fibers as well as mental and physical stimuli such as stress. The systems maintain a balance, which when dysregulated can lead to diseases and complications.

The complex interactions that transpire between host cells and microbial cells are indeed bi-directional. For example, epithelial cells that line the gastrointestinal tract receive signals from the luminal milieu in the form of secreted metabolites, pH changes, bacterial glycoproteins, and in turn may influence the composition of the local microbial community via host secretions. In the same way, bacteria and other microbes can regulate intestinal permeability, alter gut motility, environmental pH, and bind to receptors on host cells. Microbial membrane associated molecules like lipopolysaccharide have been shown to trigger enteric secretion of colony stimulating factor 1 (CSF1), which acts to recruit local muscularis macrophages. Muscularis macrophages are activated by CSF1 and in turn release bone morphogenic protein 2 which affects gastric motility and smooth muscle contraction (Muller et al., 2014). This coordination of signals from microbes, nervous system, and immune system plays a role in removing pathogens from the GI tract and returning the system back to its homeostatic set-point (Figure 1). The enteric nervous systemis also responsible for negatively modulating the gastrointestinal environment by secreting catecholaminergic transmitters and neuropeptides via vagal innervation. And conversely, utilizing a system analogous to the eukaryotic noradrenergic signaling pathway, some bacterial species like enterhemmorhagic *E. coli* display QseC receptors that recognize norepinephrine secreted by vagal nerves in the gut. Binding of ligand to QseC induces downstream signaling that leads to transcription of virulence genes and flagellar development (Rhee, Pothoulakis and Mayer, 2009; Hughes and Sperandio, 2008; Reading et al., 2007; Sperandio et al., 2003) that are necessary to promote sustained colonization of pathogenic strains. Hyper-activation of autonomic inputs to the gut due to stress have been associated with dysregulation of the microbiome perhaps by enhanced catecholaminergic secretion or by changes in gastric motility and mucosal production (Lyte, 2011). Both of the aforementioned scenarios may promote virulence of microorganisms and further disturb the ecology of the microbiome. Additionally, it is well established that increases in stress are followed by activation of the hypothalamic-pituitary adrenal axis which can modulate immune response. Hypothalamic CRH secretion stimulates proopiomelanocortin (POMC) production and POMC's subsequent cleavage to ACTH, β-endorphin, and β-MSH peptides. While ACTH perpetuates the hyperglycemia, immunosuppression, and downstream catecholaminergic release associated with the fight or flight mechanism, β-endorphin acts on the paraventricular neurons (PVns) of the hypothalamus to inhibit stress programming as a negative feedback effectors. β-endorphin suppression of PVns dis-activates sympathetic control on the spleen to increase the immune system following periods of stress. Studies have shown that inhibition of the sympathetic stress response by hypothalamic supplementation of β-endorphin peptide resulted in improved natural killer cell (NK) and macrophage functions in culture as well as in vivo (Sarkar et al., 2008; Sarkar et al., 2011; Boyadjieva et al., 2009). As effectors cells of the innate immune system and the first responders, these leukocytes are critical in preserving self-recognition as well as maintaining the mucosal barrier and surveying the intestinal microenvironment for pathogens and invaders as they do not require pre-activation and actively destroy infected cells. NK cells release cytolytic factors like perforin and granzymes (pore-forming proteins and serine-proteases, respectively) which perforate the cell membrane and induce apoptotic pathways in targets, thus mounting cellular-mediated immune response. This is consistent with findings that hail the microbiota as the conductors of neuroendocrine-immune communication (El Aidy, Dinan and Cryan, 2015). Therefore, host immunity is involved in maintaining a favorable balance throughout the gutwhile chronic stress and immune over-activation may lead to dysbiosis of themicrobiome and subsequent infection or disease.

HOST IMMUNE SURVEILLANCE ON GUT MICROBIOME

The host immune system is tasked with surveilling the environment and initiating responses against pathogens so interactions between microbes and host immune responders are critical for a healthy gastrointestinal tract. In the following section we will:

- Discuss general features of mucosal barrier and innate immunity
- Discuss how proinflammation can dysregulate microbiome

The lumen of the gastrointestinal tract houses an incredibly diverse population of bacteria that aid in maintaining homeostasis in the host organism. However, the body can also succumb to infectious pathogens that comprise a minority of the microenvironment. The luminal surface of the gastrointestinal tract is technically outside the body which means that the single layer of intestinal epithelium is the only defense that separates the body from the potentially pathogenic bacteria that reside all throughout the gut. Mechanistically, these fortress-like qualities arise from strong homo/hetero-meric protein-protein interactions between adjacent cells. Tight junctions, composed of claudin-family proteins and occludin-family proteins, exist around the apical perimeters of epithelia cells and prevent leakage across the barrier in a paracellular way. Adherens junctions are formed by interactions of cadherin proteins, integral anchoring proteins, and cytoskeletal actin. Adherens junctions allow for the formation of a continual sheet of cells that make up the barrier which inhibits bacterial translocation into the chorion and systemic circulation (Furuse, 1993, 1998; Graham et al., 2009; Groschwitz and Hogan, 2009; Ikenouchi et al., 2008;Resta-Lenert and Barrett, 2009). Secondary forms of defense against possible infections include host secretions of antimicrobial peptides. In humans, two families of these defense molecules exist and are aptly named Defensin-5 and Defensin-6. The defensins are conserved cationic peptides which function as key mediators of innate immunity, especially in the gut. While defensin-5 has potent bactericidal effects, most notably on gram-positive phyla, defensin-6 lacks such activity. Interestingly, defensin-6 has been observed to 'trap' bacteria in small molecular scaffolds of defensin-6 peptides which can enhance defensin-5-induced production of IL-8, a strong chemotactic factor that can recruit proinflammatory mediators of innate immunity during infection (de Leeuw and Lu, 2007; Yang, 1999; Yang et al., 2002; (Soruri et al., 2007; Grigat et al., 2007; Bowdish and Hancock, 2005; Wehkamp, 2004; Wehkamp et al., 2006, 2007; Ghosh et al., 2002; Ericksen et al., 2004). Perhaps the most important feature of the intestinal barrier is the mucosal layer that impedes the ability for bacteria to interact directly with epithelia cells. The mucous membrane, which is degraded and lost in the process of histological fixation, is understudied but highly necessary for the integrity of the gut epithelium. The mucous membrane has been found to contain high concentrations of host anti-microbial peptide among the anionic, sulfated, and sialylated glycoprotein matrix (Meyer-Hoffert et al., 2008; Dupont et al., 2014; Antoni et al., 2013). Together, these properties allow for retardation of bacterial movement towards the epithelium and efficient bacterial destruction. However, the ability for pathogenic microbes to elicit an immune response is still possible after their destruction. Surface polysaccharides and endotoxic molecules are dispersed and released following bacterial death and studies have highlighted the ability for defensins and other peptides to produce anti-inflammatory factors which can eliminate enteropathogens without triggering excessive inflammation. Among these factors, Lipopolysaccharide-Binding Protein (LBP), intestinal alkaline phosphatase or secretary IgA (sIgA) were identified within the mucus layer and were found to inactivate bacterial secretions (Vreugdenhil et al., 2000; Zarepour et al., 2013; Hamer et al., 2009). These factors may regulate a balance between commensal and pathogenic signals throughout the gut. Changes in the mucosal-epithelial barrier's permeability can arise from autonomic inputs, immunological activation, or changes in microbial communities and may contribute to gastrointestinal disease.

The mechanisms by which the immune system differentiates between commensal bacteria and pathogenic enterobacteria are not well understood as both types of bacteria share structural patterns and interact with the host epithelium and immune system using similar signaling molecules. The ability of the immune system to tolerate such a heterogeneous milieu of commensal bacteria is known as immune tolerance (IT) and acts to distinguish beneficial microbes from pathogenic ones. Studies have highlighted the roles of pattern recognition receptors such as the TOLL-family receptors (TLRs) and NOD-like receptors in innate immunity. These receptors are able to recognize secreted effectors produced by both commensal and pathogenic microorganisms. Pattern recognition receptors are known to bind membrane components of gram-negative bacteria in a soluble form as well as the membrane-bound form. While the inner peptidoglycan layer of gram negative bacteria is more like a symmetrical bi-layered lipid membrane, the outer covering of gram-negative bacteria is an asymmetrical membrane whose exterior is occupied by lipopolysaccharide, a molecule comprised of Lipid A, a core oligosaccharide, and an O-antigen. The lipid A component, a glucosamine-derived phospholipid anchors the LPS molecule to the outer membrane where it can bind to TLRs and NOD-like receptors on host cells. (Raetz and Whitfield, 2002; Page, 2012). In order for LPS to be recognized by TLRs on epithelia cells, binding of myeloid differentiation factor 2 (MD-2) in the membrane must occur before it can induce an immune response to a LPS challenge. Depending on the lipid moieties and acyl configurations of LPS, the resulting TLR4/MD2 signaling pathways will be regulated and affected. Thus, fine-tuning of the proinflammatory response is necessary to appropriately respond to commensals or pathogens. Upon LPS presentation to the gut-associated lymphoid cells, a series of cellular signaling cascades is initiated with both transcription factors NF- κB or AP-1 (MAPK signaling) activated to promote the expression of proinflammatory cytokines such as tumor necrosis factor (TNF)α and interleukin (IL)-1β to facilitate a subsequent proinflammatory reaction. In healthy tissue, this LPS presentation has been shown to also promote the activation of regulatory T-cells in the gastrointestinal-associated lymphoid tissue in order to maintain a balanced immune response (Hrncir et al., 2008) and to prepare for the elimination of invading pathogenic bacteria (Figure 2). In cases of dysbiosis it is possible that the innate immune system becomes hyper-sensitive to changes in bacterial populations which can result in too much inflammation and an opportunity for pathogenic blooms resulting from an altered luminal environment. The increase in proinflammatory factors can lead to inflamed gastrointestinal tract, increased reactive oxygen species and reactive nitrogen species production, and may favor the overgrowth of pathogenic taxa, which usually comprise a minority of any given microbial niche in the human GI tract (Turroni et al., 2013). Many hypotheses exist concerning the mechanisms by which the balance of commensal and virulent bacteria is skewed in dysbiosis and inflammatory diseases of the gut. One explanation may be that increases in reactive oxygen species due to chronic inflammation may promote the survival of several pathogenic facultative-aneaerobes while simultaneously decreasing the ability for beneficial obligate-anaerobic bacteria phyla to survive.

In a healthy microbiome, facultative anaerobes are suppressed by the obligate anaerobes inhabiting the gut, however in subjects suffering from inflammatory bowel diseases or from prolonged antibiotic-use, significant overgrowths of enteropathogens like γ-Proteobacteria and Gram positive cocci were observed (Buffie et al., 2011;Taur et al., 2012). This may be due to changes in the epithelia permeability and damage which may increase oxygen levels or provide an altered nutrition source which can be exploited by pathogenic strains. Dead epithelial cells which are shed into the lumen could provide macromolecules like phosphatidyl-ethanolamine/-choline which are broken down into valuable carbon-sources for different pathogenic or commensal bacteria (Bertin et al., 2010; Thiennimitr et al., 2011).

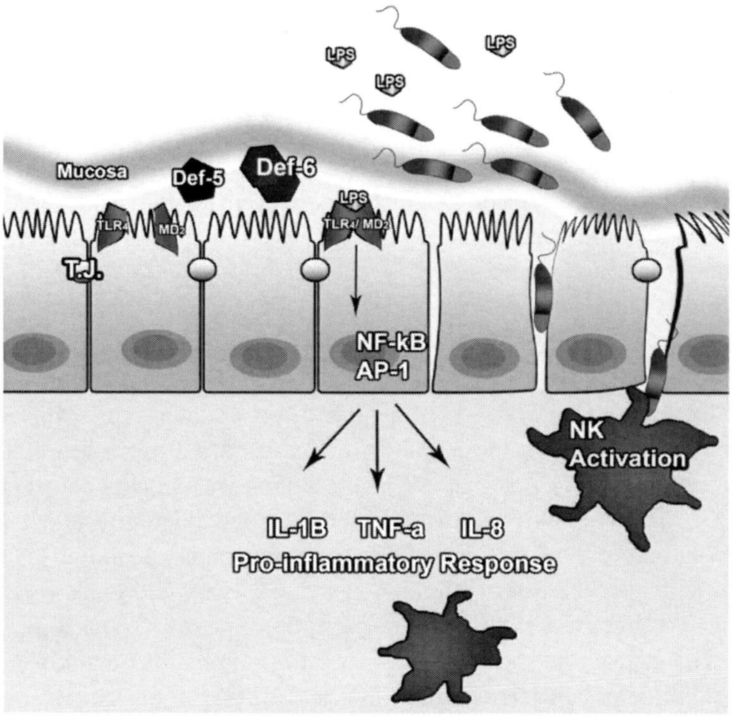

Figure 2. Changes in gut permeability can influence the ability for microbes or pathogens to invade the host. A strong mucosal layer, upregulated tight junctions (T.J.) andadherens proteins, and secreted antimicrobial peptides Defensins 5 and 6 (Def-5, Def-6) make up the layers of defense in the gut. In regions where permeability is compromised, bacteria are able to colonize the epithelium and make their way into systemic circulation. Binding of soluble or membrane bound LPS to TLR4/MD2 complexes triggers signaling cascades which stimulate NF-kB and AP-1 transcriptional activators. The resulting increase in proinflammatory cytokines can promote cellular mediated immunity and enhanced immune surveillance.

The chronic dysregulation of microbiota throughout the gut is marked by changes in bacterial populations, alterations in gut-epithelial permeability, prolonged inflammation, host behavior and changes in gut motility and function. Many links have been found between altered microbe composition in the gastrointestinal tract and metabolic complications like diabetes, obesity, and inflammatory bowel diseases. Studies have examined the impact of gastrointestinal microbes on host physiology but it is still unclear whether microbial dysbiosis causes or is the cause of major human illness. The role of gut bacteria in metabolic and gastrointestinal diseases is reviewed further below.

Obesity and Diabetes

Obesity is a very common health condition and has a valuable importance in public health. Obesity can be defined as an abnormal and unnecessary accumulation of fat in adipose tissue. Obesity is well related with many health issues such as; disability or premature death caused by type 2 diabetes mellitus or cardiovascular diseases, and wide range non-fatal conditions including; gout, respiratory conditions, gastro-esophageal reflux disease, osteoarthritis and infertility. In addition, obesity involved in some psychosocial health implications, mainly due to social bias against fatness (Ofei, 2005). An increment in food intake with decrement in energy expenditure can be considered as good predisposing factors to induce obesity and accumulation of body fat which contributes to many of an organism's needs, such as thermogenesis, lactation, immune responses, and metabolism. Adipocytes' cytoplasm contains large triacylglycerol deposits in the form of lipid droplets and these adipocytes vary in size and distribution depending on age, sex, and nutritional status. There are two types of adipose tissue in mammals: white adipose tissue (WAT) and brown adipose tissue (BAT). WAT stores energy as fat and BAT plays a role in homeostatic maintenance of body temperature by regulation of energy expenditure (Guida and Venema, 2015).

The gut microbiota can be defined as an environmental factor that can affect the body metabolism of the host body. There are many studies have been done to show the relationship between gut microbiota and how it plays a role in obesity development. These studies have shown that the gut microbiota is changed in obese mice and humans especially those have type 2 diabetes. In addition, germ-free mice have shown reduced adiposity and obesity. Other data showed that the transplantation of fecal microbiota from healthy human's donors to humans with metabolic syndrome could improve insulin sensitivity, but the mechanism by which the microbiota can exert its effect still unclear (Parséus et al., 2016).

The relative composition of the gut microbiota during early life can be predictive of the development of obesity in humans. One study comparing fecal samples from 25 overweight or obese children and 24 normal-weight children found that fecal samples from normal-weight children showed higher bifid bacterial numbers in comparison to obese children. On the other hand, it was observed that Staphylococcus aureus in infancy was increased in children who subsequently became overweight. Remarkably, other study found that the microbiota composition in pregnant overweight and normal- weight women is different, with Bactericides and Staphylococcus relatively overrepresented in women who are overweight during pregnancy. Since the mother plays an important role in supplying infants with microbiota during breast-feeding, it is possible that this can be a way that obesity can be transported from parents to infants. The infant's fecal samples composition has been found to be associated to mother's weight during pregnancy (DiBaise et al., 2012).

Genetically obese ob/ob mice are hyperphagicdue to a mutation in the gene that affects leptin which can be considered as a satiety-promoting hormone. The microbiota found in caecum of these mice contains more Firmicutes and fewer Bacteroidetesin comparison with lean wild-type littermates even whenthe mice are fed the same low-fat, polysaccharide-rich diet. Faecal microbiota of humans who are obese have shown similar changes. Bacteroidetes levels correlated negatively with body weight. Therefore, fat- or carbohydrate-restricted diets can lead to high levels of bacteroidetes, suggesting that Bacteroidetes may be responsive for calorie intake. A related effect has also been found in humans who lost weight after a Roux-en-Ygastric bypass procedure. In Roux-en-Ygastric bypass procedure patients, the high levels of Bacteroides and Prevotella were correlated with low energy intake and adiposity. Other studies showed no big change in the Firmicutes–Bacteroidetes ratio because of different clinical criteria including: age, degree of obesity, level of body weight loss and duration of calorie restriction, geographicallocations, population size, and microbiota-profiling methodology. Even though obesity and energy intake can affect the microbial composition, the gut microbiota contribution to obesity in humans is still unclear (Tremaroli and Bäckhed, 2012).

To understand the relationship between microbiota and lipogenesis, many studies have been done. The most acceptable explanation is that the gut microbiota can modulate the obese phenotype by stimulating energy harvest, especially by degradation of polysaccharides from the diet. This increase in energy harvest relates with increased fermentation capacity of the microbiota and then increased levels of short chain fatty acids (SCFAs). Likewise, the fermentation capacity of gut microbiota of obese individuals has increased resulting in elevated SCFA production. SCFAs have unique functions and they can be utilized as energy sources for numerous organs, such as colon mucosa, liver, and muscle and adipose tissue. Gpr41 and Gpr43 are specific receptors of SCFAs. Remarkably, mice deficient in either of the SCFA receptors, Gpr41 and Gpr43, are leaner than their wild-type littermates, and that can show the involving of SCFAs in the development of obesity. Colonization of germ-free mice promotes fermentation of polysaccharides to SCFAs in addition to increased glucose uptake from the small intestine. The increased levels of SCFAs and glucose are accompanying with increased lipogenesis in the liver as well as increased VLDL production. The expression of secreted proteins from the small intestine can be modulated by gut microbiota and one such molecule is the lipoprotein lipase (LPL) inhibitor angiopoietin-likeprotein 4 (Angptl4; also known as fasting induced adipose factor). Germ-free mice suppress Angptl4 expression in the ileum, and this can lead to increase LPL activity and fat storage in white adipose tissue. Angptl4 can directly affect the adiposity phenotype of colonized mice because germ-free Angptl4-deficient mice have similar amounts of body fat to colonized mice. Collectively, these results suggest that increased microbial degradation of dietary polysaccharides and generation of lipogenic substrates, in addition to dividing into adipose tissue, can all explain how the gut microbiota promotes adiposity (Greiner, and Bäckhed, 2011).

It is well established that the microbiota can help and promote obesity. Obesity has many negative effects on the body health and one of these effects is inducing the inflammatory process. There are many recent studies have confirmed the relationship between obesity and inflammatory markers in men and women. After having meal, fatty acids will be taken by fat cells and then are released to blood during fasting, and this system was supported by the action of insulin and catecholamine's controlling the blood flow to the active metabolic organs including the active adipose tissue. Any defect in this system can lead to the inflammatory process. The increase in plasma inflammatory markers after a high-fat meal had been investigated in obese men. It was found that consuming a saturated fatty acid-rich diet resulted in increased gene expression of proinflammation, while consumption of a monounsaturated fatty acid-rich diet caused a high expression of anti-inflammatory genes. It was demonstrated by Cani and colleagues that high fat diets increase intestinal permeability and the plasma concentration of LPS and metabolic endotoxemia, leading to metabolic endotoxemia and inflammation of the gut. Thus, the proinflammatory/anti-inflammatory effects of high-fat diet may be related directly to the nature of fatty acids, since an overload of adipose tissue significantly relates with long-term inflammation and indirectly moderates metabolic endotoxemia and inflammation through effects on the microbiota (Monteiro and Azevedo, 2010).

Gut microbiota can be considered as one of the factors that control early events initiating inflammation associated with obesity and metabolic dysfunction. All of that related events can lead to many changes in microbiota resulting in activation of the bacterial immune system and that in turn, will stimulate the innate and adaptive immunity and increases the inflammatory tone. TLRs, innate immune receptors, are up-regulated in the tissue affected by most inflammatory disorders and activated by both specific microbial components and dietary lipids. This up-regulation can trigger many transduction pathways such as JNK and IKKβ/NF-κB. The inflammatory pathways can produce many cytokine and chemokine such as; TNF-α, IL-1, and MCP1 that may affect the normal insulin function and trigger insulin resistance. Activated TLR and produces cytokines that regulate T-cell differentiation, into effectors inflammatory or regulatory T cells, which in turn depends upon gut microbiota-diet interactions (Sanz and Moya-Pérez, 2014).

Obesity, insulin resistance, and development of type 2 diabetes are associated with systemic and adipose tissue inflammation. The gut microbiota is a good source of lipopolysaccharide and peptidoglycan that may lead to induce inflammation in peripheral body tissues. Experimentally, colonization of germ-free mice with E. coli is adequate to increase macrophage infiltration of adipose tissue and polarize macrophages towards the expression of proinflammatory cytokines. Plasma collected from patients with type 2 diabetes has high lipopolysaccharide levels and feeding lipopolysaccharide to mice for 4 weeks increase adipose tissue inflammation and reduces insulin sensitivity. These results suggest that the gut microbiota may affect host metabolism by altering adipose tissue inflammation. Higher numbers of T cells and mast cells, and lower numbers of regulatory T cells are also involved, but the mechanism of action by which the gut microbiota affects these cells and how it contributes to metabolic disorders is still unclear (Tremaroli and Bäckhed, 2012).

Crohn's Disease and Ulcerative Colitis

Crohn's Disease (CD) and Ulcerative Colitis (UC) are the two major types of inflammatory bowel disease (IBD), which are characterized by chronic recurring inflammation of the gastrointestinal tract. There are numerous factors that converge and contribute to the development of CD and UC including: genetic heritability, diet, gut mucosal barrier, immune regulation, and the microbiota (Butto et al., 2015; Michielan and D'Incà, 2015). Prevalence rates of CD and UC in North America and Europe range from 21 to 246 per 100,000 and 8–214 per 100,000 with an incidence of 3.1 to 14.6 cases per 100,000 person-year and 2.2 to 14.3 cases per 100,000 person-years, respectively (Michielan and D'Incà, 2015; Loddo and Romano, 2015; Loftus, 2004).

An increase in the permeability of the gut mucosal barrier can contribute to the development of CD and UC by promoting interactions between the microbiota and enteric immune system, leading to chronic inflammation (Michielan and D'Incà, 2015, Mankertz and Schulzke, 2007; Nuding et al. 2014). Evidence for a genetic predisposition for mucosal permeability can be found in familial studies where there is altered mucosal permeability of the small intestine in almost 40% of relatives (Halme et al., 2002; Fries et al., 2005; Hollander et al., 1986). Furthermore, a study by D'Incà et al. in 2006 found a relation between NOD2/CARD15 mutations and abnormal mucosal permeability in ileal CD, along with more frequent cases of familial CD than random cases of CD. Additionally, deficits in Muc2, a major mucin produced in the gut that is colonized by bacteria, has been shown to induce the direct contact of gut bacteria and the epithelial lining of the gut. Without the protective barrier produced by mucin there is a greater susceptibility to chronic inflammation of the colon in UC and cancer. Likewise, there is a relation between Muc19 gene and both CD and UC development (Ohkusa and Koido, 2015; Rehman et al., 2010. Thus, a predisposition to altered mucosal barrier permeability and deficits in the mucin may lead to chronic inflammation and the development of CD and UC.

Diet is thought to play an important role in the development of CD and UC. Diets provide carbohydrates necessary for the production of SCFAs, which are important to colon health because they provide anti-inflammatory and anti-cancer properties, helps maintain the epithelial barrier, lower the pH of the lumen, and provide nourishment for colon cells. A diet high in meat may result in the production of hydrogen sulfide from sulfate-reducing bacteria, which have been found to be pervasive in UC. Hydrogen sulfide is toxic and inhibits phagocytosis and butyrate utilization. Another product of a high-meat diet is iron. Iron alters the microbiota by increasing iron-dependent bacteria and worsens UC by inducing an immune response. Vitamin D is beneficial to the gut because it plays a role in maintaining the intestinal barrier and signaling between the microbiota and host. Therefore a deficiency in Vitamin D could lead to the development of CD and UC (Serban, 2015).

Alteration in the activity of the immune systems is another contributing factor to CD and UC. Changes in NOD2/CARD15 affect innate immunity because it encodes for a cytoplasmic pathogen-recognition receptor that recognizes muramyl dipeptide, which is found to be a part of both Gram-negative and Gram-positive cell walls. Hundreds of polymorphisms have been found to be associated with CD, affecting monocytes, macrophages, intestinal epithelial and Paneth cells and confers a 1.5- to 40-fold risk when the allele one or two alleles present, respectively (Michielan and D'Incà, 2015; Bonen and Chou, 2003; Butto et al., 2015; Latz et al., 2013). A polymorphism in the IL-23R gene is very common to CD and UC, which acts as a soluble receptor antagonist to IL-23 and provides protection from these IBDs. IL-23 acts in a very broad manner, activating innate immune cells and T-cells. Furthermore, attenuated IL-23 signaling has been shown, in mice, to ameliorate colitis (Alexander et al., 2014; Elson et al., 2013; Barret et al., 2008). Other genes that play a role in IBD-susceptibility are autophagy-related protein 16-1 (ATG16L1) and immunity-related GTPase M (IRGM). ATG16L1 is a part of a large protein complex that is critical for proper autophagy and phagocytosis of the microbial contents of the gut. IRGM also plays an important role in innate immunity because it encodes a protein that regulates autophagy machinery in response to pathogens. Deficits in ATG16L1 and IRGM can lead to errors in proper autophagy function and promote susceptibility to CD and UC (Butto et al., 2015; Prescott et al., 2007; Glas et al., 2013).

Interactions between the microbiota and adaptive immunity are also very critical. An augmented T cell response towards the microbiota may induce the degradation of the microbiota. In CD following activation by antigen presenting cells, Th1/Th17 cells begin to release proinflammatory cytokines, such as IFN-γ, IL-17, IL-22, and TNF-α, which are hallmarks of the inflammatory profile observed in CD (Butto et al., 2015; Strober and Fuss, 2011). A form of regulation for these T cells in the gut occurs through innate lymphoid cells (ILC). These cells have three categories and the CCR6+ RORγ t+ Tbet− IFNγ−subset of the group 3 ILCs express major histocompatibility complex class II (MHC-II) and are able to present antigen in vivo. Importantly, this subset lacks the requisite co stimulatory molecules to induce T-cell proliferation. This tremendously limits the proinflammatory response of T cells through a MHC-II dependent and IL-23 independent mechanism (Alexander et al.,

2014). Studies also suggest that poorly regulated B cell functioning may lead to inflammation of the gut. In CD and UC patients, B cells tend to upregulate TLR-2, augment spontaneous IL-8 release, and block T-regulatory cell function. Furthermore, B cells dysregulation may lead to the production of epithelial cell-specific antibodies directed towards the host and promote UC pathology. B cells also can re-circulate and affect local and systemic immunity, which can lead to IBD symptoms like fever and gut inflammation. Upregulation of TLR-2 suggests that B cells may play a role in surveying the gut and microbiota. Augmented stimulation of B cells by the microbiota or attenuation in the regulation of B cell activation may lead to an increased response to the microbiota, the production of autoantibodies that may deteriorate the mucosal barrier, upregulation of IL-8 release and further inflammation, and worsening of IBD. Conversely, normal B cell activity may be beneficial (Noronha et al., 2009; Goetz et al., 2007).

Following alterations in the gut mucosal barrier, diet, and exaggerated immune response, patients with CD and UC tend to exhibit an imbalance in the ecological balance of the GI microbiota or dysbiosis. In CD and UC, dysbiosis tends to reflect an overall decrease in the number, stability, and biodiversity of mucosal bacteria relative to healthy controls (Serban, 2015; Sartor, 2014). A recent study with children that were recently diagnosed with CD showed an increase in the abundance of Enterobacteriaceae, Pasteurellacaea, Veillonellaceae, and Fusobacteriaceae, and a decrease in Erysipelotrichales, Bacteroidales, and Clostridiales in mucosal biopsies. Similar correlations were found in UC with most of the increased bacteria found in CD. Several of the organisms identified in this study are known to have the ability to worsen inflammation and/or invade intestinal epithelial cells, such as Fusobacterium. Enterobacteriaceae have been shown to by potentially harmful due to their ability to augment oxidative stress and thrive in oxidative stressful environments (Gevers et al., 2014; Serban, 2015). Moreover, Enterobacteriaceae are increased in obese/overweight children relative to controls (Brown et al., 2012). Veillonellaceae have the ability to produce lipopolysaccharides that may lead to the over activation of the immune system. The loss or reduction of Bacteroidales and Clostridiales are linked with a loss in basic biosynthesis and conversion towards a pathobiont-like auxotrophy, increasing aerobic or aerotolerant taxa like Pasteurellaceae. Clostridiales also appear to be beneficial to the host. Furthermore, a microbial dysbiosis index (Pediatric Crohn's Disease Activity Index [PCDAI]) was generated and showed that there is a negative correlation with microbiota diversity and a strong positive correlation with microbial dysbiosis with CD activity (Gevers et al., 2014, Serban, 2015). Another study found that the changes in the microbiota in patients with UC coincided with a reduction in carbohydrate and nucleotide metabolism in favor of increased lipid and amino acid metabolism. An alteration in metabolism could lead to a reduction in SCFA production in the gut, which, as mentioned earlier, is critically important to colon health, has anti-inflammatory and anti-cancer properties, and helps maintain the epithelial barrier (Serban, 2015).

CONCLUSION

In conclusion, a normal and functioning microbiota is vital for proper gastrointestinal homeostasis. Moreover, several factors play a role in maintaining or disturbing the microbiota, such as genetic predisposition, immune regulation, diet, gut permeability, microbiota diversity, and microbiota function. Changes in any of these factors can induce the development of diabetes mellitus, obesity, Crohn's disease, or ulcerative colitis. Additionally, these factors are being used as biomarkers to develop treatment and predict the onset of gastrointestinal disease. However, more research needs to be conducted to further establish the mechanisms through which these factors interact and alter the microbiota.

REFERENCES

Abrams, G. and Bishop, J. (1967). Effect of the Normal Microbial Flora on Gastrointestinal Motility. *Experimental Biology and Medicine*, 126(1), pp. 301-304.

Alexander, K. L., Targan, S. R. and Elson, C. O. (2014). Microbiota activation and regulation of innate and adaptive immunity. *Immunol Rev*, 260(1), 206-220. doi:10.1111/imr.12180.

Antoni L, Nuding S, Wehkamp J, Stange EF. Intestinal barrier in inflammatory bowel disease. *W J Gastroenterol* 2014; 20:1165-1179 [PMID: 24574793 DOI: 10.3748/wjg.v20.i5.1165].

Antoni L, Nuding S, Weller D, Gersemann M, Ott G, Wehkamp J, Stange EF. Human colonic mucus is a reservoir for antimicrobial peptides. J Crohns Colitis 2013;7:e652-64; PMID:23787054; http://dx.doi.org/10.1016/j.crohns.2013.05.006.

Ava Parséus, Nina Sommer, Felix Sommer, Robert Caesar, Antonio Molinaro, Marcus Ståhlman, Thomas U Greiner, Rosie Perkins, Fredrik Bäckhed. (2016). Microbiota-induced obesity requires farnesoid X receptor. *Gut* 2016;0:1–9. doi:10.1136/gutjnl-2015-310283.

Barrett JC, et al., Genome-wide association defines more than 30 distinct susceptibility loci for Crohn's disease. *Nat Genet*. 2008; 40:955–962. [PubMed: 18587394].

Bertin Y, Girardeau JP, Chaucheyras-Durand F, Lyan B, Pujos-Guillot E, Harel J, Martin C. 2011. Enterohaemorrhagic Escherichia coli gain a competitive advantage by using ethanolamine as a nitrogen source in the bovine intestinal content. *Environ Microbiol* 13:365–377.

Bonen DK, Cho JH. The genetics of inflammatory bowel disease. *Gastroenterol* 2003; 124: 521-536 [PMID: 12557156.

Bowdish, D. and Hancock, R. (2005). Anti-endotoxin properties of cationic host defence peptides and proteins. *J Endotoxin Res*, 11(4), pp. 230-236.

Boyadjieva NI, Ortigüela M, Arjona A, Cheng X, Sarkar DK. ß-endorphin neuronal cell transplant reduces corticotropin releasing hormone hyper response to lipopolysaccharide and eliminates natural killer cell functional deficiencies in fetal alcohol exposed rats. *Alcohol Clin Exp Res*. 2009; 33:931–37.

Brown, K., DeCoffe, D., Molcan, E. and Gibson, D. L. (2012). Diet-Induced Dysbiosis of the Intestinal Microbiota and the Effects on Immunity and Disease. *Nutrients,* 4(8), 1095. doi:10.3390/nu4081095.

Buffie CG, Jarchum I, Equinda M, Lipuma L, Gobourne A, Viale A, Ubeda-Morant C, Xavier J, Pamer EG. 2012. Profound alterations of intestinal microbiota following a single dose of Clindamycin results in sustained susceptibility to C. difficile-induced colitis. *Infect Immun* 80:62–73.

Buttó, L. F., Schaubeck, M. and Haller, D. (2015). Mechanisms of Microbe-Host Interaction in Crohn's Disease: Dysbiosis vs. Pathobiont Selection. *Frontiers In Immunology*, *6*555.

Caenepeel P, Janssens J, Vantrappen G, Eyssen H, Coremans G. Interdigestive myoelectric complex in germ-free rats. *Dig Dis Sci* 1989; 34:1180-1184.

Collins, J., Borojevic, R., Verdu, E., Huizinga, J. and Ratcliffe, E. (2014). Intestinal microbiota influences the early postnatal development of the enteric nervous system. *Neurogastroenterol. Motil.*, 26(1), pp.98-107.

Cordonnier, C., Le Bihan, G., Emond-Rheault, J., Garrivier, A., Harel, J. and Jubelin, G. (2016). Vitamin B12 Uptake by the Gut Commensal Bacteria Bacteroides the taiotaomicron limits the Production of Shiga Toxin by Enterohemorrhagic Escherichia coli. *Toxins,* 8(1), p. 14.

D'Incà R, Annese V, di Leo V, Latiano A, Quaino V, Abazia C, Vettorato MG, Sturniolo GC. Increased intestinal permeability and NOD2 variants in familial and sporadic Crohn's disease. *Aliment Pharmacol Ther* 2006; 23: 1455-1461 [PMID: 16669960].

deLeeuw, E. and Lu, W. (2007). Human Defensins: Turning Defense into Offense?. IDDT, 7(1), pp. 67-70.

Dethlefsen L, Relman DA. 2011. Incomplete recovery and individualized responses of the human distal gut microbiota to repeated antibiotic perturbation. *Proc Natl Acad Sci USA* 108(Suppl 1):4554–4561.

DiBaise, J. K., Frank, D. N. and Mathur, R. (2012). Impact of the gut microbiota on the development of obesity: Current concepts. *Am J Gastroenterol Suppl, 1*(1), 22-27.

Duerr RH, Taylor KD, Brant SR, Rioux JD, Silverberg MS, Daly MJ, et al., A genome wide association study identifies IL23R as an inflammatory bowel disease gene. *Science* (2006) 314:1461–3.doi:10.1126/science.1135245.

Dupont A, Kaconis Y, Yang I, Albers T, Woltemate S, Heinbockel L, Andersson M, Suerbaum S, Brandenburg K, Hornef MW. Intestinal mucus affinity and biological activity of an orally administered antibacterial and anti-inflammatory peptide. *Gut* 2014; 07 May; PMID:24811998; http://dx.doi.org/10.1136/gutjnl2014-307150.

El Aidy, S., Dinan, T. and Cryan, J. (2015). Gut Microbiota: The Conductor in the Orchestra of Immune–Neuroendocrine Communication. *ClinicalTherapeutics,* 37(5), pp.954-967.

Elson C, et al., Monoclonal anti-interleukin 23 reverses active colitis in a T cell-mediated model in mice. *Gastroenterol.* 2007; 132:2359–2370. [PubMed: 17570211].

Ericksen, B., Wu, Z., Lu, W. and Lehrer, R. (2004). Antibacterial Activity and Specificity of the Six Human -Defensins. Antimicrobial Agents *Chemotherapy,* 49(1), pp.269-275.

Fries W, Renda MC, Lo Presti MA, Raso A, Orlando A, Oliva L, Giofré MR, Maggio A, Mattaliano A, Macaluso A, Cottone M. Intestinal permeability and genetic determinants in patients, first-degree relatives, and controls in a high-incidence area of Crohn's disease in Southern Italy. *Am J Gastroenterol* 2005; 100:2730-2736 [PMID: 16393227].

Furness, J. B. (2012). The enteric nervous system and neurogastroenterology. *Nat. Rev. Gastroenterol. Hepatol.* 9, 286–294. doi: 10.1038/nrgastro.2012.32.

Geuking, M., Cahenzli, J., Lawson, M., Ng, D., Slack, E., Hapfelmeier, S., McCoy, K. and Macpherson, A. (2011). Intestinal Bacterial Colonization Induces Mutualistic Regulatory T cell Responses. *Immunity*, 34(5), pp.794-806.

Gevers D, Kugathasan S, Denson LA, et al., The treatment-naive microbiome in new-onset Crohn's disease. *Cell Host Microbe.* 2014; 15:382-392.

Ghosh, D., Porter, E., Shen, B., Lee, S., Wilk, D., Drazba, J., Yadav, S., Crabb, J., Ganz, T. and Bevins, C. (2002). Paneth cell trypsin is the processing enzyme for human defensin-5. *Nature Immunology*, 3(6), pp.583-590.

Glas J, Seiderer J, Bues S, Stallhofer J, Fries C, Olszak T, et al., IRGM variants and susceptibility to inflammatory bowel disease in the German population. *PLoS One* (2013) 8:e54338. doi:10.1371/journal.pone.0054338.

Goetz M, Atreya R, Ghalibafian M, Galle P R, Neurath M F. Exacerbation of ulcerative colitis after rituximab salvage therapy. *Inflamm Bowel Dis*. 2007; 13:1365–1368. [PubMed: 17604367].

Greiner, T. and Bäckhed, F. (2011). Effects of the gut microbiota on obesity and glucose homeostasis. *Trends in Endocrinol Metabol*, *22*(4), 117-123.

Grigat, J., Soruri, A., Forssmann, U., Riggert, J. and Zwirner, J. (2007). Chemoattraction of Macrophages, T Lymphocytes, and Mast Cells Is Evolutionarily Conserved within the Human -Defensin Family. *The Journal of Immunology*, 179(6), pp.3958-3965.

Guarner, F. and Malagelada, J. (2003). Gut flora in health and disease. *The Lancet, 361*(9356), pp.512-519.

Guida, S. and Venema, K. (2015). Gut microbiota and obesity: Involvement of the adipose tissue. *J Functi Foods*, *14*, 407-423.

Halme L, Turunen U, Heliö T, Paavola P, Walle T, Miettinen A, Järvinen H, Kontula K, Färkkilä M. Familial and sporadic inflammatory bowel disease: comparison of clinical features and serological markers in a genetically homogeneous population. *Scand J Gastroenterol* 2002; 37: 692-698 [PMID: 12126248].

Hamer HM, Jonkers DM, Loof A, Vanhoutvin SA, Troost FJ, Venema K, Kodde A, Koek GH, Schipper RG, van Heerde WL, et al., Analyses of human colonic mucus obtained by an in vivo sampling technique. Dig Liver Dis 2009; 41:559-64; PMID:19213618; http://dx.doi.org/10.1016/j.dld.2008.12.100.

Hansen, C., Nielsen, D., Kverka, M., Zakostelska, Z., Klimesova, K., Hudcovic, T., Tlaskalova-Hogenova, H. and Hansen, A. (2012). Patterns of Early Gut Colonization Shape Future Immune Responses of the Host. *PLoS One*, 7(3), p.e34043.

Hapfelmeier, S., Lawson, M., Slack, E., Kirundi, J., Stoel, M., Heikenwalder, M., Cahenzli, J., Velykoredko, Y., Balmer, M., Endt, K., Geuking, M., Curtiss, R., McCoy, K. and Macpherson, A. (2010). Reversible Microbial Colonization of Germ-Free Mice Reveals the Dynamics of IgA Immune Responses. *Science,* 328(5986), pp.1705-1709.

Hill DA, Hoffmann C, Abt MC, Du Y, Kobuley D, Kirn TJ, Bushman FD, Artis D. 2010. Metagenomic analyses reveal antibiotic-induced temporal and spatial changes in intestinal microbiota with associated alterations in immune cell homeostasis. *Mucosal Immunol* 3:148–158.

Hollander D, Vadheim CM, Brettholz E, Petersen GM, Delahunty T, Rotter JI. Increased intestinal permeability in patients with Crohn's disease and their relatives. A possible etiologic factor. *Ann Intern Med* 1986; 105: 883-885 [PMID: 3777713].

Hrncir, T., Stepankova, R., Kozakova, H., Hudcovic, T. and Tlaskalova-Hogenova, H. (2008). Gut microbiota and lipopolysaccharide content of the diet influence development of regulatory T cells: studies in germ-free mice. *BMC Immunol*, 9(1), p.65.

Hughes DT, Sperandio V. Inter-kingdom signaling: communication between bacteria and their hosts. *Nat. Rev. Microbiol*. 2008; 6:111–120.

Iwai H, Ishihara Y, Yamanaka J, Ito T. Effects of bacterial flora on cecal size and transit rate of intestinal contents in mice. *Jpn J Exp Med* 1973;43:297-305.

Kunii, J., Takahashi, K., Kasakura, K., Tsuda, M., Nakano, K., Hosono, A. and Kaminogawa, S. (2011). Commensal bacteria promote migration of mast cells into the intestine. *Immunobiology*, 216(6), pp.692-697.

Latz E, Xiao TS, Stutz A. Activation and regulation of the inflammasomes. *Nat Rev Immunol* (2013) 13:397–411. doi:10.1038/nri3452.

Loddo, I., Romano, C., Mora, J. R. and Martin, F. (2015). Inflammatory bowel disease: genetics, epigenetics, and pathogennesis. *Frontiers In Immunology*, *6*1-6. doi:10.3389/fimmu.2015.00551.

Loftus EV, Jr. Clinical epidemiology of inflammatory bowel disease: Incidence, prevalence, and environmental influences. *Gastroenterol*. 2004; 126:1504-17.

Lomax, A. E., Sharkey, K. A., and Furness, J. B. (2010). The participation of the sympathetic innervation of the gastrointestinal tract in disease states. *Neurogastroenterol. Motil.* 22, 7–18. doi: 10.1111/j.1365-2982.2009.01381.x.

Lopez, P., Gonzalez-Rodriguez, I., Sanchez, B., Ruas-Madiedo, P., Suarez, A., Margolles, A. and Gueimonde, M. (2012). Interaction of Bifidobacterium bifidum LMG13195 with HT29 Cells Influences Regulatory-T-Cell-Associated Chemokine Receptor Expression. *Applied and Environmental Microbiology,* 78(8), pp.2850-2857.

Lyte M, Vulchanova L and Brown DR (2011). Stress at the intestinal surface: catecholamines and mucosa–bacteria interactions. *Cell Tissue Res* 343, 23–32.

Macpherson, A., Geuking, M. and McCoy, K. (2012). Homeland Security: IgA immunity at the frontiers of the body. *Trends in Immunology*, 33(4), pp.160-167.

Mankertz J, Schulzke JD. Altered permeability in inflammatory bowel disease: pathophysiology and clinical implications. *Curr Opin Gastroenterol* 2007; 23: 379-383 [PMID: 17545772].

Mazmanian, S., Round, J. and Kasper, D. (2008). A microbial symbiosis factor prevents intestinal inflammatory disease. *Nature*, 453(7195), pp.620-625.

McVey Neufeld, K., Mao, Y., Bienenstock, J., Foster, J. and Kunze, W. (2012). The microbiome is essential for normal gut intrinsic primary afferent neuron excitability in the mouse. *Neurogastroenterology& Motility*, 25(2), pp. 183-e88.

Meyer-Hoffert U, Hornef MW, Henriques-Normark B, Axelsson LG, Midvedt T, P€utsep K, Andersson M. Secreted enteric antimicrobial activity localises to the mucus surface layer. *Gut* 2008; 57:764-71; PMID:18250125; http://dx.doi.org/10.1136/gut.2007.1414812.

Michielan, A. and D'Incà, R. (2015). Host-microbiome interaction in Crohn's disease: A familiar or familial issue?. *W Gastrointesti Pathophysiol*, *6*(4), 159-168.

Monteiro, R., &Azevedo, I. (2010). Chronic inflammation in obesity and the metabolic syndrome. *Med Inflam, 2010.*

Muller, P. A., Koscsó, B., Rajani, G. M., Stevanovic, K., Berres, M. L., Hashimoto, D., et al., (2014). Crosstalk between muscularis macrophages and enteric neurons regulates gastrointestinal motility. *Cell* 158, 300–313. doi: 10.1016/j.cell.2014.04.050.

National Institutes of Health, (2013). Structure, Function and Diversity of the Healthy Human Microbiome. *Nature,* pp.207-214.

Noronha, A, Liang, Y, Hetzel, J, Ganley-Leal, L, Farraye, F, Stucchi, A, Zhang, Y, Nikolajczyk, B, Hasturk, H, and Kantarci, A. (2009). Hyperactivated B cells in human inflammatory bowel disease. *J Leukocyte Biol*, 86(4), 1007-1016. doi:10.1189/ jlb.0309203.

Ofei, F. (2005). Obesity-a preventable disease. *Ghana medical journal,39*(3), 98.

Ohkusa, T., &Koido, S. (2015). Review article: Intestinal microbiota and ulcerative colitis. *J Infection Chem, 21*761-768. doi:10.1016/j.jiac.2015.07.010.

Olszak, T., An, D., Zeissig, S., Vera, M., Richter, J., Franke, A., Glickman, J., Siebert, R., Baron, R., Kasper, D. and Blumberg, R. (2012). Microbial Exposure During Early Life Has Persistent Effects on Natural Killer T Cell Function. *Science*, 336(6080), pp.489-493.

Page MG. The role of the outer membrane of Gram-negative bacteria in antibiotic resistance: Ajax'shieldor Achilles'heel? *Handb Exp Pharmacol* 2012. p. 67–86.

Prescott NJ, Fisher SA, Franke A, Hampe J, Onnie CM, Soars D, et al,. A nonsynonymous SNP in ATG16L1 predisposes to ileal Crohn's disease and is independent of CARD15 and IBD5. *Gastroenterology* (2007) 132:1665–71. doi:10.1053/j.gastro.2007.03.034.

Raetz, C. and Whitfield, C. (2002). L IPOPOLYSACCHARIDE E NDOTOXINS. *Annu. Rev. Biochem.*, 71(1), pp.635-700.

Reading, N., Torres, A., Kendall, M., Hughes, D., Yamamoto, K. and Sperandio, V. (2007). A Novel Two-Component Signaling System That Activates Transcription of an Enterohemorrhagic Escherichia coli Effectors Involved in Remodeling of Host Actin. *J Bacteriol*, 189(6), pp. 2468-2476.

Rehman A, Lepage P, Nolte A, Hellmig S, Schreiber S, Ott SJ. Transcriptional activity of the dominant gut mucosal microbiota in chronic inflammatory bowel disease patients. *J Med Microbiol* 2010; 59:1114e22.

Rogers, K. (2015). Human Microbiome. In:*Encyclopedia Britannica*, 1st ed.

Salzman, N. H., Underwood, M. A., and Bevins, C. L. (2007). Paneth cells, defensins, and the commensal microbiota: a hypothesis on intimate interplay at the intestinal mucosa. *Semin. Immunol.* 19, 70–83. doi: 10.1016/j.smim.2007.04.002.

Sanz, Y. and Moya-Pérez, A. (2014). Microbiota, inflammation and obesity. In *Microbial Endocrinology: The Microbiota-Gut-Brain Axis in Health and Disease* (pp. 291-317). Springer New York.

Sarkar DK, Boyadjieva NI, Chen CP, Ortigüela M, Reuhl K, Clement KM, et al., Cyclic adenosine monophosphate differentiated beta-endorphin neurons promote immune function and prevent prostate cancer growth. *Proc Natl Acad Sci U S A.* 2008; 105: 9105–10.

Sarkar DK, Zhang C, Murugan S, Dokur M, Boyadjieva NI, et al., Transplantation of {beta}endorphin neurons into the hypothalamus promotes immune function and restricts the growth and metastasis of mammary carcinoma. *Cancer Res.* 2011; 71:6282–91.

Sartor, R. B. (2014). The intestinal microbiota in inflammatory bowel diseases. *Nestlé Nutrition Institute Workshop Series*, 7929-39. doi:10.1159/000360674.

Sekirov, I., Russell, S. L., Antunes, L. C., and Finlay, B. B. (2010). Gut microbiota in health and disease. *Physiol. Rev.* 90, 859–904. doi: 10.1152/physrev.00045.2009.

Serban, D. E. (2015). Microbiota in Inflammatory Bowel Disease Pathogenesis and Therapy: Is It All About Diet?. *Nutrition In Clinical Practice: Official Publication of the American Society For Parenteral And Enteral Nutrition, 30*(6), 760-779. doi:10.1177/ 0884533615606898.

Sharkey, K. A., and Savidge, T. C. (2014). Role of enteric neurotransmission in host defense and protection of the gastrointestinal tract. *Auton. Neurosci.* 182, 70–82. doi: 10.1016/j.autneu.2014.03.004.

Slack, E., Hapfelmeier, S., Stecher, B., Velykoredko, Y., Stoel, M., Lawson, M., Geuking, M., Beutler, B., Tedder, T., Hardt, W., Bercik, P., Verdu, E., McCoy, K. and Macpherson, A. (2009). Innate and Adaptive Immunity Cooperate Flexibly to Maintain Host-Microbiota Mutualism. *Science,* 325(5940), pp. 617-620.

Sommer F and Backhed F (2013). The gut microbiota – masters of host development and physiology. *Nat Rev Microbiol* 11, 227–238.

Soruri, A., Grigat, J., Forssmann, U., Riggert, J. and Zwirner, J. (2007). β-Defensins chemoattract macrophages and mast cells but not lymphocytes and dendritic cells: CCR6 is not involved. *European Journal ofImmunology,* 37(9), pp.2474-2486.

Sperandio, V., Torres, A., Jarvis, B., Nataro, J. and Kaper, J. (2003). Bacteria-host communication: The language of hormones. *Proc Natl Acad Sci,* 100(15), pp.8951-8956.

Strober, W. and Fuss, I. J. (2011). Proinflammatory Cytokines in the Pathogenesis of Inflammatory Bowel Diseases. *Gastroenterology,* 140 (Inflammatory Bowel Disease: An Update on Fundamental Biology and Clinical Management), 1756-1767.e1. doi:10.1053/j.gastro.2011.02.016.

Taur Y, Xavier JB, Lipuma L, Ubeda C, Goldberg J, Gobourne A, Lee YJ, Dubin KA, Socci ND, Viale A, Perales MA, Jenq RR, van den Brink MR, Pamer EG. 2012. Intestinal domination and the risk of bacteremia in patients undergoing allogeneic hematopoietic stem cell transplantation. *Clin Infect* Dis 55:905–914.

Thiennimitr P, Winter SE, Winter MG, Xavier MN, Tolstikov V, Huseby DL, Sterzenbach T, Tsolis RM, Roth JR, Baumler AJ. 2011. Intestinal inflammation allows Salmonell at ouse ethanolamine to compete with the microbiota. *Proc Natl Acad Sci USA* 108:17480–17485.

Tremaroli, V. and Bäckhed, F. (2012). Functional interactions between the gut microbiota and host metabolism. *Nature*, *489*(7415), 242-249.

Tremaroli, V. and Bäckhed, F. (2012). Functional interactions between the gut microbiota and host metabolism. *Nature*, *489*(7415), 242-249.

Turroni, F., Serafini, F., Foroni, E., Duranti, S., O'Connell Motherway, M., Taverniti, V., Mangifesta, M., Milani, C., Viappiani, A., Roversi, T., Sanchez, B., Santoni, A., Gioiosa, L., Ferrarini, A., Delledonne, M., Margolles, A., Piazza, L., Palanza, P., Bolchi, A., Guglielmetti, S., van Sinderen, D. and Ventura, M. (2013). Role of sortase-dependent pili of Bifidobacterium bifidum PRL2010 in modulating bacterium-host interactions. *Proc Natl Acad Sci*, 110(27), pp.11151-11156.

Vreugdenhil ACE, Snoek AMP, Greve JWM, Buurman WA. Lipopolysaccharide-binding protein is vector ally secreted and transported by cultured intestinal epithelial cells and is present in the intestinal mucus of mice. *J Immunol* 2000; 165:4561-66; PMID:11035097; http://dx.doi.org/10.4049/jimmunol.165.8.4561.

Walker AW, Ince J, Duncan SH, Webster LM, Holtrop G, Ze X, Brown D, Stares MD, Scott P, Bergerat A, Louis P, McIntosh F, Johnstone AM, Lobley GE, Parkhill J, Flint HJ. 2011. Dominant and diet responsive groups of bacteria within the human colonic microbiota. *ISME J* 5:220–230.

Wehkamp, J. (2004). Defensin deficiency, intestinal microbes, and the clinical phenotypes of Crohn's disease. *J Leukocyte Biol*, 77(4), pp.460-465.

Wehkamp, J., Salzman, N., Porter, E., Nuding, S., Weichenthal, M., Petras, R., Shen, B., Schaeffeler, E., Schwab, M., Linzmeier, R., Feathers, R., Chu, H., Lima, H., Fellermann, K., Ganz, T., Stange, E. and Bevins, C. (2006). Reduced Paneth Cell α-Defensins and Antimicrobial Activity in Ileal Crohn's Disease. *Inflammatory Bowel Diseases*, 12, p.S20.

Wehkamp, J., Wang, G., Kubler, I., Nuding, S., Gregorieff, A., Schnabel, A., Kays, R., Fellermann, K., Burk, O., Schwab, M., Clevers, H., Bevins, C. and Stange, E. (2007). The Paneth Cell -Defensin Deficiency of Ileal Crohn’s Disease Is Linked to Wnt/Tcf-4. *J Immunol*, 179(5), pp. 3109-3118.

Wu GD, Chen J, Hoffmann C, Bittinger K, Chen YY, Keilbaugh SA, Bewtra M, Knights D, Walters WA, Knight R, Sinha R, Gilroy E, Gupta K, Baldassano R, Nessel L, Li H, Bushman FD, Lewis JD. 2011. Linking long-term dietary patterns with gut microbial enterotypes. *Science* 334: 105–108.

Yang, D. (1999). -Defensins: Linking Innate and Adaptive Immunity Through Dendritic and T Cell CCR6. *Science,* 286(5439), pp. 525-528.

Yang, D., Biragyn, A., Kwak, L. and Oppenheim, J. (2002). Mammalian defensins in immunity: more than just microbicidal. *Trends in Immunol*, 23(6), pp. 291-296.

Zarepour M, Bhullar K, Montero M, Ma C, Huang T, Velcich A, Xia L, Vallance B. The mucin Muc2 limits pathogen burdens and epithelial barrier dysfunction during Salmonella entericaserovar Typhimurium colitis. *Infect Immun* 2013; 81:3672-83; PMID:23876803; http://dx.doi.org/10.1128/IAI.00854-13.

In: Disorders of Gastrointestinal Systems ... ISBN: 978-1-63485-366-8
Editors:S. Rajagopal, S. Murugan and S. Ramachandran ©2016 Nova Science Publishers, Inc.

Chapter 5

ANIMAL MODELS USED IN STUDYING INFLAMMATORY BOWEL DISEASES

Basavarajaiah Swethakumar[1], Manoj Paul[1], Kesturu S. Girish[1,2,*] and Kempaiah Kemparaju[1,†]
[1]Department of studies in Biochemistry, University of Mysore, Manasagangothri, Mysore, India
[2]Department of Studies and Research in Biochemistry, Tumkur University, Tumkur, India

ABSTRACT

Of late, a myriad of pathological diseases and disorders have infested human life, affecting not only their life expectancy, but also lifestyle, economic and social statuses. To combat the diseases and disorders, it is essential to have a prior knowledge of their origin, progression and outcome. In this view, the current book chapter focuses on Inflammatory Bowel Disease (IBD), which affects individuals of all groups worldwide and thus has attained global significance. In understanding the pathology and pathophysiology of the disease and to develop new drugs, animal models have played a crucial role as they replace human subjects. Therefore, the article gives a detailed description of various types of animal models used in the study of IBD including, chemically induced, spontaneous, genetically engineered and transgenic models. Further, it also describes how each of these models work, their advantages and disadvantages, morphological, histopathological and symptomatical features, as well as the conditions under which these models are preferred. The given information may serve as a basis of knowledge to further develop not only new animal models with the desired features, but also as a pool of instructions for the researchers who are working on IBD.

* Corresponding author: Kesturu S. Girish, PhD., Department of Studies and Research in Biochemistry, Tumkur University, Tumkur-572 103, India. Tel.: +91-9964080540; E-mail: ksgbaboo@gmail.com.
† Corresponding author: KempaiahKemparaju, PhD., DOS in Biochemistry, University of Mysore, Mysore-570 006, India. Tel.: +91-9945996543; E-mail: kemparajuom@gmail.com.

Keywords: adoptive transfer model, animal model, chemically induced model, Crohn's disease, genetically induced model, inflammatory bowel disease, spontaneous model, ulcerative colitis

1. INTRODUCTION

Inflammatory Bowel Disease (IBD), a disorder arising at the gastrointestinal tract, is an idiopathic, chronic and relapsing intestinal autoimmune disorder which is characterized by exaggerated inflammation. Lately, IBD has been receiving worldwide attention due to the fact that it affects almost all age groups including the pediatric population. However, the prevalence of IBD is more in Europe and North America and an increasing number of cases are being observed in Asia as well. In Europe the annual incidence rate is 0.6-24.3 per 100,000 with the prevalence of 4.9-505 per 100,000; and in North America, the annual incidence rate is 0-19.2 per 100,000 with the prevalence of 37.5-248.6 per 100,000 (Ananthakrishnan, 2015). An elevated incidence of IBD is observed to be more in the countries with increased industrialization and westernized/hygienic lifestyle (Ananthakrishnan, 2015).

IBD comprises two types of conditions, namely Crohn's disease (CD) and Ulcerative colitis (UC). CD can occur at any part of the gastrointestinal tract and the symptoms include fatigue, abdominal pain, weight loss, fever and prolonged diarrhea with or without gross bleeding. However, UC involves inflammation of the colon and rectum with symptoms that are usually lower abdominal pain, rectal bleeding, frequent stools, tenesmus and mucus discharge from the rectum (Fakhoury et al., 2014).

Even though the basic etiology is still unknown, recent studies have provided a rough insight into the numerous factors responsible for the development and progression of IBD, which include increased level of reactive oxygen species (ROS) and reactive nitrogen species, mutation in NOD2 gene, imbalances in pro and anti-inflammatory cytokines, destruction of epithelial barrier, and alteration in microbiota composition. Thus, the interactions of genetic, environmental and immunological factors lead to the expression/progression of IBD (Sartor, 2006; You et al., 2009). The deduction of the pathways/factors that are responsible is made possible due to the use of animal models that mimic human physiology. Thus, animal models have been and are being extensively used to investigate the reasons underlying the pathogenesis of the disease, involving complexity and to develop novel therapeutic drugs to combat IBD.

Animal model for IBD was introduced for the first time by Kirsner in 1959 by sensitizing rabbits with crystalline egg albumin along with small rectal instillation of dilute formalin (Kirsner et al., 1959). Subsequently, multiple formats of animal models for IBD were developed by various researchers with different techniques using different animals. Consequently, animal models have become useful research tools in IBD studies which have improved our ability to interpret the complexity of the disease, to understand the histopathological and morphological changes in the gastrointestinal tract, impact of intestinal microorganisms and to study the mechanism of how extra intestinal manifestation arises during the pathogenesis of the disease.

2. Different Animals Used in IBD Research

2.1. Mice

Mice (*Musmusculus*) are the most commonly used experimental animals which share 98% similarities to humans in terms of anatomy, physiology, and genetics (organization of DNA, the process of gene expression). Their short lifespan, small size, less maintenance cost and uncomplicated diet have made them easy to handle and have helped investigators to speed up the progress of research. In IBD research, mice are used to study both acute and chronic intestinal inflammation because of their resemblance to physiology, anatomical structures, microbiome and immune responses of the gastrointestinal tract to humans. A variety of genetically engineered mice has allowed investigators to study several aspects of colitis like adaptive and innate immune responses during intestinal inflammation, the role of transcription factors and microbiota in the development of IBD. Even though mice provide numerous advantages, the lesions found in mice are not exactly identical with the lesions present in people suffering from IBD. Besides, the increased expression of Toll-like receptors (TLR) in mice macrophages of chemical models has not been observed in humans, as TLR expression is limited to dendritic cells and myelomonocytic cells (Jiminez et al., 2015).

2.2. Rats

Rats (*Rattusnorvegicus*) share 90% of the genome with humans and hence are extensively used as model organisms by researchers for their studies. Rats are the preferred choice to investigate the pathophysiology of IBD over mice because of their larger body size and alimentary canal allowing researchers to perform better at the time of necropsy and to collect larger organ/tissue samples for biochemical analysis which fulfill their needs. 2, 4, 6 Trinitrobenzenesulphonic acid (TNBS) for the first time was used as a colitogenic substance to induce IBD in rats which was further developed as TNBS model. The key disadvantage of rats as animal model includes the absence of proper gene knockout (KO) and transgenic techniques when compared to mice.

2.3. Pigs

The analogous arrangement of stomach and small intestine of both pigs (*Susscrofa*) and humans with functionally and anatomically similar gastrointestinal tract makes pigs an excellent model to study IBD (Patterson et al., 2008). The use of pigs has the advantage of collecting a larger amount of tissue and the disadvantages include slower growth and reproductive rates, larger housing space, and higher maintenance cost when compared to rodents and invertebrate models (Jiminez et al., 2015).

2.4. Guinea Pigs

Guinea pig (*Caviaporcellus*) is a rodent and in spite of its common name, the animal does not belong to the pig family. The use of Guinea pig in research was common during 19th and early 20th centuries and was gradually replaced by mice/rats which were cheaper and smaller. To study IBD, guinea pigs were initially used by Marcus and Watt in 1971 using carrageenan (Watt and Marcus, 1971a). The lesions developed in guinea pig IBD models resemble human IBD in many ways like crypt abscesses, neutrophilic infiltration, and epithelial necrosis and it is a readily reproducible model. It is observed that guinea pig IBD model is more physiologically and immunologically similar to humans than any other small animal models (Padilla-Carlin et al., 2008). The main drawbacks of guinea pig model are that it is more expensive and there is a complete absence of gene KO and transgenic techniques.

2.5. Non-Human Primates (NHPs)

NHPs are better animal models for scientific research as compared to rodents or any other animals because they have closely evolved with humans during evolution and they share greater similarities in psychology, physiology, anatomy, immune system, organ system and musculoskeletal system. The NHPs includes chimpanzees, gibbons, gorillas, macaques, lemurs, baboons, marmosets and cotton-top tamarin. Among NHPs, macaques and cotton-top tamarins are most commonly used animals in IBD research to investigate the pathogenesis and for the discovery of new therapeutic drugs (Jiminez et al., 2015). Gozalo et al., reported that in cotton-top tamarins there is a spontaneous development of ileitis with infiltration of mononuclear inflammatory cells and thickening of terminal ileum which has similar characteristics of CD (Gozalo et al., 2002). Another study by Ramesh et al., suggests that enterocolitis in rhesus macaques resembles both clinically and immunologically to human IBD (Ramesh et al., 2005). Even though NHPs are very good animal models, these animals are considered to be endangered and their use as models in scientific research has been banned in many countries. Moreover, due to their large size and aggressive behavior, it is a tough task for the researchers to maintain them in the animal house.

2.6. Sheep

Sheep is a convenient experimental model in scientific research because of its availability, ease of handling, feeding, and animal housing. Sheep have been in IBD research used to study intestinal problems. Even though sheep has a bigger intestine than rodents, the presence of rumen differentiates them from humans at their digestive anatomy. Besides, colonic microbiota in sheep and humans vary greatly which makes them a less ideal IBD model.

2.7. Other Animals

Rabbits, hamsters, and zebrafish have also been used commonly in IBD research. Rabbits are phylogenetically nearer to primates than rodents and also provide a higher genetic diversity than rodent strains. In IBD research, rabbit is a commonly used animal to investigate the mechanism of colonic inflammation and ulceration because of its comparatively large sized colon and greater pharmacological resemblance to humans which makes *in vivo* examination less difficult (Anthony et al., 1995). Hamster is another rodent which has been used to study colitis by many investigators because it has a longer digestive tract than mice. Ohkusa, 1985) has reported the use of hamster in studying IBD using Dextran sulfate sodium (DSS) as an inducer. Zebrafish, an invertebrate has also been used by researchers to study intestinal inflammation because of its intestinal resemblance to humans in having similar cell types such as intestinal absorptive cells, goblet cells, brush border with microvilli, and an epithelium (Jiminez et al., 2015).

3. Types of Animal Models

3.1. Chemically Induced Models of Intestinal Inflammation

Table 1. Characteristics of chemically induced models of IBD

Chemically induced models of IBD			
Models	Features	Disadvantages	Disease type
DSS model	• Orally administered through drinking water • Devoid of Anesthesia • Loss of epithelial barrier function • In combination with Azoxymethane produces colorectal cancer	• Long duration of experiments	UC
TNBS model	• Intra-rectal administration in combination with ethanol • Rapid onset of disease with single dose • Loss of immune tolerance	• Absence of spontaneous relapse • Both ethanol and TNBS induce epithelial damage	CD
Oxazolone model	• Intra-rectal administration in combination with ethanol • Inflammation lasts for several days • Driven by natural killer T-cells	• Both ethanol and TNBS induce epithelial damage	UC
Carageenan model	• Orally administered through drinking water • Degraded form induces inflammation rather that native form	• Lack of remission and exacerbations	UC
Acetic acid model	• Intrarectal administration • Production of ROS which makes ideal to study the efficacy of drugs which interferes with ROS generation	• Devoid of immunogenic property within first 24 h of administration	UC

Chemically induced models are the best explained and most widely used models because of their ease of use and flexibility. In 1969, Marcus and Watt observed that a variety of laboratory animals which were fed with extracts of various red seaweeds showed the symptoms which resembled human IBD (Marcus and Watt, 1969). Further development and alteration of this observation led to an origin of numerous types of chemically induced models. Administration of different colitogenic chemical substances like DSS, TNBS, oxazolone, carrageenan and acetic acid are known to induce intestinal damage in different experimental animals. Researchers have used various routes and specific concentrations to introduce these chemicals into the body of the animal. The commencement and duration of inflammation is immediate and controllable and it lacks genetic manipulations just as in human IBD. The only observed disadvantage of the chemically induced model is that it does not involve spontaneous remission which is seen in human IBD (Table 1).

3.2. Dextran Sulfate Sodium (DSS) Model

DSS is a high molecular weight sulfated polysaccharide ranging from 5 to 1400 kDa. Dextran sulfate is a polyanionic derivative of dextran produced by etherification of dextran with chlorosulphonic acid and it is prepared as sodium salts to make it stable and water soluble. Structurally it is a polymer of anhydroglucose with straight and branched chains with α (1→6) and α (1→3) glycosidic bond. The most effective molecular weight range of DSS to induce severe colitis in animals is 40 to 50 kDa. DSS-induced model is a widely accepted model because of its simplicity, reproducibility, low cost and was introduced for the first time by (Ohkusa, 1985) in hamsters.

DSS is variously used to induce both acute and chronic types of colitis in different animals like mice, hamsters, rats, guinea pigs, and zebrafish, with guinea pigs being more susceptible. Among mice, males are more susceptible, with C3H/HeJ and Balb/c being the strains with higher susceptibility (Goyal et al., 2014). Acute colitis is induced by providing high concentrations (3-10%) of DSS continuously for shorter periods (4-10 Days) while chronic colitis is induced by continuous administration of a low concentration (1-2%) of DSS for longer periods (15-30 days). Preparation of DSS to induce colitis in animals is quite simple as DSS is dissolved in drinking water and administered orally, hence unlike most chemically induced models, no general anesthesia is required. It is thus one of the most commonly used models for studying IBD. Administration of DSS into experimental animals induces severe intestinal damage with symptoms of diarrhea, body weight loss, the presence of blood in stools, reduction in colon length, and ulcerations. This is because of its direct toxicity to colonic epithelium causing epithelial cell injury, resulting in immune response which alters mucosal barrier function throughout the colonic epithelium which resembles UC of humans. Histologically, acute DSS-induced colitis is characterized by mucosal edema, goblet cell loss, crypt distortion and abscesses, infiltration of neutrophils and macrophages in mucosal and submucosal regions. Chronic DSS colitis is characterized by signs of erosions, epithelial regeneration, mucosal fibrosis, dysplasia, and adenocarcinoma. Colitis-associated colorectal cancer is induced by administering DSS in combination with a single dose of genotoxic colon carcinogen azoxymethane (AOM) in experimental animals (Clapper et al., 2007).

Although the mechanism by which DSS-induced colitis is unclear, recent studies have provided insight into the mechanism of DSS-induced colitis. Studies by Laroui et al., suggest that DSS combines with medium-chain length fatty acids (MCFAs) to form 200 nm sized vesicles in the colonic lumen that fuse colonocyte membranes prior to induction of colitis and these vesicles enter the epithelial cell cytoplasm and destructs intestinal barrier functions that initiate chronic inflammatory response (Laroui et al., 2012). In another study by Bauer et al., it has been reported that DSS triggers inflammation via the activation of the NLRP3 (NACHT, LRR and PYD domains-containing protein) and NLRP6 inflammasome, leading to caspase-1and NF-κB (nuclear factor kappa-light-chain-enhancer of activated B-cells) activation (Bauer et al., 2010; Elinav et al., 2011). Another suggested mechanism is that DSS treatment causes damage to zona occludin-1 protein of tight junctions in the epithelial barrier of the colon which causes increased permeability (Poritz et al., 2007). Further, Oh et al., show that luminal bacteria play an important role in the development of colitis (Oh et al., 2014).

The limitations of this model include long duration of experiments which is time-consuming. Together, inflammation by DSS treatment involves through innate immunity as T- and B-cell-deficient mice also develop severe intestinal inflammation suggesting that adaptive immune system does not play a major role in this model (Wirtz et al., 2007).

3.2.1. 2, 4, 6 TrinitrobenzeneSulphonic Acid (TNBS) Model

TNBS (picryl sulfonic acid), a nitroaryl oxidizing acid which is used as a hapten, when bound to protein, it turns into an antigen and elicits immunological responses. TNBS model was originally described by Morris et al., in rabbits (Morris et al., 1989). The TNBS model is used by many researchers since it is easily inducible, inexpensive, highly reproducible, and also needs short duration for the experiments. The model is characterized by long-lasting damage with inflammatory cell infiltration and ulcers and allows the study of early events in the development of mucosal inflammation. Thus, the model is rather suitable for the assessment of the effects of potential therapeutic agents and to study the immunological mechanism that has a role in the pathogenesis of IBD. TNBS induced model is widely applicable to vertebrates, including mice, rats, guinea pigs and rabbits. In mice, the susceptibility to TNBS-induced colitis varies between different strains: SJL, C3HeJ and BALB/c are more susceptible, whereas C57BL/6 and DBA/2 are the moreresistant ones. TNBS can be used either to induce acute colitis with a single dose (0.5 to 4 mg in 45-50% ethanol) or chronic colitis with repeated administration (Goyal et al., 2014). TNBS, in combination with ethanol, is administered intrarectally to the experimental animals. Alcohol is required to disrupt the mucosal barrier, whereas trinitrophenol (TNP) group of TNBS covalently binds to the lysinyl ε-amino group of microbial proteins, rendering them immunogenic to the host immune system. TNBS induces transmural inflammation with the activation of Type 1 T helper cell (Th1)-mediated immune response manifested by dense infiltration of CD4 T cells, neutrophils and macrophages as well as thickening of the colon wall. Inflammation in TNBS colitis is accompanied by increased levels of IFN-γ, however studies with IFN- KO mice showed that in these mice TNBS colitis may be associated with Type 2 T helper cell (Th2) mediated immune response (Dohi et al., 2000). The overall phenotypic and histopathological features of this model resemble CD. Another study by Grisham et al., has shown that TNBS induced inflammation is partly mediated by cytotoxic ROS generated by the oxidative metabolism of TNBS (Grisham et al., 1991). Further, increased level of platelet activating factor (PAF) has been observed 1-3 weeks after TNBS administration suggesting that PAF plays a key role in TNBS induced inflammation (Wallace, 1988). The disadvantages of this model include absence of spontaneous relapse which is the hallmark of human IBD, and ethanol itself causes severe intestinal inflammation which makes it tough to distinguish between the ethanol-induced inflammation and hapten-induced inflammation (Tran et al., 2012).

3.2.2. Oxazolone Model

Oxazolone (4-ethoxymethylene-2-phenyl-2-oxazolin-5-one) is another type of hapten that induces colonic inflammation and delayed type of hypersensitivity reaction in the skin. Several models have been developed to study Th1-mediated intestinal inflammation whereas, only a limited number of models exist for Th2-mediated colitis; amongst which oxazolone model is one. Boirivant et al., were the first to report that the administration of oxazolone with ethanol would induce colitis in SJL/J mice (Boirivant et al., 1998). Intrarectal administration of a single dose (1% in 50% ethanol) of oxazolone leads to the rapid development of acute inflammation limited to the distal colon region with characterized body weight loss, diarrhea, ulceration, loss of epithelial cells, infiltration of inflammatory cells, edema of lamina propria and superficial inflammation of the mucosa. Installation of oxazolone without prior sensitization leads to the rapid development of inflammation which lasts for3-4 days following rapid recovery or death of the mice whereas, chronic inflammation which persists for 1-2 weeks can be induced by sensitizing mice before intrarectal administration of oxazolone (Strober et al., 2002).

Oxazolone colitis can be easily induced in SJL/J, C57BL/10 or BALB/C mice, but the mortality rate is higher in SJL/J when compared to BALB/C strains (Kojima et al., 2004). Studies on oxazolone-induced model by Boirivant, have shown that inflammation by T cell is IL-4/IL-5 driven (Boirivant et al., 1998). Further Heller et al., have shown that natural killer T cell (NKT)-produced cytokine IL-13 plays a major role in triggering inflammation as oxazolone failed to induce colonic inflammation in NKT cell-deficient mice (Heller et al., 2002). Heller et al., have reported that the destruction of epithelial cell tight junctions with increased mucosal permeability was caused by elevated levels of IL-13 which lead to the invasion of bacteria and inflammation (Heller et al., 2002). A recent investigation by Zhu et al., has shown that CCL25 and CCR9 chemokines are highly expressed and their interactions may promote the induction and function of invariant natural killer T cells (iNKT cells) during oxazolone-induced colitis (Zhu et al., 2014).

Oxazolone model is highly reproducible and simple. Further, the model resembles human UC with respect to morphology, immunopathogenesis and the inflammation that has developed lasts for several days, which makes the model ideal to screen potential therapeutic agents.

3.2.3. Carrageenan-Induced Model

Carrageenans (CGN) are highly sulfated linearpolysaccharides obtained from several species of red seaweeds (*Rhodophyceae*) including *Gigartina*, *Chondrus* and *Eucheuma,* and structurally it is a polymer made up of alternating disaccharide units of D-galactose and 3,6-anhydro-galactose linked by α-1, 3 to β-1, 4 galactosidic linkages (Borthakur et al., 2007). There are three forms of CGN which are kappa (κ), iota (ι) and lambda (λ) with similar structures but differing in number and position of the sulfated groups, and the extent of branching and solubility. In contrast to κ- or ι-CGN, λ- CGN is the least branched and is readily soluble at cold temperatures. Marcus and Watt developed a novel method for inducing intestinal inflammation in guinea pigs by administering degraded CGN in drinking water (Watt and Marcus, 1971b). Further, colitis was induced in rats, mice, rhesus monkeys and rabbits; however, other animals like hamster, squirrel monkey and ferret have failed to produce colitis (Benitz et al., 1973; Grasso et al., 1973). The degraded CGN can be prepared by acid treatment at high temperature (80 °C) which triggers CGN hydrolysis (Watt, 1979). A recent investigation by Benard et al., has shown that 40 kDa degraded CGN is the most effective in causing intestinal inflammation (Benard et al., 2010). Oral administration of 2-10% degraded CGN through drinking water for 10 days in experimental animals induces intestinal inflammation with diarrhea, anemia, presence of blood in stools, and body weight loss. The histological features of this model include thedestruction of crypt architecture, infiltration of inflammatory cells in the lamina propria and ulceration (Goyal et al., 2014). The absence of lesions in the small bowel and the lack of remission and exacerbation are the distinguishing features of the CGN model (Tobacman, 2001).

Research on this model has provided numerous mechanisms that how degraded CGN causes inflammation. CGN exposure triggers inflammatory cascades which involve TLR4- and BCL10-dependent activation of NF-κB which leads to elevated levels of Interleukin (IL)-8 (Borthakur et al., 2007). In another study by Bhattacharyya et al., it is reported that CGN activates ROS-mediated pathway that is associated with the decrease in phospho Heat shock protein (HSP)-27, which in turn enhances the activation of NF-κB pathway (Bhattacharyya et al., 2008).

3.2.4. Acetic Acid Model

Acetic acid causes inflammation in the colon of the experimental animals and as a result it is being used to induce IBD. MacPherson and Pfeiffer reported this model first, where they administered 10-50% of acetic acid in rats (MacPherson and Pfeiffer, 1978). Acetic acid-inducedmodel of inflammation is limited to the colon and mimics UC in terms of histopathology, eicosanoid production and clinical features. The main advantage of this model is that acetic acid is easily available and economical. Mice, rats, guinea pigs, dogs and rabbits are known to be susceptible to acetic acid induced colitis. The characteristic feature of the acetic acid induced IBD model is the production of ROS which plays an important role in the progression of IBD. Therefore, this model is ideal to study the efficacy of drugs which interfere with ROS generation (Randhawa et al., 2014; Low et al., 2013). The histological features include non-transmural inflammation, goblet cell loss, inflammatory cell infiltration, edema, ulceration, and massive necrosis of mucosal and submucosal layers. Colonic inflammation can be induced by administering 10-50% acetic acid intra-rectally to the experimental animals under mild ether anesthesia. A soft and flexible medical-grade polyurethane tube has to be inserted into the anus to inject acetic acid and the experimental animals should be maintained in a head-down position for 2 minutes to prevent the leakage of the solution from the rectum. Acetic acid is predicted to induce inflammation through the release of protons which accumulate within the intracellular space and thereby cause intracellular acidification leading to epithelial destruction (Das et al., 2013). In addition, acetic acid has also been shown to elicit colonic inflammation in the experimental animals by activating NF-κB pathway (Niu et al., 2013). The disadvantage of this model is that the epithelial destruction observed with in the first 24 h of acetic acid administration is devoid of immunogenic property, which makes the test drugs that target the immune system unusable in that period (Goyal et al., 2014).

3.3. Genetically Engineered Models

Improvement in genetic engineering has given a crucial turning point in research involving IBD as it has allowed the discovery of a large number of gene variants which are hidden in people with IBD. Genome-wide association study (GWAS) has investigated and identified 163 susceptibility genes which are responsible for the progression of IBD (Bianco et al., 2015). In 1993 the discovery of three KO mice; IL-10 KO (Kühn et al., 1993), IL-2 KO (Sadlack et al., 1993) and T-cell receptor (TCR)-α KO (Mombaerts et al., 1993) mice was a major milestone in IBD research. Since then numerous genetically engineered models have been gradually established. These models have provided remarkable contributions in understanding the mechanism of disease and developing new drugs for IBD. Genetically engineered models are classified in to gene KO and transgenic models (Table 2).

Table 2. Characteristics of Genetically induced models of IBD

Genetically induced models of IBD		
Models	Features	Disease type
Conventional Gene Knockout		
IL-10$^{-/-}$	• Early onset of enterocolitis	CD
NOD2$^{-/-}$	• Susceptible gene for CD	CD
IL-2$^{-/-}$	• Develops inflammation with the signs of hemolytic anemia and lymphocytic hyperplasia	UC
TCR$^{-/-}$	• IL-4 is responsible for the development of colitis	UC
Conditional Gene Knockout		
XBP1$^{-/-}$	• Depletion of goblet cells and Paneth cells	UC
NEMO$^{-/-}$	• Reduced expression of antimicrobial defensin	CD
Conventional transgenic mice		
IL-7Tg	• Useful model to study the mechanism of T-cell involved pathogenesis of colitis	UC
STAT4Tg	• Develops severe transmural colitis after immunization with dinitrophenyl-keyhole limpet hemocyanin	CD
Conditional transgenic mice		
SOCS1Tg	• Development of colitis after 15 weeks of age with rectal prolapse	CD
CD40LTg	• Produces transmural, granulomatous colitis between 3 and 6 weeks of age with glomerulonephritis	CD

3.3.1. Gene Knockout Models

A gene knockout (KO) model is a genetically engineered organism in which a gene of interest is inactivated using various techniques. The differences in the characteristics of KO and wild-type animals have made researchers to draw information about the functionality of the gene and how it contributes to the disease. The gene KO can be of 2 ways namely, the conventional gene KO and conditional gene KO. Conventional KO animals are genetically engineered by replacing the gene of interest with an artificial piece of DNA in all the tissues or cells whereas, in conditional KO a specific target gene is inactivated from a single organ or specific cell types rather than the whole body (Mizoguchi et al., 2015). The main disadvantage of conventional KO method is that, a greater percentage of the genetically altered embryos by this method cannot grow into an adult; whereas, conditional KO method lacks embryonic lethality owing researchers to use conditional KO over conventional KO. Mice are the experimental animals which are the most closely related species to humans in which the KO technique can be easily performed, so they are a favorite model organism for KO experiments.

3.4. Conventional Knockout Models

3.4.1. IL-10$^{-/-}$

IL-10 is an anti-inflammatory cytokine that regulates physiological inflammatory condition in the gastrointestinal tract by maintaining a check on pro-inflammatory response to normal antigens and microbiota. It is observed that mice disrupted in the gene encoding IL-10 and IL-10 receptor component CRF2-4 develops enterocolitis suggesting that IL-10 is an essential regulator of the mucosal immune system (Kuhn et al., 1993; Spencer et al., 1998). The IL10$^{-/-}$ experimental model is a well-established Th1-mediated model of colitis and resembles CD in features like crypt hyperplasia, the rare occurrence of granulomas, fibrosis, the absence of fissures/fistulae, and transmural with discontinuous inflammation throughout the intestinal tract (Gomes-Santos et al., 2012). IL-10 deficient mice exhibit anemia, weight loss, infiltration of inflammatory cells, epithelial destruction and crypt distortion (Barnett and Fraser, 2011). The C3H/HeJsubstrain is more susceptible, whereas the C57BL/6J strain is resistant to this type of colitis (Jones-Hall and Grisham, 2014). IL-10 deficient mice do not develope colitis when kept under germ-free environment indicating that stimulation of mucosal immune system by commensal microflora is a critical event in the development of colitis in IL-10$^{-/-}$ model (Kiesler et al., 2015). It has been reported that there is a lesser number of caecal bacteria observed before colitis (7 weeks of age) in IL10$^{-/-}$ compared to C57Bl/6J mice suggesting that the altered microbiota in IL10$^{-/-}$ KO mice has a role in the progression of colitis (Tran et al., 2012). Sturlan et al., have reported that IL-10 deficient mice may be considered as an appropriate model only for a short period of time to study IBD because of the possible development of dysplasia and cancer (Sturlan et al., 2001).

3.4.2. NOD2-/-

NOD2 (nucleotide-binding oligomerization domain 2) is a cytoplasmic pattern recognition receptor which recognizes microbial cell wall components and regulates inflammatory response and apoptosis. NOD2 is also called Caspase recruitment domain-containing protein 15 (CARD 15) and it is expressed in all antigen presenting cells and epithelial cells. NOD2 initiates a signaling pathway that leads to the translocation of NFκB from the cytoplasm to the nucleus which leads to the activation of innate and adaptive immune responses (Barnett and Fraser, 2011). This gene was identified as susceptible to CD in 2001 (Hugot et al., 2001). A recent study by Petnicki-Ocwieja et al., has shown that NOD2 is required for regulating homeostasis between microbiota and host immune system (Petnicki-Ocwieja et al., 2009).

3.4.3. IL-2$^{-/-}$

IL-2 is a regulatory cytokine which is important for the proliferation of T and B lymphocytes and maintains tolerance between self and non-self proteins. It promotes the differentiation of immature T-cells into regulatory T-cells and prevents the development of autoimmune diseases. Sadlack et al., for the first time reported that mice with inactivated IL-2 gene develop intestinal inflammation together with the signs of hemolytic anemia, lymphocytic hyperplasia and disturbance in bone marrow hematopoietic cells (Sadlack et al., 1993). They developed symptoms of intestinal inflammation was confined to colon at the age of 6 weeks with a mortality rate of 50% (Sadlack et al., 1993). The histopathological features of this model include crypt abscesses, ulceration, mucin depletion, epithelial dysplasia and infiltration of activated T and B lymphocytes. Unlike IL-10 KO, IL-2 KO mice develop colitis in germ-free condition suggesting that the inflammation is fully mediated by an autoimmune mechanism (Mizoguchi, 2012).

3.4.4. T-Cell Receptor-α$^{-/-}$

T-cell receptor (TCR) is a membrane bound protein found on the surface of T-lymphocytes and recognizes antigenic peptides bound to major histocompatibility complex. TCR is made up of a combination of either an α and a β chain or a δ and a γ chain. Mombaerts et al., for the first time reported that, inactivation of TCR-α gene in mice results in spontaneous development of colitis at the age of 12-16 weeks (Mombaerts et al., 1993). C57BL/6 strain is known to be highly susceptible to colitis as compared to Balb/c and C3H/HeJ strains (Mizoguchi, 2012). Symptoms include superficial inflammation through the entire length of the colon, loose stools and hypertrophy. Histologically, there will be a decreased number of goblet cells, crypt distortion and infiltration of lymphocytes and neutrophils. The inflammation in this model is mediated by Th-2 type immune response. The absence of TCR-α chains results in the formation of TCR composed of only β chains which enhance the production of effector cytokine IL-4. The released IL-4 is responsible for the development of Th-2 mediated colitis which closely resembles UC (Mombaerts et al., 1993).

3.5. Conditional Genes Knockout Models

3.5.1. XBP1$^{-/-}$

X-box binding protein (XBP1) is a transcription factor that functions during endoplasmic reticulum (ER) stress by regulating unfolded protein response and together helps in the proper functioning of the immune system. XBP1 is a key component in the development of secretory cells such as Paneth and goblet cells which are located in the epithelial lining of the small intestine. Deficiency of XBP1 within the small intestinal epithelium leads to the decreased size and depletion of goblet cells, increased apoptosis of Paneth cells and reduction in crypt ratio of the villus, which suggests that XBP1 KO mice are susceptible for colitis (Kaser et al., 2008).

3.5.2. NEMO$^{-/-}$

NF-κB essential modulator (NEMO), a regulatory subunit of inhibitor of kappa B (IκB) complex that activates Nf-κB, is a key component of the Nf-κB pathway. Continuous activation of Nf-κB in immune cells promotes the expression of pro-inflammatory cytokines which is involved in IBD pathogenesis (Wirtz and Neurath, 2007). Further, Nenci et al., have shown that the inactivation of NEMO gene in the intestinal epithelial cells of mouse results in complete inhibition of Nf-κB and causes apoptosis of the cells, thus leading to the destruction of epithelial barrier (Nenci et al., 2007). The loss of epithelial barrier integrity along with the reduced expression of antimicrobial defensin, allows translocation of luminal antigens and bacteria into the colonic mucosa, which in turn triggers an inappropriate immune response and T-cell mediated inflammation. Histopathological features include transmural inflammation, goblet cell loss, infiltration of mononuclear cells, and crypt abscesses (Nenci et al., 2007). As reports suggest that both continuous activation as well ascomplete inhibition of Nf-κB contribute to the development of IBD, investigators who target Nf-κB to develop new therapeutic drugs for IBD have to consider its dual role in different cells of the gastrointestinal tract.

3.5.3. Transgenic Models (Tg)

In contrast to the deletion of genes in KO models, transgenic models offer the introduction of a gene of interest into the animal using recombinant DNA technology, resulting in overexpression of that gene. Rudolf Jaenisch and Beatrice Mintz in 1974 were the first to develop transgenic mice, however the transfer of foreign DNA into their off springs by the transgenic mice was not made until 1981(Jaenisch and Mintz, 1974). In 1980 Gordon and Ruddle created transgenic mice by using recombinant DNA technology and the first report of successful germ-line transmission of foreign DNA into the experimental mice was made in 1981 by Lacy (Costantini and Lacy, 1981; Gordon et al., 1980). Further, transgenic models are also classified into conventional and conditional transgenic models.

3.6. Conventional Transgenic Models

3.6.1. IL-7 Tg

IL-7 expressed by intestinal epithelial and goblet cells, functions as a regulatory factor for the proliferation and differentiation of lymphocytes with in the gut mucosa. It has been reported that the development of T-cell in the thymus is influenced by serum IL-7 in UC patients (Watanabe et al., 1995). IL-7 Tg mice express high levels of IL-7 which causes infiltration of neutrophils, CD4 T cells and γδ T cells in the intestine resulting in acute colitis at the age of 1-3 weeks. At 8-12 weeks IL-7 Tg mice display signs of proctoptosis with anal bleeding, crypt abscesses and reduced goblet cells. IL-7 Tg model is very useful to study the mechanism of T-cells involved in the pathogenesis of colitis, and also helps in the discovery of new drugs which target T-cells.

3.6.2. STAT4 Tg

STAT (signal transducer and activator of transcription)-4 is a transcription factor belonging to the family of signal transducer and activator of transcription, which is activated by IL-12 and IL-23. STAT4 is critical in the differentiation of naive T cells towards Th1 type which is responsible for the production of pro-inflammatory cytokines like IFN (Interferon)-γ, IL-2 and TNF (Tumor necrosis factor)-α. Mice overexpressing STAT4 develop severe transmural colitis within 7-14 days after immunization with dinitrophenyl-keyhole limpet hemocyanin which activates cytomegalovirus promoter system (Wirtz et al., 1999). The colitis developed in STAT4 transgenic mice displays close resemblance with human CD.

3.7. Conditional Transgenic Models

3.7.1. SOCS1 Tg

SOCS1 (Suppressor of cytokine signaling)-1 is a protein which is a negative regulator of cytokine signaling and is also an inhibitor of the JAK (Janus kinase) /STAT and TLR/NFκB pathway. SOCS1 contains an SH2 domain and a conservative motif SOCS box. Mice with excessively expressed SOCS1 protein in intestinal T-cells have shown to develop colitis. Even though young SOCS1 Tg mice shows no symptoms of colitis, 40% of SOCS1 Tg mice develop colitis after 15 weeks of age with rectal prolapse, and with the progression of age there will be dilation and thickening of the colon, elongation of crypts, ulcers, and soft stool (Inagaki-Ohara et al., 2006).

3.7.2. CD40L Tg

CD40 ligand, also called CD154, is a transmembrane protein expressed primarily by activated T-cells and it belongs to the member of TNF superfamily. CD40, which is a co-stimulatory receptor present in antigen presenting cells such as B-cells, dendritic cells and macrophages, exerts its effect by binding to CD40 ligand. Mice excessively expressing CD40 ligand in T-cells produce transmural, granulomatous colitis between 3 and 6 weeks of age (Clegg et al., 1997). Even though the CD40L expression is absent in B-cells, ectopic overexpression of CD40L on B-cell develops intestinal inflammation and glomerulonephritis at 8-15 weeks of age (Kawamura et al., 2004).

3.8. Adoptive Transfer Model

Adoptive transfer model includes a selective transfer of certain cells (mainly T-cells) from a healthy donor animal to a recipient animal that lacks T and B cells, resulting in the development of colitis. Adoptive transfer model was initially developed by Powrie and coworkers in 1994 (Powrie et al., 1994a). In T-cell adoptive transfer model $CD4^+$ T-cells from immunocompetent wild-type donor mice (isolated from spleen or lymph nodes) are fractionated into $CD4^+CD45RB^{high}$ T cell and $CD4^+CD45RB^{low}$ T- cell population using flow cytometric cell sorting technique. Further, $CD4^+CD45RB^{high}$ T cells will be transferred to severe combined immunodeficiency (SCID) mice or recombination activating gene 2 ($Rag2^{-/-}$) KO mice, which will develop gut inflammation after 5-10 weeks of treatment (Powrie et al., 1994a, 1994b). The transfer of matured $CD4^+CD45RB^{low}$ T- cells alone or co-transfer with $CD4^+CD45RB^{high}$ T-cells into the recipient mice failed to develop colitis because of the presence of T-regulatory cells ($Foxp3^+$Treg cells) in $CD4^+CD45RB^{low}$ T- cells that suppress inflammation by producing IL-10 and TGF (Transforming growth factor)-β (Kiesler et al., 2015). The main advantage of this model is that it is simple, highly reproducible and helps researchers to evaluate the role of different T cell populations that contribute to the progression of IBD; and the disadvantage of this model is the underlying immunodeficiency of the recipient mouse which is not observed in human IBD condition. The incidence of colitis is high in this model as 85 to 90% of recipient immunodeficient mice that receive $CD4^+CD45RB^{high}$ T-cells, exhibit histopathological symptoms similar to IBD at the time of necropsy (Maxwell et al., 2009). Lesions in this model include transmural inflammation, infiltration of inflammatory cells in lamina propria, crypt dilation with abscesses, mucin depletion, loss of goblet cells, and epithelial cell hyperplasia. The $CD4^+CD45RB^{high}$ T cell population which lacks T-regulatory cells is known to cause intestinal inflammation through the activation of pro-inflammatory IL-12 driven Th-1 response. The severity and onset of the disease in this model depends on the type of strains used for both donor and recipient mice (Goyal et al., 2014). Germ-free mice failed to develop colitis in adoptive transfer model, which indicates that commensal bacteria or bacterial antigens in the gut play a major role in the progression of the disease. In 1999, Steinhoff reported the alternative adoptive transfer model which includes the transfer of an HSP-60 specific $CD8^+$T-cell clone to immunodeficient TCR-β KO mice, resulting in the development of small bowel inflammation. The HSP-60 specific $CD8^+$T-cells induced inflammation was antigen specific and MHC (Major histocompatibility complex) class 1 dependent and surprisingly, the development of colitis was observed in the absence of normal intestinal flora (Steinhoff et al., 1999) (Table 3).

Table 3. Characteristics of Adoptive transfer and spontaneous models

Adoptive transfer and spontaneous models		
Models	Features	Disease type
Adoptive transfer models		
CD45RB-high cells into RAG/SCID mice	Ideal model to evaluate the role of different T cell populations which contributes to the progression of IBD.	CD
Hsp60 CD8+ T cells	Intestinal inflammation is MHC class I dependent and develops primarily in the small intestine.	CD
Spontaneous models		
Cotton-top tamarin	The unique feature is that it exhibits secondary complications such as colonic adenocarcinoma and sclerosing cholangitis.	UC
SAMP1/Yit	Intestinal inflammation is triggered by gut microbial antigens.	CD
C3H/HeJBir	Development of spontaneous colitis restricted to cecum and right side of the colon.	CD

3.9. Spontaneous Models

Animals such as cotton-top tamarins develop colitis spontaneously without any apparent exogenous manipulation and the intestinal inflammation developed is similar to human IBD condition (Chalifoux and Bronson, 1981; Mansfield et al., 2001). The spontaneous gut inflammation in cotton-top tamarin shows clinical, endoscopic and histopathological features, resembling human UC; and in contrast to other models, cotton-top tamarin exhibits secondary complications such as colonic adenocarcinoma and sclerosing cholangitis in humans, which is also a unique feature in this model (Watkins et al., 1997). The cotton-top tamarins have only a single MHC class I molecule from HLA (Human leukocyte antigen)-G cluster, which along with environmental factors, is alleged to be the contributing factor for the development of IBD together. (Wirtz and Neurath, 2000). Even though spontaneous cotton-top tamarin model is more relevant than mice, rat and other models, these primates are in limited use as they are listed as endangered species.

3.9.1. SAMP1/Yit

Senescence-accelerated mouse (SAM) P1/Yit is one of the most studied models of spontaneous CD. Takeda, a researcher from Japan, while studying accelerated senescence generated SAMP1/Yit mice from AKR mice using extensive interbreeding. However, these mice accidentally developed enteric inflammation in the terminal ileum and caecum, along with infiltration of inflammatory cells after 10 weeks of age and with 100% penetrance by 30 weeks of age (Matsumoto et al., 1998; Takeda et al., 1981). Intestinal inflammation in this model is driven by Th-1 mediated response and triggered by intestinal microbial antigens, resulting in the dysregulation of mucosal immunity. The developed inflammation is also been observed to be mediated by Th-2 as indicated by increased expression of IL-5 and IL-13 (Mizoguchi, 2012). Recently, Mikulski et al. reported that SAMP1/Yit mice develop ileitis due to the loss of CCL (Chemokine C-C motif ligand) 21 which is required for dendritic cell migration to establish immune tolerance (Mikulski et al., 2015). The lesions include transmural inflammation, granulomas, development of cryptitis, and changes in the epithelial architecture.

3.9.2. C3H/HeJBir

C3H/HeJBir mice are a substrain of C3H/HeJ, produced by selective breeding, which develops spontaneous colitis restricted to the cecum and right side of the colon at 3-4 weeks of age with the disappearance of symptoms at 10-12 weeks (Goyal et al., 2014). This model resembles CD because of the involvement of Th-1 type cells which produces high levels of IFN-γ and IL-2, and the histopathological symptoms include ulcers, crypt abscesses and epithelial regeneration. The susceptibility gene locus in this substrain was mapped on chromosome 3 and identified as CdCs1 gene, which makes C3H/HeJBir mouse susceptible to colitis (Mizoguchi, 2012) (Table 3).

CONCLUSION

With the advent of animal models in IBD research, there has been a tremendous change in understanding the pathology and pathophysiology of the disease, which has led to the effective management of the disease and to develop new, effective and safe drugs. Though none of the models completely resemble human IBD, multiple modes have provided an opportunity for the researcher to select the ideal IBD model according to the needs of the study. Future investigations are deemed to provide still better models for understanding the disease, wherein it could be possible to reduce the incidence and progress of the disease.

ACKNOWLEDGMENTS

Authors thank Dr. Hemshekhar M and Dr. Thushara R Mohan for proof reading the chapter. K.S.G. acknowledges the funding from the DST (DST-SERB/LS-952/2012).

REFERENCES

Ananthakrishnan, A.N., 2015. Epidemiology and risk factors for IBD. *Nat. Rev. Gastroenterol. Hepatol.* 12, 205–217.

Anthony, D., Savage, F., Sams, V., Boulos, P., 1995. The characterization of a rabbit model of inflammatory bowel disease. *Int. J. Exp. Pathol.* 76, 215–224.

Barnett, M., Fraser, A., 2011. Animal Models of Colitis : Lessons Learned, and Their Relevance to the Clinic. Ulcerative Colitis - Treat. *Spec. Popul. Futur.* 161–178.

Bauer, C., Duewell, P., Mayer, C., Lehr, H.A., Fitzgerald, K.A., Dauer, M., Tschopp, J., Endres, S., Latz, E., Schnurr, M., 2010. Colitis induced in mice with dextran sulfate sodium (DSS) is mediated by the NLRP3 inflammasome. *Gut* 59, 1192–1199.

Benard, C., Cultrone, A., Michel, C., Rosales, C., Segain, J.-P., Lahaye, M., Galmiche, J.-P., Cherbut, C., Blottière, H.M., 2010. Degraded carrageenan causing colitis in rats induces TNF secretion and ICAM-1 upregulation in monocytes through NF-kappaB activation. *PLoS One* 5, e8666.

Benitz, K.F., Golberg, L., Coulston, F., 1973. Intestinal effects of carrageenans in the rhesus monkey (Macaca mulatta). *Food Cosmet.* Toxicol. 11, 565–575.

Bhattacharyya, S., Gill, R., Chen, M.L., Zhang, F., Linhardt, R.J., Dudeja, P.K., Tobacman, J.K., 2008. Toll-like Receptor 4 Mediates Induction of the Bcl10-NF B-Interleukin-8 Inflammatory Pathway by Carrageenan in Human Intestinal Epithelial Cells. *J. Biol. Chem.* 283, 10550–10558.

Bianco, A.M., Girardelli, M., Tommasini, A., Bianco, A.M., Girardelli, M., Tommasini, A., 2015. 2015 Advances in Inflammatory Bowel Disease Genetics of inflammatory bowel disease from multifactorial to monogenic forms 21, 12296–12310.

Boirivant, M., Fuss, I.J., Chu, a, Strober, W., 1998. Oxazolone colitis: A murine model of T helper cell type 2 colitis treatable with antibodies to interleukin 4. *J. Exp. Med.* 188, 1929–1939.

Borthakur, A., Bhattacharyya, S., Dudeja, P.K., Tobacman, J.K., 2007. Carrageenan induces interleukin-8 production through distinct Bcl10 pathway in normal human colonic epithelial cells. Am. J. Physiol. Gastrointest. *Liver Physiol.* 292, G829–G838.

Chalifoux, L. V, Bronson, R.T., 1981. Colonic adenocarcinoma associated with chronic colitis in cotton top marmosets, Saguinus oedipus. *Gastroenterology* 80, 942–946.

Clapper, M.L., Cooper, H.S., Chang, W.-C.L., 2007. Dextran sulfate sodium-induced colitis-associated neoplasia: a promising model for the development of chemopreventive interventions. *Acta Pharmacol. Sin.* 28, 1450–1459.

Clegg, C.H., Rulffes, J.T., Haugen, H.S., Hoggatt, I.H., Aruffo, a, Durham, S.K., Farr, a G., Hollenbaugh, D., 1997. Thymus dysfunction and chronic inflammatory disease in gp39 transgenic mice. *Int Immunol* 9, 1111–1122.

Costantini, F., Lacy, E., 1981. Introduction of a rabbit beta-globin gene into the mouse germ line. *Nature* 294, 92–94.

Das, S., Kanodia, L., Mukherjee, A., Hakim, A., 2013. Effect of ethanolic extract of leaves of Paederia foetida Linn. on acetic acid induced colitis in albino rats. *Indian J. Pharmacol.* 45, 453–457.

Dohi, T., Fujihashi, K., Kiyono, H., Elson, C.O., McGhee, J.R., 2000. Mice deficient in Th1- and Th2-type cytokines develop distinct forms of hapten-induced colitis. *Gastroenterology* 119, 724–33.

Elinav, E., Strowig, T., Kau, A.L., Henao-Mejia, J., Thaiss, C.A., Booth, C.J., Peaper, D.R., Bertin, J., Eisenbarth, S.C., Gordon, J.I., Flavell, R.A., 2011. NLRP6 inflammasome regulates colonic microbial ecology and risk for colitis. *Cell* 145, 745–757.

Fakhoury, M., Negrulj, R., Mooranian, A., Al-Salami, H., 2014. Inflammatory bowel disease: clinical aspects and treatments. *J. Inflamm.* Res. 7, 113–20.

Gomes-Santos, A.C., Moreira, T.G., Castro-Junior, A.B., Horta, B.C., Lemos, L., Cruz, D.N., Guimaraes, M.A.F., Cara, D.C., McCafferty, D.-M., Faria, A.M.C., 2012. New insights into the immunological changes in IL-10-deficient mice during the course of spontaneous inflammation in the gut mucosa. *Clin. Dev. Immunol.* 2012, 560817.

Gordon, J.W., Scangos, G.A., Plotkin, D.J., Barbosa, J.A., Ruddle, F.H., 1980. Genetic transformation of mouse embryos by microinjection of purified DNA. *Proc. Natl. Acad. Sci. U. S. A.* 77, 7380–7384.

Goyal, N., Rana, A., Ahlawat, A., Bijjem, K.R. V, Kumar, P., 2014. Animal models of inflammatory bowel disease: A review. *Inflammopharmacology* 22, 219–233.

Grasso, P., Sharratt, M., Carpanini, F.M., Gangolli, S.D., 1973. Studies on carrageenan and large-bowel ulceration in mammals. *Food Cosmet.* Toxicol. 11, 555–564.

Grisham, M.B., Volkmer, C., Tso, P., Yamada, T., 1991. Metabolism of trinitrobenzene sulfonic acid by the rat colon produces reactive oxygen species. *Gastroenterology* 101, 540–547.

Heller, F., Fuss, I.J., Nieuwenhuis, E.E., Blumberg, R.S., Strober, W., 2002. Oxazolone colitis, a Th2 colitis model resembling ulcerative colitis, is mediated by IL-13-producing NK-T cells. *Immunity* 17, 629–638.

Hugot, J.P., Chamaillard, M., Zouali, H., Lesage, S., Cézard, J.P., Belaiche, J., Almer, S., Tysk, C., O'Morain, C. a, Gassull, M., Binder, V., Finkel, Y., Cortot, a, Modigliani, R., Laurent-Puig, P., Gower-Rousseau, C., Macry, J., Colombel, J.F., Sahbatou, M., Thomas, G., 2001. Association of NOD2 leucine-rich repeat variants with susceptibility to Crohn's disease. N*ature* 411, 599–603.

Inagaki-Ohara, K., Sasaki, a, Matsuzaki, G., Ikeda, T., Hotokezaka, M., Chijiiwa, K., Kubo, M., Yoshida, H., Nawa, Y., Yoshimura, a, 2006. Suppressor of cytokine signalling 1 in lymphocytes regulates the development of intestinal inflammation in mice. *Gut* 55, 212–9.

Jaenisch, R., Mintz, B., 1974. Simian virus 40 DNA sequences in DNA of healthy adult mice derived from preimplantation blastocysts injected with viral DNA. *Proc. Natl. Acad. Sci. U. S. A.* 71, 1250–1254.

Jiminez, J. a., Uwiera, T.C., Douglas Inglis, G., Uwiera, R.R.E., 2015. Animal models to study acute and chronic intestinal inflammation in mammals. *Gut Pathog*. 7, 29.

Jones-Hall, Y.L., Grisham, M.B., 2014. Immunopathological characterization of selected mouse models of inflammatory bowel disease: Comparison to human disease. *Pathophysiology* 21, 1–22.

Kaser, a, Lee, a H., Franke, a, Glickman, J.N., Zeissig, S., Tilg, H., Nieuwenhuis, E.E., Higgins, D.E., Schreiber, S., Glimcher, L.H., Blumberg, R.S., 2008. XBP1 links ER stress to intestinal inflammation and confers genetic risk for human inflammatory bowel disease. *Cell* 134, 743–756.

Kawamura, T., Kanai, T., Dohi, T., Uraushihara, K., Totsuka, T., Iiyama, R., Taneda, C., Yamazaki, M., Nakamura, T., Higuchi, T., Aiba, Y., Tsubata, T., Watanabe, M., 2004. Ectopic CD40 ligand expression on B cells triggers intestinal inflammation. J. Immunol. 172, 6388–97.

Kiesler, P., Fuss, I.J., Strober, W., 2015. Experimental Models of Inflammatory Bowel Diseases. Cell. Mol. *Gastroenterol. Hepatol*. 1, 154–170.

Kirsner, J.B., Elchlepp, J.G., Goldgraber, M.B., Ablaza, J., Ford, H., 1959. Production of an experimental ulcerative "colitis" in rabbits. *Arch. Pathol.* 68, 392–408.

Kojima, R., Kuroda, S., Ohkishi, T., Nakamaru, K., Hatakeyama, S., 2004. Oxazolone-induced colitis in BALB/C mice: a new method to evaluate the efficacy of therapeutic agents for ulcerative colitis. *J. Pharmacol. Sci.* 96, 307–313.

Kuhn, R., Lohler, J., Rennick, D., Rajewsky, K., Muller, W., 1993. Interleukin-10-deficient mice develop chronic enterocolitis. *Cell* 75, 263–274.

Kühn, R., Löhler, J., Rennick, D., Rajewsky, K., Müller, W., 1993. Interleukin-10-deficient mice develop chronic enterocolitis. *Cell* 75, 263–74.

Laroui, H., Ingersoll, S.A., Liu, H.C., Baker, M.T., Ayyadurai, S., Charania, M.A., Laroui, F., Yan, Y., Sitaraman, S. V., Merlin, D., 2012. Dextran Sodium Sulfate (DSS) Induces Colitis in Mice by Forming Nano-Lipocomplexes with Medium-Chain-Length Fatty Acids in the Colon. *PLoS One* 7, e32084.

Low, D., Nguyen, D.D., Mizoguchi, E., 2013. Animal models of ulcerative colitis and their application in drug research. *Drug Des. Devel. The*r. 7, 1341–57.

MacPherson, B.R., Pfeiffer, C.J., 1978. Experimental production of diffuse colitis in rats. *Digestion* 17, 135–150.

Mansfield, K.G., Lin, K.C., Xia, D., Newman, J. V, Schauer, D.B., MacKey, J., Lackner, A.A., Carville, A., 2001. Enteropathogenic Escherichia coli and ulcerative colitis in cotton-top tamarins (Saguinus oedipus). *J. Infect. Dis*. 184, 803–807.

Marcus, R., Watt, J., 1969. Seaweeds and ulcerative colitis in laboratory animals. Lancet (London, England) 2, 489–490.

Matsumoto, S., Okabe, Y., Setoyama, H., Takayama, K., Ohtsuka, J., Funahashi, H., Imaoka, A., Okada, Y., Umesaki, Y., 1998. Inflammatory bowel disease-like enteritis and caecitis in a senescence accelerated mouse P1/Yit strain. *Gut* 43, 71–78.

Maxwell, J.R., Brown, W.A., Smith, C.L., Byrne, F.R., Viney, J.L., 2009. Methods of inducing inflammatory bowel disease in mice. *Curr. Protoc. Pharmacol.* doi: 10.1002/0471141755.ph0558s47.

Mikulski, Z., Johnson, R., Shaked, I., Kim, G., Nowyhed, H., Goodman, W., Chodaczek, G., Pizarro, T.T., Cominelli, F., Ley, K., 2015. SAMP1/YitFc mice develop ileitis via loss of CCL21 and defects in dendritic cell migration. *Gastroenterology* 148, 783–793.e5.

Mizoguchi, A., 2012. Animal models of inflammatory bowel disease. *Prog. Mol. Biol. Transl. Sci.* 105, 263–320.

Mizoguchi, A., Takeuchi, T., Himuro, H., Okada, T., Mizoguchi, E., 2015. Genetically Engineered Mouse Models for Studying Inflammatory Bowel Disease. *J. Pathol.* 1–15.

Mombaerts, P., Mizoguchi, E., Grusby, M.J., Glimcher, L.H., Bhan, A.K., Tonegawa, S., 1993. Spontaneous development of inflammatory bowel disease in T cell receptor mutant mice. *Cell* 75, 274–282.

Morris, G.P., Beck, P.L., Herridge, M.S., Depew, W.T., Szewczuk, M.R., Wallace, J.L., 1989. Hapten-induced model of chronic inflammation and ulceration in the rat colon. *Gastroenterology* 96, 795–803.

Nenci, A., Becker, C., Wullaert, A., Gareus, R., van Loo, G., Danese, S., Huth, M., Nikolaev, A., Neufert, C., Madison, B., Gumucio, D., Neurath, M.F., Pasparakis, M., 2007. Epithelial NEMO links innate immunity to chronic intestinal inflammation. *Nature* 446, 557–561.

Niu, X., Fan, T., Li, W., Huang, H., Zhang, Y., Xing, W., 2013. Protective effect of sanguinarine against acetic acid-induced ulcerative colitis in mice. *Toxicol. Appl. Pharmacol.* 267, 256–265.

Oh, S.Y., Cho, K.-A., Kang, J.L., Kim, K.H., Woo, S.-Y., 2014. Comparison of experimental mouse models of inflammatory bowel disease. *Int. J. Mol. Med.* 33, 333–340.

Ohkusa, T., 1985. [Production of experimental ulcerative colitis in hamsters by dextran sulfate sodium and changes in intestinal microflora]. *Nihon Shokakibyo Gakkai Zasshi* 82, 1327–1336.

Padilla-Carlin, D.J., McMurray, D.N., Hickey, A.J., 2008. The Guinea Pig as a Model of Infectious Diseases. *Comp. Med.* 58, 324–340.

Patterson, J.K., Lei, X.G., Miller, D.D., 2008. The pig as an experimental model for elucidating the mechanisms governing dietary influence on mineral absorption. *Exp. Biol. Med.* (Maywood). 233, 651–664.

Petnicki-Ocwieja, T., Hrncir, T., Liu, Y.-J., Biswas, A., Hudcovic, T., Tlaskalova-Hogenova, H., Kobayashi, K.S., 2009. Nod2 is required for the regulation of commensal microbiota in the intestine. *Proc. Natl. Acad. Sci. U. S. A.* 106, 15813–15818.

Poritz, L.S., Garver, K.I., Green, C., Fitzpatrick, L., Ruggiero, F., Koltun, W.A., 2007. Loss of the tight junction protein ZO-1 in dextran sulfate sodium induced colitis. *J. Surg. Res.* 140, 12–19.

Powrie, F., Coffman, R.L., Correa-Oliveira, R., 1994a. Transfer of $CD4^+$ T cells to C.B-17 SCID mice: a model to study Th1 and Th2 cell differentiation and regulation in vivo. *Res. Immunol.* 145, 347–353.

Powrie, F., Leach, M.W., Mauze, S., Menon, S., Caddle, L.B., Coffman, R.L., 1994b. Inhibition of Th1 responses prevents inflammatory bowel disease in scid mice reconstituted with CD45RBhi $CD4^+$ T cells. *Immunity* 1, 553–562.

Ramesh, G., Alvarez, X., Borda, J.T., Pyone, P., Lackner, A. a, Sestak, K., Aye, P.P., 2005. Visualizing Cytokine-Secreting Cells In Situ in the Rhesus Macaque Model of Chronic Gut Inflammation Visualizing Cytokine-Secreting Cells In Situ in the Rhesus Macaque Model of Chronic Gut Inflammation. *Clin. Diagn. Lab. Immunol.* 12, 192–197.

Randhawa, P.K., Singh, K., Singh, N., Jaggi, A.S., 2014. A review on chemical-induced inflammatory bowel disease models in rodents. Korean *J. Physiol. Pharmacol.* 18, 279–88.

Sadlack, B., Merz, H., Schorle, H., Schimpl, A., Feller, A.C., Horak, I., 1993. Ulcerative colitis-like disease in mice with a disrupted interleukin-2 gene. *Cell* 75, 253–261.

Sartor, R.B., 2006. Mechanisms of Disease: pathogenesis of Crohn's disease and ulcerative colitis. *Nat. Clin. Pract. Gastroenterol.* & Hepatol. 3, 390–407.

Spencer, S.D., Di Marco, F., Hooley, J., Pitts-Meek, S., Bauer, M., Ryan, A.M., Sordat, B., Gibbs, V.C., Aguet, M., 1998. The orphan receptor CRF2-4 is an essential subunit of the interleukin 10 receptor. *J. Exp. Med.* 187, 571–578.

Steinhoff, U., Brinkmann, V., Klemm, U., Aichele, P., Seiler, P., Brandt, U., Bland, P.W., Prinz, I., Zügel, U., Kaufmann, S.H.., 1999. Autoimmune Intestinal Pathology Induced by hsp60-Specific CD8 T Cells. *Immunity* 11, 349–358.

Strober, W., Fuss, I.J., Blumberg, R.S., 2002. The immunology of mucosal models of inflammation. Annu. Rev. Immunol. 20, 495–549.

Sturlan, S., Oberhuber, G., Beinhauer, B.G., Tichy, B., Kappel, S., Wang, J., Rogy, M. a, 2001. Interleukin-10-deficient mice and inflammatory bowel disease associated cancer development. *Carcinogenesis* 22, 665–71.

Takeda, T., Hosokawa, M., Takeshita, S., Irino, M., Higuchi, K., Matsushita, T., Tomita, Y., Yasuhira, K., Hamamoto, H., Shimizu, K., Ishii, M., Yamamuro, T., 1981. A new murine model of accelerated senescence. *Mech. Ageing Dev.* 17, 183–194.

Tobacman, J.K., 2001. Review of harmful gastrointestinal effects of carrageenan in animal experiments. *Environ. Health Perspect.* 109, 983–94.

Tran, C.D., Katsikeros, R., Abimosleh, S.M., 2012. Current and novel treatments for ulcerative colitis. Ulcerative Collitis Genet. *Complicat.* 189–222.

Wallace, J.L., 1988. Release of platelet-activating factor (PAF) and accelerated healing induced by a PAF antagonist in an animal model of chronic colitis. *Can. J. Physiol. Pharmacol.* 66, 422–425.

Watanabe, M., Ueno, Y., Yajima, T., Iwao, Y., Tsuchiya, M., Ishikawa, H., Aiso, S., Hibi, T., Ishii, H., 1995. Interleukin 7 is produced by human intestinal epithelial cells and regulates the proliferation of intestinal mucosal lymphocytes. *J. Clin. Invest.* 95, 2945–2953.

Watkins, P.E., Warren, B.F., Stephens, S., Ward, P., Foulkes, R., 1997. Treatment of ulcerative colitis in the cottontop tamarin using antibody to tumour necrosis factor alpha. *Gut* 40, 628–33.

Watt, J., Marcus, R., 1971. Carrageenan-induced ulceration of the large intestine in the guinea pig. *Gut* 12, 164–171.

Wirtz, S., Finotto, S., Kanzler, S., Lohse, A.W., Blessing, M., Lehr, H.A., Galle, P.R., Neurath, M.F., 1999. Cutting edge: chronic intestinal inflammation in STAT-4 transgenic mice: characterization of disease and adoptive transfer by TNF- plus IFN-gamma-producing $CD4^+$ T cells that respond to bacterial antigens. *J. Immunol.* 162, 1884–1888.

Wirtz, S., Neufert, C., Weigmann, B., Neurath, M.F., 2007. Chemically induced mouse models of intestinal inflammation. *Nat. Protoc.* 2, 541–546.

Wirtz, S., Neurath, M.F., 2007. Mouse models of inflammatory bowel disease. *Adv Drug Deliv Rev* 59, 1073–1083.

Wirtz, S., Neurath, M.F., 2000. Animal models of intestinal inflammation: new insights into the molecular pathogenesis and immunotherapy of inflammatory bowel disease. *Int. J. Colorectal Dis.* 15, 144–160.

You, Y., Fu, J.J., Meng, J., Huang, G.D., Liu, Y.H., 2009. Effect of N-acetylcysteine on the murine model of colitis induced by dextran sodium sulfate through up-regulating PON1 activity. *Dig. Dis. Sci.* 54, 1643–1650.

Zhu, S., Bing, Y., Wang, X., Yu, Q., Wang, Y., Xu, S., Song, L., Wang, X., Xia, B., Zhu, Y., Zhou, R., 2014. CCL25/CCR9 interactions regulate the function of iNKT cells in oxazolone-induced colitis in mice. *PLoS One* 9, e100167.

In: Disorders of Gastrointestinal Systems … ISBN: 978-1-63485-366-8
Editors:S. Rajagopal, S. Murugan and S. Ramachandran ©2016 Nova Science Publishers, Inc.

Chapter 6

NANOTECHNOLOGY BASED DIAGNOSIS AND THERAPEUTICS FOR GASTROINTESTINAL DISORDERS

Buddolla Viswanath[1], Uday Sankar Allam[2], Aleem Basha Pinjari[3], Senthilkumar Rajagopal[3], PhD, Devarapogu Rajakumari[4], Pathan Shajahan Begum[5], Dowlathabad Muralidhara Rao[6] and Meerza Abdul Razak[3,*]

[1]Department of Bionanotechnology, Gachon University, Sujeong Gu, Seongnam Si, Gyeonggi Do. Republic of Korea
[2]Department of Biotechnology, Vikrama Simhapuri University, Nellore, A.P, India
[3]Department of Biotechnology, Rayalaseema University, Kurnool, A.P, India
[4]Department of Zoology, Sri Venkateswara University, Tirupati, A.P, India
[5]Department of Zoology, K.V.R. Govt College for Women, Kurnool, A.P, India
[6]Department of Biotechnology, Sri Krishnadevaraya University, Anantapur, A.P, India

ABSTRACT

In spite of advances in the diagnosis and treatment of gastrointestinal disorders (GI), they remain one of the major causes of death throughout the globe symbolizing a rising health crisis. The key barriers in fighting these diseases are the restrictions of existing diagnostic techniques and the high instability, low availability and vagueness of pharmacological treatment. Current trends and advances in nanotechnology present new hope for disease prevention, detection and treatment of GI disorders. At present, the increasing awareness in the utilization of nanoparticles for diagnosis and treatment of GI disorders has gained research attention and good funding in the area of nanomedicine. Fascinating, effective and very promising application of nanotechnology in diagnosis of GI disorders are such as magnetic localization, photodynamic therapy and molecular

* Corresponding author: Dr. Meerza Abdul Razak, PhD., DST-SERB Young Scientist, Department of Biotechnology, Rayalaseema University, Kurnool-518002, Andhra Pradesh, INDIA. Email:meerza99@yahoo.com.

targeting. Nanoparticles and nanotechnology-based strategies are under active progress towards the design of diagnostic and therapeutic tools for GI disorders. Nanotechnology has revolutionized medicine, coupling the nanoparticle with chemotherapeutic agents decrease in toxicity and therapeutic dose, prevention of drug degradation, reduction of drug level in healthy tissue. The objective of this chapter is to review the clinical use of nanotechnology for GI diagnosis and treatment and to provide an overview of the influence of nanotechnology on the management of GI disorder. Even though different issues and barriers are hindering the progress of nanotechnology, the potential application of nanotechnology as multimodal nanotheranostic agents will open the way to combat against GI disorders and support the progress of promising therapy for early diagnosis and treatment of GI diseases. We can expect few of our unachieved goals in diagnostics and treatment of GI disorders can be achieved by utilizing nanotechnology.

Keywords: gastrointestinal disorders, nanotechnology, nanotheranostics, nanomedicine

INTRODUCTION

Nanotechnology is science field where chemistry, biology, medicine and engineering sciences are amalgamated. A variety of nanotechological based diagnosis, therapeutics and applications are employed in gastrointestinal disorders for early recognition, prevention and in curing. Nanomedicine is a fast developing field in which targeted therapeutic strategies using nanotechnology depended on the pathophysiology of gastrointestinal disorders and diseases are being developed. Conventional methods usually do not meet the patients' expectations because of very low specificity and poor patient stratification. Specifically targeted and highly modified treatments are required (Song, 2007). Towards this requirement, nanomedicine and nanotechnology have been discovered so that they can be potentially employed in advanced therapeutic strategies.

The usage of nanomedicine in gastrointestinal disorders and diseases has afford new trust within the scientific society for the growth of new therapeutic strategies to cure gastrointestinal disorders (Cai et al., 2008), as a result scientists have find out novel exquisite and extremely sophisticated approaches to synthesis nanoscale particles with diverse sizes, compositions, and geometries to use in nanomedicine (Elsersawi, 2010). A wide variety of nanoparticles are employed in therapeutics and diagnosis of different gastrointestinal disorders and diseases. Nanoparticles support in screening tumors and delivering drugs in systematic pattern with minimum side effects and toxicity. Some of the nanoparticles which are used in the diagnosis and therapeutics for gastrointestinal disorders include carbon nanotubes, gold nanoparticles, liposomes, quantum dots, paramagnetic nanoparticles and novel nanoparticles for extremely specific recognition of protein and DNA. (Kircher et al., 2003, Nam et al., 2004, Ferrari M, 2005, Neuwelt et al., 2004, Jamieson et al., 2007).

Current progress in the field of nanomedicine had led to the development of bioaffinity, nanoparticles probes for cellular and molecular imaging, integrated for very early detection and screening of gastrointestinal cancers and targeted nanoparticles for gastrointestinal disorders. These progresses in nanomedicine put forward thrilling offers for the advancement of modified therapy, in which the molecular summary of an individual's protein and genetic biomarkers may be utilized in diagnoses and therapeutics of patient's gastrointestinal disorders and cancers.

Table 1. Examples of nanomaterials used in diagnosis and therapeutics of gastrointestinal disorders

Shape	Size range	Material	Properties	Properties Applicability	Reference
Complex, branched polymer	10–200 nm	Dendrimers		Drug delivery systems	(Kambhampati and Kannan 2013, Gras et al., 2012, Fleming, et al., 2011)
Spherical	1–10 nm	Quantum dots	Cd/Zn-selenides	*In vitro* diagnostic Imaging	(Ma et al., 2012, Poselt et al., 2012, Erogbogboet al., 2011)
Spherical	3–100 nm	Magnetic nanoparticles	Magnetic properties	Magnetic immunoassays, drug delivery, cell separation, purification, and tissue repair	(Sensenig et al., 2012, Hsieh et al., 2012, Fan et al., 2012)
Spherical	3–100 nm	Gold nanoparticles	Electronic, optical, and thermal properties	Diagnostics and detection of biological molecules at low concentration	(Ma, X, Sim, S.J, 2013, Mancuso et al., 2013, Zhuet al., 2013)
Spherical	1–1000 nm	Carbon nanotubes	Biodegradable Biocompatible Smart material (external stimuli degradation pH temperature)	Drug/gene delivery	(Larouiet al., 2010, Laroui et al., 2007, Laroui et al., 2011, Theiss et al., 2011, Zhao et al., 2012, Shi et al., 2012, Acharya et al., 2012)
Nanotubes	nm	Fullerene	Carbon nanomaterials in molecular electronics	Nanowire and biosensor for diagnosis	(Balasubramanian et al., 2006, Gruner et al., G, 2006)

Examples of some nanoparticles synthesized of different materials which display different physico-chemical properties are applied in diagnosis and therapeutics of gastrointestinal disorders are illustrated in Table 1.

Methods Used to Deliver Nanoparticles in Gastrointestinal Tract

The urgent necessity in treatment of gastrointestinal disorders is exploring novel methods for targeted delivery of drug loaded nanoparticle to the colon and terminal ileum which are affected by colon cancer and inflammatory diseases. Four different types of targeted delivery of drug loaded nanoparticle in gastrointestinal tract are present; these methods are based on the enzyme environment, pH, ambient pressure and relative stable transit time in the digestive tract.

Enzyme-Based Approach

Enzyme-based approach is completely based on the degradation of nanoparticle by gastrointestinal bacteria and release of the drug into the GI tract. As GI contains bacteria, this approach is very potential to deliver drugs specifically to the GI tract. The bacteria residing in the GI tract produces specific enzymes which can be seen only in the GI tract. Based on this enzyme based approach, Laroui et al., successfully delivered the anti-inflammatory tripeptide in the colon by loading them in polylactic acid nanoparticles (Larouiet al., 2010) [30]. This anti-inflammatory tripeptide loaded polylactic acid nanoparticles were encapsulated in a hydrogel made up of chitosan and alginate. This alignate and chitosan of hydrogel were degraded by the specific colonic enzymes. Like alignate and chitosan different polysaccharides such as amylopectin and amylase can be used in the preparation of hydrogel since they can be degraded by specific enzymes of colonic bacteria (Crocianiet al., 1994, Larouiet al., 2011, McConnell et al., 2008).

Pressure-Dependent Approach

The feces present in the colon are evacuated by the sturdy muscular contraction of the colon. This muscular contraction acts as the driving force for the motion of colon contents. As a result of this motion inside the colon, it creates mechanical pressure which is higher when compared to other parts of the gastrointestinal tract. Capsules coated with ethyl cellulose, a polymer which is insoluble in water are named as Intestinal pressure-controlled colon delivery capsules (PCDCs). These capsules are majorly used for delivering drug in the colon (Hu et al., 2000, Hu et al., 2000, Shibata et al., 2001, Takaya et al., 1995). PCDCs works as ethyl cellulose balloon after oral taken by patient. The suppository base of PCDCs liquefies at body temperature as they enter the gastrointestinal tract. As the upper gastrointestinal tract consists of fluid present in the stomach and small intestine, PCDCs are not openly exposed to the luminal pressures. But once they enter the colon, viscosity of the luminal contents is more because of reabsorption of the water in the colon (Debongnieet al., 1978). Therefore increased intestinal pressure straight away changes the system through colonic peristalsis. In reaction to the increased pressure, PCDCs break and discharge the drug in the colon. The same mechanism can be applied for the delivery of drug through nanoparticles in the colon.

Time-Dependent Approach

Time dependent approach is completely depended on the transit time in the gastrointestinal tract. In this type of approach, first the outer layer of the drug delivery system is cracked and later the drug is released. In this type of strategy, the physico-chemical properties of the nanoparticles can be exploited for drug delivery, for example degree of swelling of a polymer matrix or the pH alteration. Dorkoosh et al. investigated to change the release time profile by using the modification in enteric coating and the thickness and concentration of the polymer layer. By employing this procedure, we can aim any site of the colon or intestine (Dorkoosh et al., 2001). Laroui et al. applied the same technique to aim the colon, in his research he investigated on the performance of diverse concentrations of a combination of two polysaccharides (alginate and chitosan). In his investigation he observed that elevated drug release profile was seen from the nanoparticles in the targeted area of the gastrointestinal tract. The charged polymers or erosion rate of the polymer coating or osmotic activity of the salt altered the kinetics of the release (Laroui et al., 2010).

pH-Dependent Approach

The gastrointestinal tracts have a different pH values at different sites such as pH 7 in the colon, pH 2–3 in the stomach and pH 5–6 in the small intestine. Researchers have developed commercially available nanoparticles that release drugs based on the pH. Eudragit poly (meth-) acrylate polymers are examples for nanoparticles that release drugs based on pH. Eudragit poly (meth-) acrylate polymers contain alkaline or acidic groups that facilitate the pH based delivery of the drugs. Polyacrylamide is a polymer which is extremely susceptible to pH. Generally it is degraded at neutral pH but it remains stable at acidic pH. This property makes it very appropriate for drug protection at the time of GI tract passage. By taking advantage of pH-dependent constancy, polysaccharides such as alginate, chitosan, and pectin have been utilized for the drug delivery purposes (Onishi et al., 2010, Sajeesh et al., 2010). A small alteration in the pH will produce striking change on the kinetics of drug delivery. Mostly microspheres are used for the drug delivery based on pH dependent strategy. Lamprecht et al. demonstrated that Eudragit P-4581F microspheres can be effectively used to release 5-fluorouracil in time by altering the pH (Lamprecht et al., 2003). As the microspheres are highly sensitive even to small change in pH they are used as excellent colonic delivery systems. Even the small change in pH can convert prodrug from its inactive form to an active form in the required targeted site (Jung and Kim, 2010). In one of the other approaches, the encapsulated prodrug is chemically changed into the active drug by alteration in the pH or by grafting the drug with polysaccharide to aim at required site.

Application of Nanoparticles in Diagnosis of Gastrointestinal Disorders

Gastrointestinal tract has different parts and each part has its own distinct properties and application of therapeutics and diagnosis is not easy. The delivery of drugs to the targeted site in the gastrointestinal tract is still far from perfection. Knowing the characteristics of nanoparticles and utilizing nanotechnology in gastrointestinal tract gives new hope and seems promising. Nanotechnology has been applied in many gastrointestinal disorders with diverse success.

Quantum Dots in Diagnostic Applications

Quantum dots (QDs) are crystal like semiconductor nanoparticles; they possess the features which are transitional between the properties of distinct molecules and vast semiconductors. Generally the diameter of quantum dots range from 2 to 10 nm. Quantum dots exhibits the dimension based fluorescent properties and quantized energy levels. Dimension based fluorescent properties of quantum dots make them suitable for imaging and drug delivery applications (Alivisatos A.P, 1996). Many of the gastrointestinal disorders can be identified by utilizing cautiously synthesized QDs. QDs exhibiting specific emission spectra are tagged with particular DNA tags so that emission spectra is coupled with unique and particular immobilized DNA tag. These DNA tag-labeled QDs are then mixed with a DNA sample which has to be tested, and then the DNA tags generally get coupled to the DNA sequence in the test sample which is associated with the oncogene or gastrointestinal disorders. The unique bar code emitted by the photo illumination of QDs-tagged DNA helps in recognition of the disease associated DNA sequence. A method was developed from this technology to recognize different molecular markers at a time in a single tissue specimen (Larson et al., 2003). Semiconductor quantum dots have more retention and improved permeability at the gastrointestinal diseased site. Gao et al. has demonstrated the targeted accumulation of quantum dots *in vivo* in a xenograft model using a human prostate cancer cell line in nude mice (Gao et al., 2004, Navarro et al., 2012).

Different regions of the DNA can be identified by unique labels which are created based on the full spectrum of quantum dots. The uniqueness and diversity of quantum dot based methods is crucial for the identification of cancer and gastrointestinal disorders, which are resulted due to the accumulation of several independent DNA mutations within the cell. When compared with other nanoparticles, quantum dots are very advantageous because the formulation of quantum dots is non-invasive and avoids the need for a biopsy. But the nanotoxicity of quantum dots is main problem for application in gastrointestinal disorders (Yan et al., 2011, Chen et al., 2012, Akbarzadeh et al., 2012, Tang et al., 2010, Akbarzadeh et al., 2012, Wang et al., 2010).

Nanowires in Diagnostics Application

Nanowire devices facilitate easy ultrasensitive direct electrical recognition of chemical and biological species. Generally nanowires are placed across the micro fluidic channel. Sensors of nanowire identify the molecular signatures of chemical and biological species and pass on the message to a signal analyzer. Nanowire has the ability to detect the presence of mutated genes associated with the diseases; as a result scientist can easily find the correct location of these genetic mutations. At a time identification of several cancer biomarkers in a single diverse detection platform can be done by using silicon nanowire biosensor array (Jabir et al., 2012). Silicon nanowire biosensor array coupled with three cognate antibodies is used to detect three cancer markers such as mucin-1 antigen, carcinoembryonic antigen and prostate-specific antigen. Single time high sensitivity analysis of several biomarkers by silicon nanowire biosensor array facilitates detection of cancer at early stages. Coupled ZnO nanowire arrays using a vapor–solid process are successfully used in the scanning electron microscopy. The aligned arrays of nanowires have significant application in nanobiotechnology and they are also used in the conversion of mechanical energy into electricity in nanodevices, cellular manipulation and biosensing (Zheng et al., 2005).

Using surface receptors and nanowires, a highly sophisticated nanodevice named silicon (Si) nanowire field-effect device was developed. The ability of silicon nanowire field-effect device for screening of protein markers in patients sample with high accuracy and selectiveness offers the capacity for treatment and diagnosis of gastrointestinal disorders and cancers. Other nanodevices named as Single-walled carbon nanotubes display unique spectroscopic and electrical properties along with strong resonant Raman scattering and near-infrared photoluminescence which may be utilized in imaging and biological sample identification.

CANTILEVERS IN DIAGNOSTIC APPLICATIONS

The novel nanocantilever supports the quantitative estimation of even small levels of particular molecules. Microscopic flexible beams present in the nanoscale cantilever look like a line of diving boards and they support fast and accurate identification. Due to binding of molecules, the physical properties of the nanocantilevers get altered and can be seen in real-time. The resonant frequency and deflection of nanocantilevers are easily changed by attachment of surface immobilized affinity reagent to biomarker nucleic acid or protein (Sun et al., 2002). Molecular products produced by diseased or cancer cells specifically bind to antibody coated cantilever. This detection is attached to modern communication devices, so that patients can detect in real time their own inflammatory level. Atomic force microscopy (AFM) also consists of cantilevers. The instruments of cantilever consist of cantilever with pointed tip, which is used to scan specimen surface. Generally cantilever is made up of silicon nitride or silicon with tip radius of curvature at nanometers scale. Cantilevers in atomic force microscopy are used to screen very low concentrations of cancer-associated molecules. Therefore cantilevers are very powerful nanodevices for early detection of gastrointestinal disorders and cancers (Yue et al., 2004, Majumdar A, 2002).

APPLICATION OF LIPOSOMES IN DIAGNOSIS AND THERAPEUTICS OF GASTROINTESTINAL DISORDERS

Liposomes had showed surprising potentially in therapeutic and diagnostic application of gastrointestinal disorders. Generally liposomes are synthesized with special surface characteristics within the size range of 50–700nm. Liposomes are round vesicles with aqueous core enclosed by a phospholipids bilayer in association with cholesterol (Lasic et al., 1995, Razak et al., 2015). The circulation time of the liposomes can be increased by linking polyethylene glycol molecules to their surface so that PEG molecules defend the liposome and avoid their clearance. In the field of drug delivery and imaging liposomes have very potential applications; particularly super paramagnetic liposomes are very excellent MRI contrast agents. In regard of magnetic resonance angiography, liposomes are found to be extremely efficient contrast agents, here liposomes are injected into the body intravenously and after 24 hours of administration images were collected (Martina et al., 2005). Liposomes are also used as the efficient gene transfer delivery systems. As gene delivery systems liposomes have many advantages such as facile alteration with a targeting agent and facile control over size. The disadvantage of using liposomes as gene delivery carriers is very poor efficiency in regard of DNA encapsulation. The drawback of very poor encapsulation efficiency can be avoided by using cationic liposomes consisting of lipid bilayers with positive charge which can associate with negatively charged DNA through hydrophobic and electrostatic interactions. By associating liposomes with cholesterol and altering them with functional ligands we can increase the transfection efficiency of liposomes (Lasic, 1998).

Application of Dendrimers in Diagnosis and Therapeutics of Gastrointestinal Disorders

Dendrimers are big complex branched polymers with a good- distinct structure enclosing an inner core. The branching length, shape and size and surface properties of a dendrimer can be restricted towards the synthesis of functional nanoparticles (Svenson and Tomalia, 2005). Polyamidoamines are a group of dendrimers generally used as therapeutic agents and for the delivery of drugs. For a dendrimer, drug molecules are attached to the outside edge or loaded in the inner core. One of the most advanced applications of dendrimer is in the field of NIR or MIR contrast agents for cancer treatment. The antibodies attached to the periphery of dendrimer can make available contrast agents which have been evaluated by using confocal and flow cytometry methods.

PAMAM is the most commonly and efficient dendrimer used for gene delivery, because it display high transfection efficiency. The PAMAM transfection efficiency can be improved by treatment with butanol or water (Tomalia et al., 2007). The dendrimer most commonly used in gene delivery applications is PAMAM, which shows high transfection efficiency. The transfection efficiency can be further enhanced by heat treatment in water or butanol. Heat treatment enhances the dendrimer flexibility, which condenses the dendrimer upon conjugating with DNA (Tang et al., 1996).

Delivery of Anti-inflammatory Nanoparticles in Gastrointestinal Tract to Cure Inflammatory Bowel Disease

There are several advantages in using nanostructure vectors as drug delivery systems. Some of the surprising properties of nanostructured vectors are enhancing the interaction specificity between target and drug and decrease the harshness and occurrence of side effects by reducing the required dose (Laroui et al., 2011).

In diseases like inflammatory bowel disease, Crohn's disease and ulcerative colitis the targeted organ is colon. The molecules such as siRNA, proteins and tripeptides are loaded alone or encapsulated with some other different molecules inside nanoparticles. Nanoparticles loaded with anti-inflammatory compounds and their delivery to the colon is one the most efficient method to cure the gastrointestinal disorders. A potential and successful technique was developed to deliver particular nanoparticles to specific regions of the gastrointestinal tract by using hydrogel which is held together by electrostatic interactions between negative and positive polysaccharides. The amalgamation of nanostructures and hydrogels enhanced efficient loading, decrease of dose and delivery to the colon, where the drug delivery prevented colon inflammation (Laroui et al., 2012).

Table 2. Nanotechnology-based Clinical Trials in Gastrointestinal Tumors (http://www.clinicaltrials.gov)

Company/Authors	Tumors	Drug	Code
Calando Pharmaceuticals Ribas, A., Tolcher, A. W., Yen, Y.	Solid tumor	siRNA (CALAA-01) against M2subunit of ribonucleotidereductase (R2) protected with Nps	NCT00689065
Peking University Lin, L.	Gastric adenocarcinoma	Albumin-Bound PCT (ABI-007)	NCT01336062
Zhang, Y. Affiliated hospital of Harbin Medical University	Gastric adenocarcinoma	Albumin-Bound PCT (ABI-007)plus capecitabine	NCT01641783
University of California and National Cancer Institute Moasser, M. M.	Bladder Cancer, Brain and Central Nervous, System Tumors, Breast Cancer, Esophageal Cancer, Gastric Cancer, Lung Cancer Ovarian Cancer Prostate Cancer Extragonadal Germ,	PCT albumin-stabilized Np formulation plus lapatinib	NCT00313599
Anhui Medical University and Technion, Israel Institute of Technology Liu, H.	Gastric cancer, Gastritis, Gastriculcer Normal	Gold Nps and carbon nanotubes for cancer diagnosis using breath analysis	NCT01420588
University of Miami Sylvester Comprehensive Cancer Center Lopes, G.	Pancreatic cancer	PCT albumin-stabilized nanoparticle formulation	NCT00691054
University of California, San Francisco and Celgene Corporation Ko, A.	Pancreatic neoplasms, Pancreatic cancer, Adenocarcinoma	PCT albumin-stabilized Np plusGEM and Capecitabine	NCT01161186
Anderson Cancer Center and National Cancer Institute Javle, M.	Pancreatic cancer	Cholesterol liposome-based Np (BikDD)	NCT00968604
Massachusetts General Hospital Weissleder, R.	Pancreatic cancer	USPIO for cancer detection by MRI	NCT00920023
University of Kansas Williamson, S.	Pancreatic cancer	Fe/Fe3O4 Nps for cancer diagnosis(detection of active proteases)	NCT01707758
Rambam Health Care Campus, Technion, Israel Institute of Technology Galimidi, Z., Segol, O.	Breast and colon cancer	NaNose system for cancer diagnosis using breath analysis	NCT01292369
National Cancer Institute(NCI) and National Institutes of Health Clinical Center (CC) Uldrick, T. S.	Hepatic metastases from colorectal cancer, pancreas cancer, gastric cancer, breast cancer and ovarian cancer	Lipid Nps containing siRNA (TKM 080301) against the PLK1 gene product	NCT01437007

Application of Nanogel in Diagnosis and Therapeutics of Gastrointestinal Disorders

Nanogels often called as Nano-size hydrogels are swollen nano-sized networks formed by covalent cross linking of polymer chains or non-covalent interactions. Some of the specific characteristics of nanogels are reactive to environmental stimulus, good drug loading ability, controlled drug delivery, size tunability and large surface to volume ratio. Now a day nanogels have gained good research interest due to its targeted drug delivery, decreasing side effects and imaging labels (Arunrajet al., 2014). Nanogels with 5-fluorouracil (5-FU) were synthesized which displayed effectively reduced toxicity and pH-sensitive release property; they are used as novel colon targeting drug carrier and delivery systems (Ashwanikumar et al., 2012).

Nanogels have been proved to be efficient and successful oral drug delivery systems. The 5-FU nucleoside floxuridine prepared into polymeric nanogels can be utilized as a novel oral drug form, which shows an excellent antitumor effect on drug resistant tumors (Senanayake et al., 2013). Senanayake et al., synthesized a novel nanoencapsulated drug associated with gemcitabine for oral use in cancer chemotherapy. This innovative medical technology enhanced gemcitabine to effectively cross the generally impermeable gastrointestinal barrier and arrive at the site of interest, as per the results of permeability studies.

An excellent antitumor effect was also demonstrated *in vivo* in nude mice against several drug resistant human tumors (Senanayake et al., 2013). In recent years there is growing number of clinical trials on nanoparticle based approaches against gastrointestinal tumors and disorders. Table 2 lists some of the nanoparticle based strategies against gastrointestinal tumors.

Conclusion

Nanomedicine and the progress of novel nanoparticles have made a major growth in the diagnosis and therapeutics of gastrointestinal disorders and cancers. The major advantages of these novel nanoparticle strategies include enhancing prognosis, we can expect good results in patients with gastrointestinal tumors that do not respond to conventional treatments, such as gastric cancer and those with tumors that are diagnosed late due to the lack of markers, such as pancreatic cancer, permitting its advance detection. The property of nanoparticles to bind to particular tumour cell ligand facilitates the selective treatment. The investigation of clinical trials in gastrointestional disorders and tumors has showed that employing nanotechnology in treatment will improve the effects of standard medicine, boost their protection against degradation and finally enhance the response of patients. In coming years, nanotechnology will certainly change diagnosis and medical approach. Nanoscale sensors and devices may allow a personal and cost-effective continuous medical monitoring of patient's health. It is essential to pass the time for a few more years to develop advanced and novel nanotechnology research that can fetch decisive progress in the treatment of these patients.

REFERENCES

Acharya, G, Lee, CH, Lee, Y, 2012. Optimization of cardiovascular stent against resteno- sis, factorial design-based statistical analysis of polymer coating conditions. *PLoS ONE*. 7, e43100.

Akbarzadeh, A, Mikaeili, H, Zarghami, N, 2012. Preparation and *in vitro* evaluation of doxorubicin-loaded Fe (3) O (4) magnetic nanoparticles modi- fied with biocompatible copolymers. *International Journal of Nanomedicine*. 7, 511–26.

Akbarzadeh, A, Samiei M, Davaran, S, 2012. Magnetic nanoparticles, preparation, phys- ical properties, and applications in biomedicine. *Nanoscale Research Letters*. 7, 144.

Alivisatos, A.P, 1996. Semiconductor clusters, nanocrystals, and quantum dots. *Science*.271, 933–7.

Arunraj, T.R, Sanoj, Rejinold, N, Ashwin Kumar, N, Jayakumar, R, 2014. Bio-responsive chitin-poly(L-lactic acid) composite nanogels for liver cancer. *Colloids Surf B Biointerfaces*. 113, 394-402.

Ashwanikumar, N, Kumar, N.A, Nair, S.A, Kumar, G.V, 2012. Methacrylic-based nanogels for the pH-sensitive delivery of 5-fluorouracil in the colon. *Int J Nanomedicine*. 7, 5769-5779.

Balasubramanian, K, Burghard, M, 2006. Biosensors based on carbon nanotubes. *Ana- lytical and Bioanalytical Chemistry*.385, 452–68.

Cai, W.G.T, Hong, H, Sun, J, 2008. Applications of gold nanoparticles in cancer nanotechnology. *Journal of Nanotechnology, Science and Applications*.1,11.

Chen, N, He, Y, Su, Y, 2012. The cytotoxicity of cadmium-based quantum dots. *Biomaterials*.33, 1238–44.

Crociani, F, Alessandrini, A, Mucci, M.M, Biavati, B, 1994. Degradation of complex carbohydrates by Bifidobacterium spp. *Int J Food Microbiol*. 24, 199–210.

Debongnie, J.C, Phillips, S.F, 1978. Capacity of the human colon to absorb fluid. *Gastroenterology*. 74, 698–703.

Dorkoosh, F.A, Verhoef, J.C, Borchard, G, Rafiee-Tehrani, M, Junginger, H.E, 2001. Development and characterization of a novel peroral peptide drug delivery system. *J Control Release*. 71, 307–318.

Elsersawi, A, 2010. World of nanobioengineering, potential big ideas for the future. In, Bloom- ington, editor. Author House.

Erogbogbo, F, Yong, K.T, Roy, I, 2011. *In vivo* targeted cancer imaging, sentinel lymph node mapping and multi-channel imaging with biocompatible silicon nanocrystals. *ACS Nano*. 5, 413–23.

Fan, Z, Senapati, D, Singh, A.K, 2012. Theranostic magnetic core-plasmonic shell star shape nanoparticle for the isolation of targeted rare tumor cells from whole blood, fluorescence imaging, and photothermal destruction of cancer. *Molecular Pharmaceutics*.

Ferrari, M, 2005. Cancer nanotechnology, opportunities and challenges. *Nature Reviews Cancer*.5, 161–71.

Fleming, C.J, Yin, N.N, Riechers, S.L, 2011. High-resolution imaging of the intramolecular structure of indomethacin-carrying dendrimers by scanning tunneling microscopy. *ACS Nano*. 5, 1685–92.

Gao, X.H, Cui, Y.Y, Levenson, R.M, 2004. *In vivo* cancer targeting and imaging with semiconductor quantum dots. *Nature Biotechnology*. 22, 969–76.

Gras, R, Relloso, M, Garcia, M.I, 2012. The inhibition of Th17 immune response *in vitro* and *in vivo* by the carbosilanedendrimer 2G-NN16. *Biomaterials*. 33, 4002–9.

Gruner, G, 2006. Carbon nanotube transistors for biosensing applications. *Analytical and Bioanalytical Chemistry*. 384, 322–35.

Hsieh, W.J, Liang, C.J, Chieh, J.J, 2012. *In vivo* tumor targeting and imaging with anti-vascular endothelial growth factor antibody-conjugated dextran-coated iron oxide nanoparticles. *International Journal of Nanomedicine*. 7, 2833–42.

Hu, Z, Mawatari, S, Shibata, N, Takada, K, Yoshikawa, H, Arakawa A, Yosida Y, 2000. Application of a biomagnetic measurement system (BMS) tothe evaluation of gastrointestinal transit of intestinal pressure-controlledcolon delivery capsules (PCDCs) in human subjects. *Pharm Res*. 17,160–167.

Hu, Z, Mawatari, S, Shimokawa, T, Kimura, G, Yoshikawa, Y, Shibata, N, Takada, K, 2000. Colon delivery efficiencies of intestinal pressure-controlledcolon delivery capsules prepared by a coating machine in human subjects. *J Pharm Pharmacol*. 52, 1187–1193.

Jabir, N.R, Tabrez, S, Ashraf, G.M, 2012. Nanotechnology-based approaches in anti- cancer research. *International Journal of Nanomedicine*. 7, 4391–408.

Jamieson, T, Bakhshi, R, Petrova, D, 2007. Biological applications of quantum dots. *Biomaterials*.28, 4717–32.

Jung, Y, Kim, Y.M,2010. What should be considered on design of a colon specific prodrug? *Expert Opin Drug Deliv*.7, 245–258.

Kambhampati, S.P, Kannan, R.M, 2013. Dendrimer nanoparticles for ocular drug deliv- ery. *Journal of Ocular Pharmacology and Therapeutics*.

Kircher, M.F, Mahmood, U, King, R.S, 2003. A multimodal nanoparticle for pre- operative magnetic resonance imaging and intraoperative optical brain tumor delineation. *Cancer Research*.63, 8122–5.

Lamprecht, A, Yamamoto, H, Takeuchi, H, Kawashima, Y, 2003. Microsphere design for the colonic delivery of 5-fluorouracil. *J Control Release*. 90, 313–322.

Laroui, H, Dalmasso, G, Nguyen, H.T, 2010. Drug-loaded nanoparticles targeted to the colon with polysaccharide hydrogel reduce colitis in a mouse model. *Gastroenterology*. 138, 843-53 e1-2.

Laroui, H, Dalmasso, G, Nguyen, H.T, Yan Y, Sitaraman, S.V, Merlin, D, 2010. Drug-loaded nanoparticles targeted to the colon with polysaccharidehydrogel reduce colitis in a mouse model. *Gastroenterology*. 138, 843– 853.e41– 42.

Laroui, H, Dalmasso, G, Nguyen, H.T, Yan, Y, Sitaraman, S.V, Merlin, D, 2010. Drug-loaded nanoparticles targeted to the colon with polysaccharide hydrogel reduce colitis in a mouse model. *Gastroenterology*. 138, 843– 853.e41– 42.

Laroui, H, Grossin, L, Leonard, M, 2007. Hyaluronate-covered nanoparticles for the therapeutic targeting of cartilage. *Biomacromolecules*. 8, 3879–85.

Laroui, H, Sitaraman, S.V, Merlin, D, 2012. Gastrointestinal delivery of anti- inflammatory nanoparticles. *Methods in Enzymology*. 509, 101–25.

Laroui, H, Theiss, A.L, Yan, Y, 2011. Functional TNFalpha gene silencing medi- ated by polyethyleneimine/TNFalphasiRNAnanocomplexes in inflamed colon. *Biomaterials*.32, 1218–28.

Laroui, H, Theiss, A.L, Yan, Y, Dalmasso, G, Nguyen, H.T, Sitaraman, S.V, Merlin, D, 2011. Functional TNF_ gene silencing mediated by polyethyl- eneimine/TNF_ siRNAnanocomplexes in inflamed colon. *Biomaterials.* 32, 1218–1228.

Laroui, H, Wilson, D.S, Dalmasso, G, 2011. Nanomedicine in GI. *American Journal of Physiology Gastrointestinal and Liver Physiology*. 300, G371–83.

Larson, D.R, Zipfel, W.R, Williams, R.M, 2003. Water-soluble quantum dots for multiphoton fluorescence imaging *in vivo*. *Science*. 300, 1434–6.

Lasic, D.D, 1998 Novel applications of liposomes. *Trends in Biotechnology*.16,307–21.

Lasic, D.D, Lipowsky, R, Sackmann, E, 1995. Structure and dynamics of membranes. In, *Handbook Biology Physics*.. p. 493–516.

Ma, Q, Nakane, Y, Mori, Y, 2012. Multilayered, core/shell nanoprobes based on magnetic ferric oxide particles and quantum dots for multimodality imaging of breast cancer tumors. *Biomaterials*.33, 8486–94.

Ma, X, Sim, S. J, 2013. Femtomolar detection of single mismatches by discriminant anal- ysis of DNA hybridization events using gold nanoparticles. *Analyst.*

Majumdar, A, 2002. Bioassays based on molecular nanomechanics. *Disease Markers*.18, 167–74.

Mancuso, M, Jiang L, Cesarman, E, 2013. Multiplexed colorimetric detection of Kaposi's sarcoma associated herpesvirus and Bartonella DNA using gold and silver nanoparticles. *Nanoscale*.5, 1678–86.

Martina, M.S, Fortin, J.P, Menager, C, 2005. Generation of superparamagneticlipo- somes revealed as highly efficient MRI contrast agents for *in vivo* imaging. *Journal of the American Chemical Society*.127, 10676–85.

McConnell, E.L, Murdan, S, Basit, AW, 2008. An investigation into the digestion of chitosan (noncrosslinked and crosslinked) by human colonic bacteria. *J Pharm Sci*. 97, 3820–3829.

Nam, J.M, Stoeva, S.I, Mirkin, C.A, 2004. Bio-bar-code-based DNA detection with PCR-like sensitivity. *Journal of the American Chemical Society*.126, 5932–3.

Navarro, D.A, Bisson, M.A, Aga, D.S, 2012. Investigating uptake of water-dispersible CdSe/ZnS quantum dot nanoparticles by Arabidopsis thaliana plants. *Journal of Hazardous Materials*. 211–212, 427–35.

Neuwelt, E.A, Varallyay P, Bago A.G, 2004. Imaging of iron oxide nanoparticles by MR and light microscopy in patients with malignant brain tumours. Neu- *ropathology and Applied Neurobiology*.30, 456–71.

Onishi, H, Koyama, K, Sakata, O, Machida, Y,2010. Preparation of chitosan/ alginate/calcium complex microparticles loaded with lactoferrin and their efficacy on carrageenan-induced edema in rats. *Drug DevInd Pharm*. 36, 879–884.

Poselt, E, Schmidtke, C, Fischer, S, 2012. Tailor-made quantum dot and iron oxide based contrast agents for *in vitro* and *in vivo* tumor imaging. *ACS Nano*.6, 3346–55.

Razak, M.A, Shankarappa Devi Prasad, Viswanath, B, 2015. Drug-Loaded Nanocarriers in Tumor Targeted Drug Delivery. *Current Biotechnology*, 4 (3), 319-344.

Sajeesh, S, Bouchemal, K, Sharma, C.P, Vauthier, C, 2010. Surface-functionalized polymethacrylic acid based hydrogel microparticles for oral drug delivery. *Eur J Pharm Biopharm*. 74, 209–218.

Senanayake, TH, Warren, G, Wei, X, Vinogradov, SV, 2013. Application of activated nucleoside analogs for the treatment of drug-resistant tumors by oral delivery of nanogel-drug conjugates. *J Control Release*.167, 200-209.

Sensenig, R, Sapir, Y, MacDonald, C, 2012. Magnetic nanoparticle-based approaches to locally target therapy and enhance tissue regeneration *in vivo*. *Nanomedicine* (London). 7, 1425–42.

Shi, S, Zhu, X, Guo, Q, 2012. Self-assembled mPEG-PCL-g-PEI micelles for simultaneous codelivery of chemotherapeutic drugs and DNA, synthe- sis and characterization *in vitro*. *International Journal of Nanomedicine*. 7, 1749–59.

Shibata, N, Ohno, T, Shimokawa, T, Hu, Z, Yoshikawa, Y, Koga, K, 2001. Murakami, M, Takada, K. Application of pressure-controlled colondelivery capsule to oral administration of glycyrrhizin in dogs. *J Pharm Pharmacol*. 53, 441–447.

Song, S.Y, 2007. Future direction of nanomedicine in gastrointestinal cancer. *Korean Journal of Gastroenterology*. 49, 271–9.

Sun, Y.P, Fu, K.F, Lin, Y, 2002. Functionalized carbon nanotubes, properties and applications. *Accounts of Chemical Research*. 35, 1096–104.

Svenson, S, Tomalia, D.A, 2005. Dendrimers in biomedical applications – reflections on the field. *Advanced Drug Delivery Reviews*. 57, 2106–29.

Takaya, T, Ikeda, C, Imagawa, N, Niwa, K, Takada, K, 1995. Development of a colon delivery capsule and the pharmacological activity of recombinant human granulocyte colony-stimulating factor (rhG-CSF) in beagle dogs. *J Pharm Pharmacol*. 47, 474–478.

Tang, M.X, Redemann, C.T, Szoka, Jr FC, 1996. *In vitro* gene delivery by degraded polyamidoaminedendrimers. *Bioconjugate Chemistry*.7, 703–14.

Tang, X.H, Xie, P, Ding, Y, 2010. Synthesis, characterization, and *in vitro* and *in vivo* evaluation of a novel pectin-adriamycin conjugate. *Bioorganic and Medicinal Chemistry*. 18, 1599–609.

Theiss, A.L, Laroui, H, Obertone, T.S, 2011. Nanoparticle-based therapeutic delivery of prohibitin to the colonic epithelial cells ameliorates acute murine colitis. *Inflammatory Bowel Diseases*. 17, 1163–76.

Tomalia, D.A, Reyna, L.A, Svenson, S, 2007. Dendrimers as multi-purpose nanodevices for oncology drug delivery and diagnostic imaging. *Biochemical Society Trans- actions*.35, 61–7.

Wang, Z.M.M, Kunets, V.P, Xie, Y.Z.Z, 2010. Multilayer self-organization of InGaAs quantum wires on GaAs surfaces. *PhysicsLetters A*. 375, 170–3.

Yan, M, Zhang, Y, Xu, K, 2011. An *in vitro* study of vascular endothelial toxicity of CdTe quantum dots. *Toxicology*. 282, 94–103.

Yue, M, Lin, H, Dedrick, D.E, 2004. A 2-D microcantilever array for multiplexedbiomolecular analysis. *Journal of MicroelectromechanicalSystems*.13, 290–9.

Zhao, Z.X, Gao, S.Y, Wang, J.C, 2012. Self-assembly nanomicelles based on cationic mPEG-PLA-b-Polyarginine (R15) triblock copolymer for siRNA delivery. *Bioma- terials*.33, 6793–807.

Zheng, G, Patolsky, F, Cui Y, 2005. Multiplexed electrical detection of can- cer markers with nanowire sensor arrays. *Nature Biotechnology*. 23, 1294–301.

Zhu, Y, Chandra, P, Shim, Y.B, 2013. Ultrasensitive and selective electrochemical diagnosis of breast cancer based on a hydrazine-au nanoparticle-aptamer bio- conjugate. *Analytical Chemistry*. 85, 1058–64.

In: Disorders of Gastrointestinal Systems … ISBN: 978-1-63485-366-8
Editors:S. Rajagopal, S. Murugan and S. Ramachandran ©2016 Nova Science Publishers, Inc.

Chapter 7

ROLE OF MICROORGANISM IN HUMAN GASTROINTESTINAL CANCER*

Dhanalakshmi Thiyagarajan, PhD
and Suruliandi Rajendran, PhD
Department of Microbiology, Nehru Arts and Science College,
Coimbatore, Tamil Nadu, India

ABSTRACT

Gastrointestinal cancer forms in the veneer of the gastrointestinal tract (GI) which includes entire digestive system such as esophagus, gallbladder, liver, pancreas, stomach, small intestine, bowel and anus. Gastrointestinal Cancer is a multifarious disease in developing countries and also in developed countries. Moreover in Asia, cancer cases increased in the recent years, especially gastrointestinal cancer including the digestive system. Conditionally gastric cancer, colorectal cancer, liver cancer, esophageal cancer and pancreatic cancer are the most common cancers. This review describes about the microorganism playing main role in causing cancers of the GI. We focus on *Helicobacter pylori* causing GI related cancers and its mechanisms, symptoms, diagnosis and prevention. Food nutrition of fruit and vegetable consumption for control or at least to reduce the risk of GI cancers are also discussed. GI cancer awareness should be given to all level of people in understandable format for prevention, if not complete eradication of GI cancers.

Keywords: diagnosis and prevention, food nutrition, GI cancer, Helicobacter pylori, mechanisms

* Corresponding author: Dr. Dhanalakshmi, PhD., Assistant Professor, Department of Microbiology, Nehru Arts and Science College, Coimbatore, Tamil Nadu, India, dhanvarshar@gmail.com; Mo: 099 65664834.

1. INTRODUCTION

The gastrointestinal (GI) tract is essential for our well being in the conditionally functional form. The GI tract is the second largest body surface area after the respiratory tract, described to be somewhere between 250 and 400 m^2, or comparable in size to a tennis court. Totally 60 tons of foods pass through this canal during lifetime, which is important for well being, but also constitutes an enormous threat to the integrity of the digestive tract and the whole body. Therefore, this organ is often affected by inflammatory diseases and cancer (Bengmark, 1998). A good understanding of the factors promoting carcinogenesis in CRC should enable a better strategy of prevention and a more efficient screening protocol. The majority of CRC occurrences are considered erratic, meaning they are due to the environmental factors rather than the genetic alteration. Among environmental factors, the western lifestyle is considered to impact on CRC occurrence mainly food habitats (Sobhani et al., 2012). Recently, all vegetables and fruits are grown with chemical fertilizers and fast foods are made with food additives. These are the factors very important to cause cancer.

2. ROLE OF MICROBES IN CRC

Microbes play major roles in biological environments. About 16% of cancers to be caused by microorganisms and numerous cancers in the liver and gastrointestinal tract are clearly detected as being microorganism related (deMartel et al., 2012). WHO Agency for Research on Cancer has reported that the *Helicobacter pylori* have been associated with gastric adenocarcinoma and lymphoma involved in the mucosa associated lymphoid tissues. Many proofs have been obtained on this association from epidemiological data, experimental results in animal trial and interventional trials by eradication of the bacterium in humans. Good understanding of the entire physiology of the gastric function has been obtained when a single microbe has made human gastric carcinogenesis. Many number of colon micro flora is a multifarious system hosting more than billions of bacteria and massive amount of functions contrast to the *H. pyroli* (Sobhani et al., 2012). So we have focused on the gastric carcinogenesis which is caused by microbes and the mechanisms that could be involved are discussed.

The relationship between the bacterial infection and cancer is that of *H. pyroli associated* in two different forms of gastric cancers such as MALT lymphoma and gastric adenocarcinoma (Marshall and Windsor, 2005). Colon cancer is caused by *Streptococcus bovis*, *Chlamydiae pneumonia* associated with lung cancer and *Bartonella* sp. with vascular tumor formation (Marshall and Windsor 2005, Littman et al., 2005, Dehio, 2005 and Ellmerich et al., 2000). Some animal studies have shown the association of *H. hepaticus* in chronic active hepatitis that developed to heptocellular carcinoma in A/JCr mice (Ward et al., 2000). *Citrobacter rodentium* is a mouse pathogen, which genetically resemble enteropathogenic *E. coli* and can result in colon cancer (Newman et al., 2001). Recent study has shown that *H. hepaticus* has been stated to initiate cancer development indirectly in mammary gland of mice (Rao et al., 2006).

3. Mechanisms of Bacterial Carcinogenesis

Some forms of cancer can be prevented and cured when carcinogenesis induced by bacteria (Malfertheiner et al., 2005). There is a controversy in the involvement of bacteria in carcinogenesis because no clear conformity has been achieved on the molecular mechanism/s by which they may promote carcinogenesis. Many scientists started hypothesis in the 21st century in two ways: (1) chronic inflammation occurred by bacterial infection when prolonged for long period may lead to carcinogenesis (Lax and Thomas, 2002, Karin and Greten, 2005, Travaglione et al., 2008); (2) Bacterial toxins and secondary metabolites may induce carcinogenesis when chronic bacterial infection occurred (Lax and Thomas, 2002). Now many scientists have accepted that chronic bacterial infection may cause many chronic diseases and cancers (Lax and Thomas, 2002, Vogelmann and Amieva, 2007). There might be different mechanism behind the carcinogenesis induced by chronic bacterial infection (Agarwal, 2005, Surh and Kundu 2007, Qiao et al., 1995, Tjandrawinata &Hughes, 1997, Jaiswal et al., 2001, Xu et al., 2002, Ghosh et al., 1998, Pikarsky et al., 2004, Quintar et al., 2010, Altimari et al., 2003). Common feature of chronic infection is a continuous process of releasing mediators (Lax &Thomas 2002, Karin and Greten, 2005). Inflammation driven carcinogenesis may be linked to the nuclear factor κB (NF- κB) family of transcription (Karin and Greten 2005). The NF- κB activation of transcription is induced by microbial infections and also by proinflammatory cytokines, such as TNF-α and IL-1and this lead to activation of IKK.

Tumor suppressor gene DNA modifies and form complex by the activation of oncogenes (Hacker and Karin, 2006) and to degrade NF-κB inhibitors, NF-κB initiators enter into the nucleus and mediate transcription of target genes. Cell cycle regulators such as cyclin D1, CDK2 kinase, and c-myc are involved to upregulate the cell cycle, mean time apoptosis responding genes, such as p21, p53 and pRb are down regulated by NF-κB. Numerous cytokines, such as IL-1β, IL6, and VEGF which are responsible for proinflammatory and proangiogenic process up regulated by NF-κB, but down regulating the TNF, enhances tumor growth. NF-κB is up regulating an invasion and metastasis responding gene and down regulation of genes involved in suppression of apoptosis, i.e., Bcl-2 family members and IAP proteins, an imperative character of cancer cells, is mostly due to deregulation by NF-κB. NF-κB also leads to suppression of cell death and not only helps in persistence of intracellular and extracellular infections, thus creating a niche for bacterial survival confronting the host immune response (Van et al., 1996, Ferrero et al., 2007). Survival of such partially transformed cells provides a chance for a higher level of transformation. Inflammatory epithelial cells produced ROS (Reactive oxygen species) and NO (nitric oxide) and these compounds increase mutations in genes responsible for controlling malignant transformation. In particularly, ROS could inhibit tyrosine phosphatases, causing over expression of Mox1 which is the catalytic subunit of NADPH oxidizes and does not inhibit the Fpg protein (Wink and Laval 1994), NO inhibits the Fpg protein, a DNA repair enzyme (Wink and Laval 1994), leading to failure of damage control. HER-s2/neu or ErbB2 stands for "human epidermal growth factor receptor 2" and is a protein conferring higher ferociousness in breast cancers. ErbB2 is a member of the ErbB protein family, generally known as the epidermal growth factor receptor family, which is involved in cell proliferation, differentiation and oncogenesis. Due to the chronic inflammation over expression of ErbB2 can be occurred. The activation of intrinsic protein kinase activity will be prolonged by binding of ErbB1 and ErbB2 to ligands and leading to activate the biochemical cascade reaction for mitogenic cell signal transduction (Quintar et al., 2010, Altimari et al., 2003). All these factors are associated with the multistage process of carcinogenesis (Coussens and Werb 2002) and these factors cause oxidative damage to DNA of the cells.

4. Bacterial Toxins Associated in Carcinogenesis

Bacterial toxins and their possible role in carcinogenesis are *Haemophilus ducreyi, Helicobacter hepaticus, Salmonella typhi* and *Actinomycetemco mitans* produce CDT (3 subunits: CdtB is a functional unit, while CdtA and CdtC serve as accessory units for delivery into target cells); *Salmonella typhi* produces cytolethal distending toxin B (Haghjoo and Galán 2004) as a genotoxin and leads the DNAse activity (Nesic et al., 2004, Li et al., 2002), and *E. coli* secrete colibactin (Nougayrède et al., 2002) and it function is unknown. *Pasturella multocida* secretes toxin which modifies Gq proliferation (Seo et al., 2000), *H. pylori* secrete CagA and vacuolating cytotoxin A which leads to binds to SHP2 and c-Met cells scattering and up regulation of VEGF expression (Oswald et al., 2005), *Bacteroides fragilis* produces toxin which cleaves E-cadherin proliferation, *E. coli, Shigella dsenteriae, Campylobacter jejuni* and *S. typhi, Helicobacter hepaticus* and *Actinomycetemco mitans* secrete cytotoxic necrotizing factor-1 which modifies Rho family protein, inflammation and inhibition of cell cycle, block cytokines (Travaglione et al., 2008). Bacterial toxins can either kill the cells or modify the cellular processes that control DNA damage, proliferation, apoptosis and differentiation. These toxins obstruct either with the key eukaryotic processes, such as cellular gesturing components or directly by attacking the DNA (Lax 2007, Schiavo et al., 2001).

The host cells damage will be mediated by two ways:

1) By direct ways: a) Enzymatic attack, b) DNA damage, c) by affecting DNA repair mechanisms.
2) By indirect ways: a) provoking a chronic inflammatory reaction, b) Producing free radicals.

5. Gallbladder Cancer and Helicobacter Species

50% of the world populations of the people are infected by Gram negative rod shaped bacteria H. pylori. In 1994 the international Agency for research on cancer listed out the H. pylori is a definite human oncogenic agent and it causes more than 60% of all stomach cancers. H. pylori are a relative risk of 3 and it was a strong risk factor for nancardia intestinal gastric adenocarcinoma. The stomach cancer will be caused by infection of H. pylori (Amieva and ElOmar 2008). In 1982, thirty species of Helicobacter have been identified from the stomach, intestinal tract and liver of mammals and birds. H. bilis, H. pillorum, H. hepaticus and H. pyroli are found in human bile and biliary tract tissue biopsies which suspected to cause biliary tract diseases. As per the earlier discussion, any Helicobacter sp. causing persistent infection in the biliary tract may induce chronic inflammation and gall-stone formation, especially due to urease production (Belzer et al., 2006, Maurer et al., 2007). Further exaggerate chronic inflammation could induce transformation, which multiplies several fold by many toxins and metabolites of known carcinogenic potential produced by the Helicobacter (Wistuba and Gazdar, 2004, Jergens et al., 2007).

6. Case Study on Detection of *Helicobacter sp.*

H. hepaticus is a chronic active infectious pathogen of biliary canaliculi progressing to liver cancer (Nevin et al., 1976). Different species of Helicobacter is detected in biliary tract cancer from 0% - 82.8% by PCR method (De et al., 2009). With species- specific primers, H. bilis was found in 35 out of 67 specimens from four different studies, whereas H. hepaticus was searched for in two studies, but only in one study were four out of 19 specimens found to be positive for the bacterium. In Nepal, Prathan et al., (2004) have shown H. hepaticus infection in 82% of nonmalignant gallbladders and in 87.5% of malignant cases. Whether it is the main cause of the type of gallstone formation that finally leads to malignancy, or is itself a risk factor for the pathogenesis of carcinoma gallbladder, is yet to be determined. Murata et al., (2004) studied that H. bilis specific sequences can be amplified in three of eleven (27.2%) gallbladder cancer cases and in one of three (33.3%) cases with biliary duct cancer. Another study conducted in Japanese and Thai populations showed that patients for H. bilis had a 6-fold higher risk of biliary tract carcinoma. However, it is untimely to make conclusion about the role of Helicobacter sp. in causing CaGB. The age and sex is a main risk for H. pylori infection to cause biliary tract cancer and the corresponding RR (relative risk) was 9.9 (95%CI: 1.4-70.5). Both H. bilis and H. pylori have been detected in bile clinical specimens and associated with risk of biliary tract cancer. Murata et al., (2004) found a positive association between H. bilis and CaGB, with a basic RR of 2.6 (95% CI: 0.6-4.6). We need several epidemiological studies before identifying Helicobacter in gallbladder cancer, but after the development and validation of specific serological tests and direct detection of these bacterial species in the gallbladder itself.

7. Diagnosis and Assessment of Stomach Cancer (Patient.Info/Health/Stomach-Gastric-Cancer)

Gastroscopy or endoscopy is the initial assessment of stomach cancer if there is a suspect of cancer in earlier stage. A gastroscope is a thin, flexible telescope. It enters through the mouth, into the oesophagus and down towards the stomach and the primary part of the duodenum. It contains fiber optic channels which permit light to shine down so inner side of the stomach and duodenum can be seen.

When any abnormal cells are seen in the results of gastroscopy, then biopsy is needed. Biopsy is to confirm the diagnosis when a small sample of tissue is taken from a part of the body. The biopsy sample is examined under the microscope to look for abnormal cells. This is done by entering thin take hold of instrument down a side channel of the gastroscope. It could be taken two weeks for the biopsy results.

Once the occurrence of stomach cancer is confirmed, further diagnosis will be extended to tests the level of cancer. The following tests can be taken, such as a barium meal X-ray, a CT scan, an MRI scan, an ultrasound, laparoscopy or other tests like DNA level diagnosis. This assessment is called staging of the cancer.

7.1. Determination of Malignancy of Cancer

The level of the tumor in the stomach has grown, whether partially or fully through the wall of the stomach, whether it spreads to local lymph nodes and whether it has spread to other areas of the body will determine its malignancy. By finding out the stage of the cancer it helps doctors to recommend on the best treatment and also gives a reasonable suggestion of outlook of the disease.

7.2. Treatment for Stomach Cancer

The aim of the treatment is to cure the cancer. Some stomach cancers can be cured at the earlier stages, particularly if they are diagnosed early. The doctors can use the word "diminution" rather than the word "cured." However, in some cases a cancer returns months or years later. So the term "cured" cannot be used. Main aim of the treatment is to control the cancer, which means to limit the growth or spread of the cancer. Sometimes there may not be any symptoms, when the treatment may aim to ease symptoms. If cure is not possible, it can be used to reduce the size of a cancer, which may ease symptoms such as pain. If a cancer is advanced, solutions such as food supplements can be recommended. Pain killers and other methods to help keep away from the pain.

Treatment choices which may be considered include surgery, therapeutic methods of chemotherapy, radiotherapy, gene therapy and stem therapy. The treatment recommendation for each case depends on the various factors like:

- Sufficient nutrition rich food and better get advice from dietician.
- Complete discussion with a specialist to get the all information likely success rate, possible side-effects and other details about the various possible treatment options.
- Information about the surgery removing the tumor at early stage of the cancer.

The usual operation is to cut out the affected area of the stomach or sometimes remove whole of the stomach and this is done by laparoscopically. A cure is not possible, if cancer is in advanced stage. Some surgical techniques may be placed to ease symptoms; a blockage may be eased by removing part of the stomach or by using laser surgery or by a bypass operation.

Chemotherapy is a one of the treatment of cancer by using anti-cancer medicines which kill cancer cells or inhibit them from multiplying. There are two kinds of chemotherapy, first one is used in addition to surgery it is known as adjuvant chemotherapy and this aims to kill any cancer cells which may have spread away from primary tumor. The second one is given before surgery, to shrink a large tumor so that surgery is easier and this is called as neoadjuvant chemotherapy.

Radiotherapy is a treatment which uses high wave length of radiation to be focused on cancerous tissue. This kills the cancer cells or inhibits cancer cells from multiplying of the cancer cells. It is not commonly used to treat stomach cancer but sometimes used to reduce the size of a particular part of the cancer.

Chemoradiotherapy is a combination of chemotherapy and radiotherapy and it offered to addition of the surgery at the particular time of the operation.

8. Anticancer Effect by Probiotics

Probiotics is defined as live microorganisms that have beneficial effect to prevent and treat the specific pathological conditions. Antitumor bacterial effect prohibition of opportunistic pathogens by commensal bacteria may be represented a natural defense against GI diseases, including CRC. Probiotic bacteria such as *Lactobacillus* sp. and *Bifidobacterium* sp. exert anticarcinogenic effects, in part by inactivating microbial enzymes. *Lactobacillus casei* and *Lactobacillus acidophilus* of lactic acid bacteria perform decreasing activity of β-glucuronidase, azoreductase and nitroreductase. *Bifidobacterium longum* decreases AOM-provoked abnormal crypt formation, which correlates with a decrease in AOM- activating β-glucuronidase activity. *Lactobacillus* sp. and *Bifidobacterium* could inhibit DNA damage and tumourigenesis induces by N-methyl-N'-nitro-N-nitrosoguanidine, 1, 2- dimethylhydrazine (Arthur and Jobin, 2011). In common, probiotic fermentation of dietary fibers directs short-chain fatty acid acetate, propionate and butyrate production. These are absorbed by coloncytes and used as a primary source of energy and they provide protection during the early stages of tumourigenesis (Scheppach, 1994). The uses of probiotics to prevent gentle inflammation in the colonic mucosa via bacteria change would be the main hopeful therapeutic in the future.

Conclusion

The prevalence of microorganisms in our environment is unavoidable and mandatory. Among the existing microorganisms, several pathogenic strains exist that can cause diseases ranging from simple flu to cancer. These organisms are very easy to isolate but difficult to analyze. Thus, remedial measures for such strains can be devised only when their genetic and proteomic content are known in detail. Several control and preventive measures which can be affordable by all groups of people include dietary supplements and natural medicines available in our nature. The cure and/or remedy for cancers caused by microorganisms can only be reduced if proper awareness is created among the public.

References

Agrawal A, Gutteridge E, Gee JM, Nicholson RI, Robertson JF. Overview of tyrosine kinase inhibitors in clinical breast cancer. *Endocr Relat Cancer.* 2005; 12 Suppl. 1: S135-S144.

Altimari A, Fiorentino M, Gabusi E, Gruppioni E, Corti B, D'Errico A, Grigioni WF. Investigation of ErbB1 and ErbB2 expression for therapeutic targeting in primary liver tu-mours. *Dig. Liver Dis.* 2003; 35: 332-338.

Amieva MR, El-Omar EM. Host-bacterial interactions in Helicobacter pylori infection. *Gastroenterology.* 2008. 134: 306-323.

Arthur, J. and Jobin, C. (2011) The struggle within: microbial influences on colorectal cancer. *Inflamm Bowel Dis.* 17: 396–409.

Belzer C, Kusters JG, Kuipers EJ, van Vliet AH. Urease in-duced calcium precipitation by Helicobacter species may initiate gallstone formation. *Gut.* 2006. 55: 1678-1679.

Bengmark.S., 1998. Ecological control of the gastrointestinal tract, the role of probiotics flora, *Leading article.*

Coussens LM, Werb Z. Inflammation and cancer. *Nature* 2002; 420: 860-867

de Martel C, Plummer M, Parsonnet J, van Doorn LJ, Franceschi S. Helicobacter species in cancers of the gallbladder and extrahepatic biliary tract. *Br. J. Cancer* 2009; 100: 194-199.

Dehio C. Bartonella-host-cell interactions and vascular tu- mour formation. Nat Rev Microbiol 2005; 3: 621-631.

deMartel, C., Ferlay, J., Franceschi, S., Vignat, J., Bray, F., Forman, D. et al. (2012) Global burden of cancers attributable to infections in 2008: a review and synthetic analysis. *Lancet Oncol.* 13: 607–615.

Ellmerich S, Schöller M, Duranton B, Gossé F, Galluser M, Klein JP, Raul F. Promotion of intestinal carcinogenesis by Streptococcus bovis. *Carcinogenesis* 2000; 21: 753-756.

Ferrero-Miliani L, Nielsen OH, Andersen PS, Girardin SE. Chronic inflammation: importance of NOD2 *and* NALP3 in interleukin-1beta generation. *Clin. Exp. Immunol.* 2007; 147: 227-235.

Flemma RJ, Flint LM, Osterhout S, Shingleton WW. Bacteriologic studies of biliary tract infection. *Ann. Surg.* 1967; 166: 563-572.

Ghosh S, May MJ, Kopp EB. NF-kappa B and Rel proteins: evolutionarily conserved mediators of immune responses. *Annu Rev. Immunol.* 1998; 16: 225-260.

Gopal Nath, Anil K Gulati, Vijay K Shukla, Role of bacteria in carcinogenesis, with special reference to carcinoma of the gallbladder. *World J. Gastroenterol.* 2010; November 21; 16(43): 5395-5404.

Gorbach SL, Plaut AG, Nahas L, Weinstein L, Spanknebel G, Levitan R. Studies of intestinal microflora. II. Microorganisms of the small intestine and their relations to oral and fecal flora. *Gastroenterology* 1967; 53: 856-867.

Häcker H, Karin M. Regulation and function of IKK and IKK-related kinases. *Sci. STKE* 2006; 2006: re13.

Haghjoo E, Galán JE. *Salmonella typhi* encodes a functional cytolethal distending toxin that is delivered into host cells by a bacterial-internalization pathway. *Proc. Natl. Acad. Sci. USA* 2004; 101: 4614-4619.

IARC Working Group on the Evaluation of Carcinogenic Risks to Humans. Schistosomes, liver flukes and Helicobacter pylori. IARC Monogr. *Eval. Carcinog. Risks Hum.*1994; 61:1–241.

Jaiswal M, LaRusso NF, Gores GJ. Nitric oxide in gastroin-testinal epithelial cell carcinogenesis: linking inflammation to oncogenesis. *Am. J. Physiol. Gastrointest. Liver Physiol.* 2001; 281: G626-G634.

Jergens AE, Wilson-Welder JH, Dorn A, Henderson A, Liu Z, Evans RB, Hostetter J, Wannemuehler MJ. Helicobacter bilis triggers persistent immune reactivity to antigens derived from the commensal bacteria in gnotobiotic C3H/HeN mice. *Gut* 2007; 56: 934-940.

Karin M, Greten FR. NF-kappaB: linking inflammation and immunity to cancer development and progression. *Nat Rev Immunol* 2005; 5: 749-759

Keighley MR, Flinn R, Alexander-Williams J. Multivariate analysis of clinical and operative findings associated with bilary sepsis. *Br. J. Surg.* 1976; 63: 528-531.

Lax AJ, Thomas W. How bacteria could cause cancer: one step at a time. *Trends Microbiol.* 2002; 10: 293-299.

Lax AJ. New genotoxin shows diversity of bacterial attack mechanisms. *Trends Mol. Med.* 2007; 13: 91-93.

Li L, Sharipo A, Chaves-Olarte E, Masucci MG, Levitsky V, Thelestam M, Frisan T. The Haemophilus ducreyi cytolethal distending toxin activates sensors of DNA damage and re-pairs complexes in proliferating and non-proliferating cells. *Cell Microbiol.* 2002; 4: 87-99.

Littman AJ, Jackson LA, Vaughan TL. Chlamydia pneu- moniae and lung cancer: epidemiologic evidence. *Cancer Epidemiol. Biomarkers Prev.* 2005; 14: 773-778.

Malfertheiner P, Sipponen P, Naumann M, Moayyedi P, Mégraud F, Xiao SD, Sugano K, Nyrén O. Helicobacter pylori eradication has the potential to prevent gastric cancer: a state-of-the-art critique. *Am. J. Gastroenterol.* 2005; 100: 2100-2115.

Marchès O, Ledger TN, Boury M, Ohara M, Tu X, Goffaux F, Mainil J, Rosenshine I, Sugai M, De Rycke J, Oswald E. Enteropathogenic and enterohaemorrhagic Escherichia coli deliver novel effectors called Cif, which blocks cell cycle G2/M transition. *Mol. Microbiol.* 2003; 50: 1553-1567.

Marshall BJ, Windsor HM. The relation of Helicobacter pylo- ri to gastric adenocarcinoma and lymphoma: pathophysiolo- gy, epidemiology, screening, clinical presentation, treatment, and prevention. *Med. Clin. North Am.* 2005; 89: 313-344, viii.

Maurer KJ, Rao VP, Ge Z, Rogers AB, Oura TJ, Carey MC, Fox JG. T-cell function is critical for murine cholesterol gall-stone formation. *Gastroenterology* 2007; 133: 1304-1315.

Murata H, Tsuji S, Tsujii M, Fu HY, Tanimura H, Tsujimoto M, Matsuura N, Kawano S, Hori M. Helicobacter bilis infection in biliary tract cancer. *Aliment Pharmacol Ther* 2004; 20 *Suppl*. 1: 90-94.

Nesić D, Hsu Y, Stebbins CE. Assembly and function of a bacterial genotoxin. *Nature* 2004; 429: 429-433.

Nevin JE, Moran TJ, Kay S, King R. Carcinoma of the gall-bladder: staging, treatment, and prognosis. *Cancer* 1976; 37: 141-148.

Newman JV, Kosaka T, Sheppard BJ, Fox JG, Schauer DB. Bacterial infection promotes colon tumorigenesis in Apc(Min/+) mice. *J. Infect. Dis.* 2001; 184: 227-230.

Nielsen ML, Asnaes S, Stage JG. Susceptibility of the liver and biliary tract to anaerobic infection in extra hepatic biliary tract obstruction. II. Liver function and morphology of the liver and biliary tract--an experimental study in rabbits. *Scand. J. Gastroenterol.* 1976; 11: 73-85.

Nougayrède JP, Homburg S, Taieb F, Boury M, Brzusz-kiewicz E, Gottschalk G, Buchrieser C, Hacker J, Dobrindt U, Oswald E. *Escherichia coli* induces DNA double-strand breaks in eukaryotic cells. *Science* 2006; 313: 848-851.

Nougayrède JP, Taieb F, De Rycke J, Oswald E. Cyclomodulins: bacterial effectors that modulate the eukaryotic cell cycle. *Trends Microbiol.* 2005; 13: 103-110.

Oswald E, Nougayrède JP, Taieb F, Sugai M. Bacterial toxins that modulate host cell-cycle progression. *Curr. Opin. Microbiol.* 2005; 8: 83-91.

Piehler JM, Crichlow RW. Primary carcinoma of the gall-bladder. *Surg Gynecol. Obstet.* 1978; 147: 929-942.

Pikarsky E, Porat RM, Stein I, Abramovitch R, Amit S, Kasem S, Gutkovich-Pyest E, Urieli-Shoval S, Galun E, Ben-Neriah Y. NF-kappaB functions as a tumour promoter in inflammation-associated cancer. *Nature* 2004; 431: 461-466.

Pradhan SB, Dali S. Relation between gallbladder neoplasm and Helicobacter hepaticus infection. *Kathmandu Univ. Med. J.* (KUMJ) 2004; 2: 331-335.

Qiao L, Kozoni V, Tsioulias GJ, Koutsos MI, Hanif R, Shiff SJ, Rigas B. Selected eicosanoids increase the proliferation rate of human colon carcinoma cell lines and mouse colono-cytes in vivo. *Biochim. Biophys. Acta* 1995; 1258: 215-223.

Quintar AA, Doll A, Leimgruber C, Palmeri CM, Roth FD, Maccioni M, Maldonado CA. Acute inflammation promotes early cellular stimulation of the epithelial and stromal com-partments of the rat prostate. *Prostate* 2010; 70: 1153-1165.

Rao VP, Poutahidis T, Ge Z, Nambiar PR, Boussahmain C, Wang YY, Horwitz BH, Fox JG, Erdman SE. Innate immune inflammatory response against enteric bacteria Helicobacter hepaticus induces mammary adenocarcinoma in mice. *Cancer Res.* 2006; 66: 7395-7400.

Scheppach, W. Effects of short chain fatty acids on gut morphology and function. *Gut* 1994; 35: S35–S38.

Schiavo G, van der Goot FG. The bacterial toxin toolkit. *Nat. Rev. Mol. Cell Biol.* 2001; 2: 530-537.

Schiller AL. Bones and joints. In: Rubin E, Farber JL, editors. Pathology. Philadelphia: *J. B. Lippincott.*, 1988: 1304-1393.

Seo B, Choy EW, Maudsley S, Miller WE, Wilson BA, Lut-trell LM. Pasteurella multocida toxin stimulates mitogen-activated protein kinase via G(q/11)-dependent transacti-vation of the epidermal growth factor receptor. *J. Biol. Chem.* 2000; 275: 2239-2245.

Sobhani Iradj, Aurelien Amiot, Yann Le Baleur, Michael Levy, Marie-Luce Auriault, Jeanne Tran Van Nhieu and Jean Charles Delchier, 2012. Microbial dysbiosis and colon carcinogenesis: could colon cancer be considered a bacteria-related disease? *Ther. Adv. Gastroenterol.* 2013;6(3) 215 –229.

Surh YJ, Kundu JK. Cancer preventive phytochemicals as speed breakers in inflammatory signaling involved in aber-rant COX-2 expression. *Curr. Cancer Drug Targets* 2007; 7: 447-458.

Surh YJ, Kundu JK. Cancer preventive phytochemicals as speed breakers in inflammatory signaling involved in aber- rant COX-2 expression. Curr Cancer Drug Targets 2007; 7: 447-458 Qiao L, Kozoni V, Tsioulias GJ, Koutsos MI, Hanif R, Shiff SJ, Rigas B.

Selected eicosanoids increase the proliferation rate of human colon carcinoma cell lines and mouse colonocytes in vivo. *Biochim. Biophys. Acta* 1995; 1258: 215-223.

Teige I, Hvid H, Svensson L, Kvist PH, Kemp K. Regulatory T cells control VEGF-dependent skin inflammation. *J Invest Dermatol* 2009; 129: 1437-1445.

Tjandrawinata RR, Hughes-Fulford M. Up-regulation of cyclooxygenase-2 by product-prostaglandin E2. *Adv. Exp. Med. Biol.* 1997; 407: 163-170

Travaglione S, Fabbri A, Fiorentini C. The Rho-activating CNF1 toxin from pathogenic E. coli: a risk factor for human cancer development? *Infect. Agent Cancer* 2008; 3: 4.

Van Antwerp DJ, Martin SJ, Kafri T, Green DR, Verma IM. Suppression of TNF-alpha-induced apoptosis by NF-kappaB. *Science* 1996; 274: 787-789.

Vogelmann R, Amieva MR. The role of bacterial pathogens in cancer. *Curr Opin. Microbiol.* 2007; 10: 76-81.

Ward JM, Fox JG, Anver MR, Haines DC, George CV, Col- lins MJ Jr, Gorelick PL, Nagashima K, Gonda MA, Gilden RV. Chronic active hepatitis and associated liver tumors in mice caused by a persistent bacterial infection with a novel *Helicobacter* species. *J. Natl. Cancer Inst.* 1994; 86: 1222-1227.

Wickham ME, Lupp C, Vázquez A, Mascarenhas M, Coburn B, Coombes BK, Karmali MA, Puente JL, Deng W, Fin-lay BB. Citrobacter rodentium virulence in mice associates with bacterial load and the type III effector NleE. *Microbes Infect.* 2007; 9: 400-407.

Wink DA, Laval J. The Fpg protein, a DNA repair enzyme, is inhibited by the biomediator nitric oxide in vitro and in vivo. *Carcinogenesis* 1994; 15: 2125-2129.

Wistuba II, Gazdar AF. Gallbladder cancer: lessons from a rare tumour. *Nat. Rev. Cancer* 2004; 4: 695-706.

Xu W, Liu LZ, Loizidou M, Ahmed M, Charles IG. The role of nitric oxide in cancer. *Cell Res.* 2002; 12: 311-320.

In: Disorders of Gastrointestinal Systems … ISBN: 978-1-63485-366-8
Editors:S. Rajagopal, S. Murugan and S. Ramachandran ©2016 Nova Science Publishers, Inc.

Chapter 8

Gall Bladder Diseases: Diet and Control

Geethalakshmi Sundararaman * ***and Saranya Natarajan***
Division of Biosciences, Nehru Arts and Science College,
Coimbatore, Tamil Nadu, India

Abstract

Gall bladder is a pear shaped organ present under the liver which stores bile. The gall bladder releases the bile into the small intestine through bile duct for digestion. The most commonly prevailing disease of gall bladder is formation of stones which blocks the flow of bile to the small intestine which may develop into cancer. Also, malfunctions like colic pain, acalculous cholecystitis, infections, polyps can also occur. Over-weighted, fertile females are more susceptible to gall bladder stones and problems. Diet control has a great impact in preventing gall bladder diseases. Practices like avoiding transfats, smoking, alcohol, refined carbohydrates and carbonated drinks can reduce gall bladder diseases. In order to avoid, rather, reduce the problem arising as a result of unhealthy food practices, healthy food practices are mandatory to have a healthy gall bladder. This review discusses the food habits and healthy practices to be followed by men, children, and especially women in forties for preventing various complications leading to removal of the gall bladder.

Keywords: gall bladder, acalculous cholecystitis, food practices, removal of the gall bladder, Diet control, gall stones

1. Introduction

The gallbladder is a pear-shaped, hollow structure located under the liver and on the right side of the abdomen and is a part of the biliary tract. The primary function of gall bladder is to store bile which is produced by the liver. The gallbladder stores bile in its absorbent lining when it is used for digestion. When food enters the small intestine, a hormone called

* Corresponding author: E-mail: s.geethalakshmi@gmail.com, Mo: 9952411764.

cholecystokinin is produced, which signals the gallbladder to contract and secrete bile into the small intestine through the common bile duct. The bile breaks fats in the food and helps it to digest. It also removes the waste product from the liver and takes it to the duodenum. An excess accumulation of cholesterol, bilirubin, or bile salts cause the formation of gallstones. Gallstones are small, hard deposits of bile formed inside the gallbladder. The symptoms of the gall stone formation cannot be felt until the stone size increases or the stone blocks the bile duct. The most common way to treat the gall stone is surgical removal of the gallbladder, called cholecystectomy (Resch et al. 2015). Majority of gallbladder diseases are due to the inflammation and irritation of the gallbladder wall, known as cholecystitis. This inflammation is caused by gallstones which block the ducts connecting the small intestine and causing bile to accumulate. It may gradually lead to necrosis or gangrene. Other diseases of the gallbladder include gallbladder polyps and gallbladder cancer.

2. Parts of the Gallbladder

The gallbladder has 3 parts:

- Fundus: The bottom of the gallbladder that is projected from bottom of the liver.
- Body: The central portion of gallbladder that lies between the fundus and cystic duct.
- Neck: The narrower part that tapers into the cystic duct.
- Cystic duct: about 3 to 4 centimeters long; carries bile into the common bile duct.

2.1. Blood Supply and Lymphatic Drainage

Cystic artery which emerges from right hepatic artery carries blood to the gallbladder. The blood drainage is done by cystic veins which drain blood from the neck part and cystic duct of the bladder.

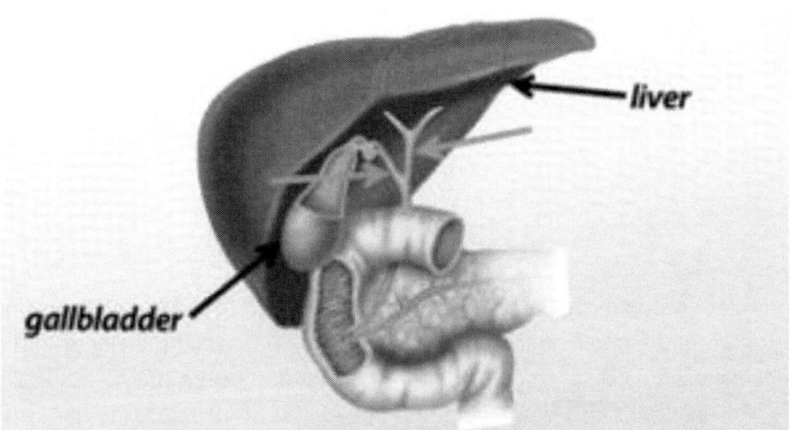

Figure 1. Location of Gall Bladder.

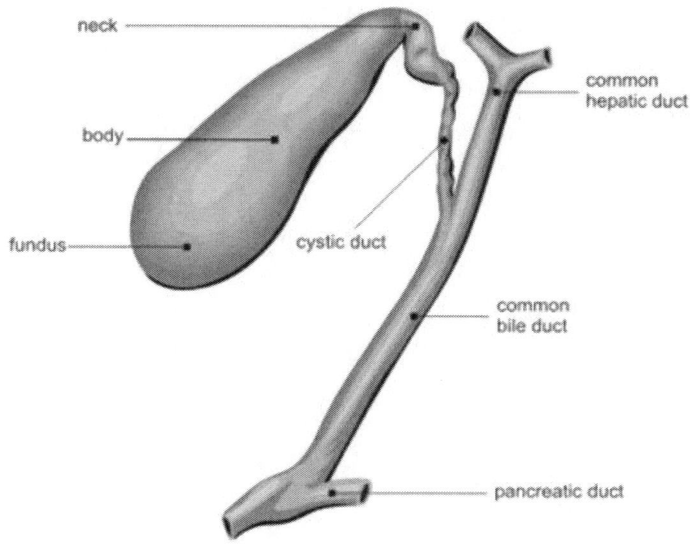

Figure 2. Parts of a Gall Bladder.

Hepatic sinusoids perform the drainage of blood from the body and fundus of the gallbladder and direct it into the visceral surface of the liver.

2.2. Functions of the Gallbladder

The primary function of the gallbladder is to store the bile and release it whenever needed.

1. The gallbladder stores bile and also concentrates the bile from the liver. This helps in storing large volume of bile and its contents in a small area.
2. It secretes bile via muscular contractions of its wall which is stimulated by both neural and hormonal factors. This stimulation is made possible by fatty foods stored in the duodenum.

2.3. Gallbladder Tests

There are several measures for analyzing the problems that arise in the gallbladder.

- *Abdominal ultrasound:* It is a common test in which a probe supplies high-frequency sound waves to the skin which reflects from the structures present in the abdominal region. It is an accurate and reliable test for gall stones and inflammation.
- *HIDA scan (cholescintigraphy):* It is a nuclear medicine test, in which a radioactive dye is injected intravenously and is transported into the bile. If the dye does not interact with bile and the scan results are negative, it means Cholecystitis is likely.
- *Endoscopic retrograde cholangiopancreatography (ERCP):* In this method, a flexible tube is inserted through the mouth, via the stomach into the small intestine.

A dye is injected through the tube into the duct. The path of the dye and its reaction can be monitored using a detector system. Using this method, gall stones can be removed using small surgical tools at the early stages.

- *Magnetic resonance cholangiopancreatography (MRCP):* It is basically an MRI scanning system which gives high-resolution images of the bile ducts, pancreas, and gallbladder. The results of this test can be useful to design the treatment measures.
- *Endoscopic ultrasound:* A flexible tube containing a small ultrasound probe on one end is inserted through the mouth into the intestine. This method can detect choledocholithiasis and gallstone pancreatitis.
- *Abdominal X-ray:* This method is used to detect gall stones only but not applicable to other gallbladder diseases.

2.4. Anatomy of Gall Bladder

2.4.1. Gross Anatomy

Gallbladder is a hollow, muscular and pear-shaped organ having 3 inches length and 1.5 inches width. The bigger, huge end of the gallbladder is located in the inferior position at the right side and the tapered end is directed superiorly and medially. The tapered end of the gallbladder shrinks and enters into a small bile duct known as the cystic duct which in turn is connected to the common hepatic duct that transports bile from the liver. These two ducts merge to form the common bile duct that elongates to merge with the wall of the duodenum (Eslick and Shaffer 2014).

2.4.2. Microscopic Anatomy

The innermost layer of gallbladder is made up of mucosa and is lined with simple columnar epithelial tissue. The columnar epithelial tissue is made up of microvilli on its surface, which enhances the surface area. This increase in surface area is favourable for absorption of water and concentrates the dilute bile. Under the columnar tissue, a thin layer called lamina propria which is made up of connective tissue and capillaries is present and it supports and adheres to the epithelial layer (Frierson et al. 1989). Below the lamina propria, a layer called muscularis layer is present which is made up of smooth muscle tissue. The bile is pushed out of the gallbladder due to the contraction of the muscularis and the bile is transferred to cystic duct. A thin layer of fibrous connective tissue surrounds the muscularis which makes the wall of the gallbladder strong. The outermost layer is called serosa which is an epithelial layer that forms a part of the peritoneum. This layer is necessary for preventing friction between the moving organs associated with gallbladder (Eslick and Shaffer 2014).

3. Diseases of Gall Bladder

3.1. Gallstones

When substances in the bile such as calcium, bile salts, cholesterol accumulate and get converted to hard particles, these are called gall stones. They block the pathway of the bile depending on their size. The gallstones are also formed when there is no proper emptying of the gallbladder. The size of the stones can vary from small grain to a large ball (Bansal et al. 2014). Many factors donate to the risk of gallstones. These include:

- Obesity
- High cholesterol containing food
- Diabetes
- Being age 60 or older
- Medicines containing estrogen
- Family history of gallstones
- Female

3.2. Choledocholithiasis

Various sized gallstones may get deposited in the neck region of the gallbladder or in the bile ducts and blocks the gallbladder. So the bile cannot flow out of the duct and accumulation of the bile can cause inflammation. This block can also lead to prevention of bile from flowing to the intestine.

Choledocholithiasis can be a reason for:

- Severe pain in the middle of the upper abdomen
- Fever
- Chillness
- Nausea
- Vomiting (Ell et al. 1990)

3.3. Cholecystitis

The most common type of gallbladder disease is Cholecystitis, which is characterized by acute or chronic inflammation of the gallbladder (Bansal et al. 2014).

3.3.1. Acute Cholecystitis

Acute cholecystitis is generally caused by gallstones. Other factors such as tumors and other complications can also result in acute cholecystitis. The symptoms include pain in the upper right side or upper middle part of the abdomen. The occurrence of pain may be more after food intake, starting as a mild ache and projecting to sharp pangs (Resch et al. 2014). Acute cholecystitis can also be a reason for:

- Fever
- Nausea
- Vomiting
- Jaundice
- Differently colored stools

3.3.2. Chronic Cholecystitis

Accumulation of several episodes of acute cholecystitis will make the gallbladder shrink and reduces its function. The symptoms of such severe conditions will be abdominal pain, nausea and vomiting (Legorretta et al. 1993).

3.4. Sclerosing Cholangitis

Sclerosing cholangitis means inflammation, scarring and injury to the bile ducts (Yang et al. 1992). The reason for this disease is not known clearly, but patients with this impediment show liver and spleen enlargement combined with loss of appetite and body mass.

3.5. Acalculous Gallbladder Disease

Acalculous gallbladder disease is also called as biliary dyskinesia. It occurs in the absence of gallstones. It results in malfunctioning of gallbladder valve and muscles and it can be persistent or severe. Abdominal pain arises on the right side of the body and radiates to the shoulder. Foods with high fat content are the reason for causing this complication (Aune et al., 2015).

Other symptoms of this complication are:

- Nausea
- Vomiting
- Bloating
- Loose stools

3.6. Gallbladder Cancer

It is a rare type of disease. It does not have specific symptoms but resemble acute cholecystitis. When untreated, the cancer can spread from the inner region of the walls of gallbladder to the outer region and can extend to the duct and other organs (Melson et al. 1976; Strom et al. 1995).

3.7. Gangrene of the Gallbladder

When there is improper blood supply to the gallbladder, it stops its function and this condition is called gangrene (Sherlock and Dooley, 1997). The improper blood supply may be due to:

- Injury
- Surgery
- Infections

- Diseases related to blood circulation
- Diabetes

The gallbladder gangrene can also cause:

- Pain in the abdominal region
- Fever
- Nausea or vomiting
- Gas
- Low blood pressure

3.8. Gallbladder Polyps

Gallbladder polyps are lesions or growths occurring on wall of the gallbladder. They are benign and does not produce any symptoms (Babu et al. 2015).

3.9. Abscess of the Gallbladder

When there is an accumulation of pus in any part of the body, there will be swelling in the gallbladder which results in abscess of the gallbladder (Xie et al. 2010). The swelling may take place along with pain in the upper right-side of the abdomen.

4. Diagnosis

Diagnosis of the gallbladder complications depends on the severity of the symptoms. The examination starts with the patient's history and a general examination of the abdomen is performed. The diagnosis also includes examination of the severity of the pain in the abdomen (Lee et al. 2014). This is followed by one or all of the following tests.

4.1. Detailed Patient History

The patient is analyzed for other symptoms and complications associated with abdominal pain. Also, the family history of the patient, any previously known cases of gallbladder complications in the family and a general health evaluation of the subject is performed to find out if any long term complications of gallbladder diseases exist.

4.2. Chest and Abdominal X-Ray

Occurrence of cholecystitis when examined by an abdominal x-ray will show stones if the stones are made up of calcium (Bortoff et al. 2000).

4.3. Ultrasonography

Ultrasonography is the most important method of diagnosis of gallbladder disease using sound waves. Ultrasonography is used to detect gallstones, thickened walls, or any other complications in the gallbladder (Numata et al. 2007; Matos et al. 2015).

4.4. Other Investigations

Other types of investigations include blood tests which reveal the increase in white blood cells and functioning of the liver.

5. TREATMENT

5.1. Medical Treatment

Initial symptoms of gallbladder pain and inflammations can be treated using antibiotics and general medicines for pain. Surgery will be recommended only when here is repeated pain and complications (Bansal et al. 2014).

5.2. Surgery

In the severe and extreme conditions of gallbladder diseases, surgery is performed to remove the gallbladder (Michailidou et al. 2014). The surgery can be performed using laparoscopy or by cutting open the abdomen. The open surgery is performed by making three holes in the abdominal region and inserting a camera. The removal is performed by monitoring the entire process on a television screen. The time of recovery of the patient is longer in open surgery compared to laparoscopic surgery. Also the scars formed are minimum in laparoscopy; hence it is preferred by most of the surgeons. But this method of laparoscopy can be performed for those patients who do not require immediate removal or any other severe complications (Andrews et al. 2014).

6. POTENTIAL LONG-TERM COMPLICATIONS OF GALLBLADDER DISEASE

For some unknown reasons, the gallbladder may function abnormally by forming an atypical passage for the flow and functioning of bile. This is abnormality is severe and goes undetectable for long term (Aune at el. 2015). Only after the symptoms get severe, it can be detected. This unusual condition is also associated with complications like:

- Stumbling block of the intestine
- Inflammation

- Holes in the gallbladder
- Contamination by bacteria
- Malignant tumor formation

7. Understanding Gallbladder Problems

The very existence of gallbladder symptoms does not mean that there is a complication. The actual problem will arise only when there is a previous history of one such complication. The gallbladder problems are rarely fatal, but they should be treated on time which otherwise would lead to extreme severity (Jain et al. 2014).

When there is a serious pain or discomfort in the abdomen, bloating, nausea and vomiting which increases with time making the subject uncomfortable, it is necessary to remove the gallbladder (Park et al. 2005).

8. Healthy Gall Bladder Diet

For optimum working of the gallbladder, it requires a healthy diet, like other parts of the body. Gallstones and other gallbladder problems can be avoided by taking a healthy and nutritious diet, maintaining the body weight, intake of high fiber and low cholesterol diet (Lim et al. 2015). Diet is the major responsible reasons for most of the gallbladder problems, along with patient's family history. Subjects with obesity, having the habit of junk foods are likely to have a gallbladder problem. The risk of the problem increases in women due to their hormonal content (Stokes et al. 2015). Gallstones can be formed by detrimental diet containing high amount of cholesterol, fat and proteins. Even food containing very low fiber is also responsible for complications. Balanced food containing plenty of fruits, vegetables and high in fiber are to be taken by people who are prone to gallbladder diseases (Jo et al. 2015, Oskarsson et al. 2015).

8.1. Diet for Healthy Gallbladder

Give below is a list of foods that can be included into the diet for a healthy gallbladder (Pandey and Shukla 2002).

1. Fresh Fruits and Vegetables are the major source of fibre and are part of a balanced diet. Avocados, berries, grapes, beets, cucumbers and apples can be taken in large amounts to avoid gallstones, as well as control diarrhoea. Carrots, onions, broccoli, cranberries and Brussels sprouts should be included in the diet.
2. Whole grains including oats, brown rice, whole-wheat bread and bran cereal, foods containing whole grains, such as breads made up of multiple grains and cereals are the major source of fiber.
3. Meats containing less fat, poultry without skin and fish, pork and lamb are the source of low-fat diet.

4. Dairy food with low-fat or fat-free, buttermilk, goat's milk, soy milk, yogurt, cheese, sour cream with low fat content can be taken.
5. Research studies have shown that alcohol and caffeine can reduce the risk of gallstones. However, there are no enough evidences for its practical functioning.

8.2. Foods to Be Avoided

There are certain food stuffs that should be avoided for a healthy gallbladder, since these food stuff will make the gallbladder to work hard, increasing the risk of gall stones (Pastides et al. 1990; Tseng et al. 1999).

1. Refined Carbohydrates including table sugar, syrup, corn syrup, food stuff made out of white flour should be avoided.
2. Sugars and sweeteners must be present less than five percent in the diet.
3. Beverages including tea, wine, soft drinks, beer, sweetened fruit juices can cause all types of gallbladder problems.
4. Frozen or Canned Fruits and Vegetables are not recommended as they may contain additives which will make the gallbladder hard.
5. White Flour Foods are made up of refined carbohydrates, which lead to gallbladder problems, obesity and high blood pressure. They also enhance the chances of developing diabetes.
6. Heavily processed snacks like potato chips, cheese containing food create complications.
7. Fried foods, red meat, dairy products like cheese or ice cream, and foods rich in high fat contribute to gallbladder problems.
8. Diets containing less than 1,000 calories daily are prone to create gallstones.

8.3. Diet after Gallbladder Surgery

Surgical removal of gallbladder is the only solution for severe complications and it needs only very short recovery time by the patient to return to their routine life. Removal of the gallbladder should be considered as major surgery and the patient needs careful attention. All medications should be followed as directed (Choices 2014).

During the first few days after surgery, liquid diet is to be taken containing fruit juices and other low fibre diet. Gradually soft foods like porridge, boiled potato and soups can be added after two weeks. Fried foods, alcohol, peanut butter, red meats, fat rich food, raw vegetables, caffeine and alcohol should be avoided (Perkins and Kehlet 2000).

Conclusion

Gallbladder diseases are most commonly occurring complications, most of them does not show any symptoms until the condition becomes worse. Factors that contribute to the gallbladder disease include gender, ethnicity, medical history, family history and diet and nutrition (Sunilkumar et al. 2015). The primary diagnosis of gallbladder disease can be done by imaging techniques which has its own advantages and disadvantages which is projected on their accuracy.

Depending on the type of diagnosis, the doctor and the disease, one method of examination will be preferred over the other; or in some cases, two or more techniques has to be combined for a better diagnosis. For complicated and severe conditions, surgery is the only remedy, but for those complications that does not show any symptoms or that does not cause discomfort, basic medications is sufficient. The performance of surgery depends on the physician as well the willingness of the patient to undergo surgery. Physicians and pharmacists can take part in creating awareness among the public by explaining them the method of treatment, the risk factors, nutrition, diet control, exercise and other measures for a healthy gallbladder (Lim et al. 2015).

REFERENCES

Andrews, S. E., Ghane, A., Legg, A. M., Tabuenca, A. and Sweeny, K., 2014. Expectations in the context of gallbladder and hernia surgery: a descriptive report. Health Expectations.

Aune, D., Norat, T. and Vatten, L. J., 2015. Body mass index, abdominal fatness and the risk of gallbladder disease. *European journal of epidemiology*, *30*(9), pp.1009-1019.

Babu, B. I., Dennison, A. R. and Garcea, G., 2015. Management and diagnosis of gallbladder polyps: a systematic review. *Langenbeck's Archives of Surgery*, *400*(4), pp.455-462.

Bansal, V. K., Misra, M. C., Rajan, K., Kilambi, R., Kumar, S., Krishna, A., Kumar, A., Pandav, C. S., Subramaniam, R., Arora, M. K. and Garg, P. K., 2014. Single-stage laparoscopic common bile duct exploration and cholecystectomy versus two-stage endoscopic stone extraction followed by laparoscopic cholecystectomy for patients with concomitant gallbladder stones and common bile duct stones: a randomized controlled trial. *Surgical endoscopy*, *28*(3), pp.875-885.

Bortoff, G. A., Chen, M. Y., Ott, D. J., Wolfman, N. T., and Routh, W. D. (2000). Gallbladder Stones: Imaging and Intervention 1. *Radiographics*, *20*(3), 751-766.

Choices, N. H. S., 2014. Do I need to change my diet after gallbladder surgery?-Health questions-NHS Choices.

Ell, C., Kerzel, W., Schneider, H. T., Benninger, J., Wirtz, P., Domschke, W., and Hahn, E. G. (1990). Piezoelectric lithotripsy: stone disintegration and follow-up results in patients with symptomatic gallbladder stones. *Gastroenterology*, *99*(5), 1439-1444.

Eslick, G. D. and Shaffer, E. A., 2014. Epidemiology of Gallstones and Biliary Tract Cancers. GI Epidemiology: Diseases and Clinical Methodology, Second Edition, pp.296-305.

Frierson Jr., H. F. (1989). The gross anatomy and histology of the gallbladder, extrahepatic bile ducts, Vaterian system, and minor papilla. *The American journal of surgical pathology*, *13*(2), 146-162.

Jain, K., Mohapatra, T., Das, P., Misra, M. C., Gupta, S. D., Ghosh, M., Kabra, M., Bansal, V. K., Kumar, S., Sreenivas, V. and Garg, P. K., 2014. Sequential occurrence of preneoplastic lesions and accumulation of loss of heterozygosity in patients with gallbladder stones suggest causal association with gallbladder cancer. *Annals of surgery*, *260*(6), pp.1073-1080.

Jo, H. B., Lee, J. K., Choi, M. Y., Han, I. W., Choi, H. S., Kang, H. W., Kim, J. H., Lim, Y. J., Koh, M. S. and Lee, J. H., 2015. Is the Prevalence of Gallbladder Polyp Different between Vegetarians and General Population? *The Korean Journal of Gastroenterology*, *66*(5), pp.268-273.

Lee, S. C., Choi, B. J. and Kim, S. J., 2014. Two-port cholecystectomy maintains safety and feasibility in benign gallbladder diseases: A comparative study. *International Journal of Surgery*, *12*(9), pp.1014-1019.

Legorreta, A. P., Silber, J. H., Costantino, G. N., Kobylinski, R. W., and Zatz, S. L. (1993). Increased cholecystectomy rate after the introduction of laparoscopic cholecystectomy. *JAMA*, *270*(12), 1429-1432.

Lim, S. H., Kim, D., Kang, J. H., Song, J. H., Yang, S. Y., Yim, J. Y., Chung, S. J., Kim, J. S. and Cho, S. H., 2015. Hepatic fat, not visceral fat, is associated with gallbladder polyps: A study of 2643 healthy subjects. *Journal of gastroenterology and hepatology*, *30*(4), pp.767-774.

Matos, C., Santiago, I., Maciel, J., Levy, A. D. and Polyps, A. G., 2015. Gallbladder Neoplasms. *Gastrointestinal Imaging*, p.474.

Melson, G. L., Reiter, F., and Evens, R. G. (1976, October). Tumorous conditions of the gallbladder. In Seminars in roentgenology (Vol. 11, No. 4, pp. 269-282). WB Saunders.

Michailidou, M., Kulvatunyou, N., Friese, R. S., Gries, L., Green, D. J., Joseph, B., O'Keeffe, T., Tang, A. L., Vercruysse, G. and Rhee, P., 2014. Time and cost analysis of gallbladder surgery under the acute care surgery model. *Journal of Trauma and Acute Care Surgery*, *76*(3), pp.710-714.

Numata, K., Oka, H., Morimoto, M., Sugimori, K., Kunisaki, R., Nihonmatsu, H., ... and Tanaka, K. (2007). Differential diagnosis of gallbladder diseases with contrast-enhanced harmonic gray scale ultrasonography. *Journal of ultrasound in medicine*, *26*(6), 763-774.

Oskarsson, V., Orsini, N., Sadr-Azodi, O. and Wolk, A., 2015. Fish consumption and risk of non–gallstone-related acute pancreatitis: a prospective cohort study. *The American journal of clinical nutrition*, *101*(1), pp.72-78.

Pandey, M., and Shukla, V. K. (2002). Diet and gallbladder cancer: a case–control study. *European journal of cancer prevention*, *11*(4), 365-368.

Park, P. O., Bergström, M., Ikeda, K., Fritscher-Ravens, A., and Swain, P. (2005). Experimental studies of transgastric gallbladder surgery: cholecystectomy and cholecystogastric anastomosis (videos). *Gastrointestinal endoscopy*, *61*(4), 601-606.

Pastides, H., Tzonou, A., Trichopoulos, D., Katsouyanni, K., Trichopoulou, A., Kefalogiannis, N., and Manousos, O. (1990). A case-control study of the relationship between smoking, diet, and gallbladder disease. *Archives of Internal Medicine*, *150*(7), 1409-1412.

Perkins, F. M., and Kehlet, H. (2000). Chronic pain as an outcome of surgery: a review of predictive factors. *Anesthesiology*, *93*(4), 1123-1133.

Resch, T., Sucher, R., Perathoner, A., Laimer, E., Mohr, E., Pratschke, J. and Mittermair, R., 2014. Single-Incision Laparoscopic Cholecystectomy: Will it Succeed as the Future Leading Technique for Gallbladder Removal? *Surgical Laparoscopy Endoscopy and Percutaneous Techniques*, *24*(6), pp.e207-e210.

Sherlock, S., and Dooley, J. (1997). Gallstones and inflammatory gallbladder diseases. *Diseases of the liver and biliary system*, 593-623.

Stokes, C. S., Gluud, L. L., Casper, M. and Lammert, F., 2014. Pharmacological interventions for the primary prevention of gallbladder stones in adults. The Cochrane Library.

Strom, B. L., Soloway, R. D., Rios-Dalenz, J. L., Rodriguez-Martinez, H. A., West, S. L., Kinman, J. L., ... and Berlin, J. A. (1995). Risk factors for gallbladder cancer. An international collaborative case–control study. *Cancer*, *76*(10), 1747-1756.

Sun, Y., Song, W., Hou, Q., Li, J. and Guo, H., 2015. Gallbladder perforation: a rare complication of postoperative chemotherapy of gastric cancer. *World journal of surgical oncology*, *13*(1), p.1.

Sunilkumar, K. B., Kulkarni, V., Suresh, K. K. and Chandrasekhar, H. R., 2015. Prevalence of Various Gallbladder lesions in Central Karnataka Region–a Four Year Prospective Study. *Indian Journal of Public Health Research and Development*, *6*(1), pp.256-260.

Tseng, M., Everhart, J. E. and Sandler, R. S., 1999. Dietary intake and gallbladder disease: a review. *Public health nutrition*, *2*(02), pp.161-172.

Xie, X. H., Xu, H. X., Xie, X. Y., Lu, M. D., Kuang, M., Xu, Z. F., ... and Lin, M. X. (2010). Differential diagnosis between benign and malignant gallbladder diseases with real-time contrast-enhanced ultrasound. *European radiology*, *20*(1), 239-248.

Xu, J. M., Guo, L. H., Xu, H. X., Zheng, S. G., Liu, L. N., Sun, L. P., Lu, M. D., Xie, X. Y., Wang, W. P., Hu, B. and Yan, K., 2014. Differential Diagnosis of Gallbladder Wall Thickening: The Usefulness of Contrast-Enhanced Ultrasound. *Ultrasound in medicine and biology*, *40*(12), pp.2794-2804.

Yang, H. L., Sun, Y. G., and Wang, Z. (1992). Polypoid lesions of the gallbladder: diagnosis and indications for surgery. *British journal of surgery*, s*79*(3), 227-229.

Zhu, J. Q., Han, D. D., Li, X. L., Kou, J. T., Fan, H. and He, Q., 2015. Predictors of incidental gallbladder cancer in elderly patients. *Hepatobiliary and Pancreatic Diseases International*, *14*(1), pp.96-100.

In: Disorders of Gastrointestinal Systems … ISBN: 978-1-63485-366-8
Editors:S. Rajagopal, S. Murugan and S. Ramachandran ©2016 Nova Science Publishers, Inc.

Chapter 9

MICROBIAL INTERACTION ON GASTRO INTESTINAL SYSTEM: UNIQUE MOLECULAR SIGNATURE IN ESTABLISHMENT OF INFECTIONS

S. Gowtham Kumar**, MSc, PhD***
Faculty of Allied Health Sciences,
Chettinad Academy of Research and Education,
Kelambakkam, India

ABSTRACT

Numerous lines of defence mechanisms were exist in the host against the intruders. Pathogens have evolved a broad range of strategies to colonize and invade human organs. The gastrointestinal (GI) area is the largest surface of the body with an epithelial surface is in constant exposure to the microorganisms. Epithelia of various organs get in touch with the extracellular environment and consequently with microbes. These organs were covered by a mucus layer that allows a defence beside intruders. The bacterial translocation facilitates the passage of sufficientbacteria from the gastrointestinal tract to extra intestinal sitesfor example the mesenteric-lymph-node complex, liver, spleen and bloodstream. Infections caused by microorganisms are very common. Disruption of the intercellular junctions is a strategy used by several microorganisms as a means of adhering to cells, entering cells, and/or exploiting host signalling to their advantage. Molecular basis for pathogenesis could eventually show the way to effective early prognostic tools. This chapter deals with gut microbiota in particular *Escherichia coli, Salmonella, Shigella and Helicobacter pylori* bacteria virulence factors and its role in the establishment of infection/disease.

Keywords: gastrointestinal infections, microbial adhesion, bacterial translocation, molecular pathogenesis

* Corresponding author: S. Gowtham Kumar, MSc, PhD., Assistant Professor: E-mail: gowtham_phd @yahoo.com, Mobile: +91 9962527952.

INTRODUCTION

The human body quay a variety of bacteria excluding their localization in healthy person is usually restricted to mucosal layers of nasal, buccal, vagina and most notably the gastrointestinal tract. The internal tissues are in general sterile. In some conditions, various opportunistic pathogens are capable to penetrate the host by taking benefit of injuries in one of the various host barriers. In addition, pathogens have developed mechanisms to defeat host barriers and accomplish deeper organs in which they multiply and lead to cruel disease for their host (Ma et al. 2012; Schommer and Gallo 2013).

The mucosa is poised of three layers: an epithelium, a layer of slack connective tissue known as lamina propria, and a slight thin layer of smooth muscles. These surfaces comprise frontier barriers limiting the invasion by mutually bacteria normal flora and pathogenic bacteria as well. Although the diverse protection mechanisms occurring at the level of these barriers, pathogenic bacteria have developed a variety of molecular strategies to stick on to these epithelia and to multiply at their surface. Epithelia of various organs in get touch with the extracellular environment, and thus with bacteria are covered by a mucus layer that allows a defence against intruder. Intestinal mucus layer plays a key function in restrictive invasion by commensal bacteria of the microbial flora or by food borne pathogenic bacteria (McGuckin et al. 2011).

The mucus is primarily composed of digestive enzymes, glycoproteins mucins, immunoglobulins, antimicrobial peptides. Bacteria are frequently originate at the top most of the intestinal mucus layer in which they interact with mucin glycoprotein. Whereas the interior layer of mucus, the amount of antimicrobial compounds is elevated is generally entirely lacking of bacteria. Mucins are secreted by goblet cells in the intestine, and their production can be amended in reaction to microbial yield or inflammation. The level of antimicrobial peptides, principally secreted by Paneth cells from intestinal basements can also be harmonized by the incidence of microorganisms. IgA antibodies, secreted by B cells in the lamina propria and secreted into the mucus through epithelial cells, are concerned in limiting bacterial relationship with the intestinal epithelium. Scaly mucus can be an added mechanism to restrict bacterial adhesion to epithelial layer, as documented in the gastric mucus colonized by the organism *Helicobacter pylori* (Johansson et al. 2008; Linden et al. 2009).

Fascinatingly, several bacterial pathogens have developed mechanisms to go throughout this mucus layer sequentially to get in touch with epithelial cells. They produce proteases enzyme and straight forwardly target host mucin layer, locomotion by flagella based motility or defend against to antimicrobial products. Interactions involving pathogenic bacteria and host mucus thus represent a challenging matter in host infection. Besides mucus, an important player in the managing invasion of pathogen is the microbial biota, which is generally comprised of commensal bacteria living on human mucosal surfaces. In the human intestine, this microbial biota plays fundamental roles in digestion, as well as in intestinal epithelial metabolism and proliferation.

Microbia metabolites plays a key role in the fighting to food borne infections by directly opposing with enteric pathogens. Certainly, inhibitory metabolites such as acetate or butyrate can be released by diverse species of commensal bacteria. These bacteria can furthermore utilize a range of nutrients of the intestinal lumen, which would then be no longer accessible for incoming pathogens (Stecher and Hardt 2011). Mucosal epithelia ascertain an edge among the exterior milieu and the inner organelles. It acts as a functional restriction that avoids external factors such as bacteria to attain the interstitial gap and the circulatory system. The process is mostly proficient by the existence of cell-cell junctions-tight junctions, desmosomes, adherens junctions and gap junctions are vital constituents of epithelial reliability. The stretched junctions are the majority apical set of cell-cell junctions that split the apical and basolateral part of the plasma membrane and particularly control the paracellular flux of ions and tiny molecules. They are poised of transmembrane proteins occludin, claudins along with junctional adhesion molecules (JAMs), cytosolic proteins zonula ocludens (ZO) 1, 2, and 3 that link transmembrane proteins with cytoskeleton. Adherens link are constrained directly under tight junctions and their most important role is to enable cell-cell adhesion. The most important constituent of the adherens junctions is *E cadherin*, which is a trans-membrane protein.

The extracellular component of *E cadherin* creates homophilic interactions with *E cadherin* molecules of nearest cells, endorsing consistency of the epithelium. *E cadherin* might excessively create heterophilic communications with the receptor tyrosine kinases EGFR and c-Met, altering their signaling processes. The cytoplasmic part of *E cadherin* is linked with β p120, and β catenins and this multipart establishes a link to the actin cytoskeleton through *Eplin*. The protein-protein interactions and the phosphorylation condition of the catenins are significant in stabilization of junction. Desmosomes make available mechanical fidelity and intercellular interactions to the adjacent cells.

Gap junctions are plaques of numerous tiny channels represented by connexins that tolerate intercellular moving through the ions and small molecules. Additionally, gap junctions have a function in control the establishing polarity, cell shape and reorganization of the cytoskeleton. Disturbance of the intercellular junctions is an approach used by numerous microorganisms as an involved of adhering to cells, penetrating cells as well as using host signalling process to their benefit. Though in mucosal epithelia the tight junctions avoid mainly microorganisms from pervasive into tissues, a few can break this barrier and make cell–cell junctions at tight junctions, called adherens junctions (Cossart and Helenius 2014).

ROLE OF FLAGELLA IN ESTABLISHMENT OF BACTERIAL INFECTION

Role of flagella have essentially been studied in bacterial pathogens and from the perspective of bacterial virulence owing to the different probable applications that exist for flagella and flagellin like in drug development and diagnostics. The flagellin constituent has been used for a generation of vaccines for *Salmonella enterica* serovar Paratyphi A, *Pseudomonas aeruginosa*, and *E. coli O157:H7*.

In spite of the protection provided by the microbial biota, various enteric pathogens are capable to proficiently colonize the gut and yet cross the intestinal fence. Elicit of inflammation can be considered as a mechanism exploited by pathogens to alter the microbiota composition, thus permitting them to outcompete luminal commensal microbes. Inflammation of the gut is distinguished by enhance in the amount of mucosal antimicrobial peptides to which bacterial pathogens could express elevated resistance compared to common microbiota. Mucosal inflammation leads to the production of glycosylated proteins or tetrathionate molecule that can be used by pathogens (Stecher et al. 2008; Winter et al. 2010).

Flagellar protein and their functions

Protein	Function	Part of Flagella/Role of Flagella
Fli D	Filament cap	Flagella
Flg K, Flg L	Hook-filament junction	Connect filament to hook
Flg J	Muramidase	Basal body
Flh E	Chaperone or plug	Export machinery
Mot A ,Mot B	Rotation of Flagella	Rotation of Flagellum
FlhC, FlhD, FlbA	Regulator	Flagellar biosynthesis regulation
CheW and CheV	Chemotaxis	Motility

These molecules is definitely used by the murine enteric bacterial pathogen such as Salmonella typhimurium, which uses it as a terminal electron acceptor in anaerobic respiration, giving to this bacterial pathogen a growth improvement over fermenting commensal bacteria in the inflamed milieu. Simultaneously, the cross talk and interactions among commensal bacteria, enteric pathogens and host are critical in the establishment and development of intestinal diseases. Additionally to mucus and to the microbial biota, epithelial cell regeneration plays a significant role in the control of bacterial colonization. Adhesion of bacteria to host surfaces is a critical feature of host colonization as it prevents the involuntary clearing of pathogens and grants a selective improvement towards bacteria of the endogenous flora (Pedron and Sansonetti 2008).

BACTERIAL PILI AS A VIRULENCE FACTOR

Hence, bacteria have evolved a very large cache of molecular approaches allowing them to target and adhere to the host cells. Bacterial pili, are polymeric hair-like organelles projecting from the exterior of bacteria, signify an unequalled of structures implicated in the binding of bacteria to host cells. The base of these structures originally discovered in gram negative bacteria is attached to the bacterial outer membrane, while the terminal part is generally an adherence factor giving the binding specificity of these structures.

The base of these structures originally discovered in gram negative bacteria, is anchored to the bacterial outer membrane but the terminal part is frequently an adherence factor presenting the binding specificity of these structures. For example, uropathogenic *Escherichia coli* (UPEC) colonizing the urinary tract and involved in urinary tract infections display pyelonephritis associated (P) pili on their surface. The tip of these pili is comprised by an adhesion factor called *Pap G* which binds to glycosphingolipids molecules of the epithelium in kidney.

Several UPEC also possess Type I pili on their surface which comprise binding specificity to D-mannosylated receptors. Type IV pili represent a further class of polymeric adhesive surface structures expressed by diverse gram negative bacteria. These pili are poised of thousands of copies of the major pilin protein that are first synthesized in the bacterial cytoplasm and after that translocated across the inner membrane and processed proteolytically. Just the processed forms of pilin are capable for polymerization.

The assembled pili then pass via the outer membrane through a channel created by the secretin protein. Once formed, these pili are competent to aggregate to form bundle like structures.

Type IV pili have the capability to pull back through the bacterial cell wall, whereas the pilus tip residue attached to its target surface allowing twitching motility, a flagella independent form of motility important for competent colonization of host surfaces (Johanna Haiko and Benita Westerlund-Wikström 2013, Melville and Craig 2013).

M cells are specific cells originate in the intestinal epithelium and other epithelia in humans. These cells have a function diverse from that of their neighbouring epithelial cells.

In intestine, they continuously sample the lumen and transfer luminal antigens transversely the epithelial barrier to the underlying lymphoid tissue thus contributing to intestinal immunity. M cells are exploited by many diverse pathogens as a mode of entry to deeper tissues of the host. Intestinal ligated loop infection models have established that *S. typhimurium* can cross the intestinal barrier by these M cells.

Undeniably targeting of M cells by *S. typhimurium* leads to M cells damage thereby introducing breaks in the intestinal barrier (Melville and Craig 2013).

Bacteria are then capable to multiply rapidly to organs before the establishment of an immune response. In a parallel manner, *S. flexneri* was shown to target and penetrate into M cells allowing translocation of bacteria across the epithelial barrier, devoid of being toxic for the epithelial cells.

Salmonella Pathogenesis-Entry and Dissemination

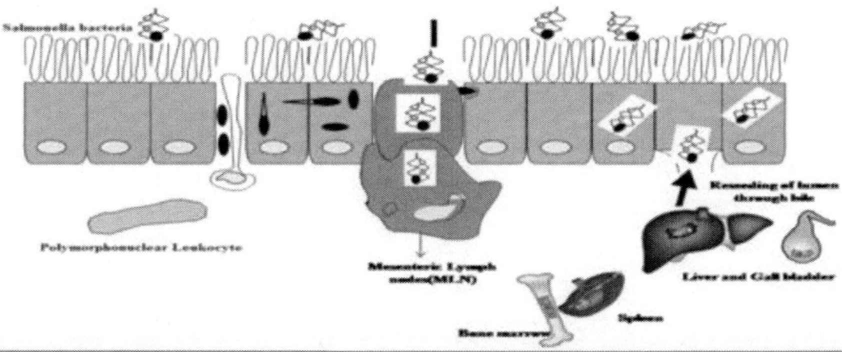

1	Salmonella bacteria enter the intestinal tract mucosal surface by invading Microfold cells, specialized epithelial cells that take up and transcytose luminal antigens for uptake by phagocytic macrophages.
2	This is follow by inflammation and phagocytosis of bacteria by neutrophils and macrophages and conscription of T and B cells. In systemic salmonella infections, bacteria may target unambiguous types of host cells, such as dendritic cells and/or macrophages that support dissemination through the lymphatics and blood stream to the mesenteric lymph nodes (MLNs) and to deeper tissues.
3	It leads to spreading to the spleen, bone marrow, liver and gall bladder.

S. flexneri then re-invade epithelial cells baso-laterally and activates an inflammatory response that disrupts the epithelium thus facilitating the translocation of additional bacteria. Dentric cells (DCs) constitute an additional cell type that sense antigens of the mucosal milieu and which participate an essential part in the immune response.

These cells are present in mucosal tissues may drift to mesenteric lymph nodes where interrelate with lymphocytes. The phagocytic action of these cells and their capability to migrate from periphery to circulation has been exploited by diverse bacterial pathogens. *S. typhimurium*, may be taken up by DCs sited in intestinal Peyer's patches, but also by inter-epithelial dentric cells that send dendrites among absorptive cells devoid of altering the epithelial cell permeability. This mechanism was projected to also contribute to the speedy crossing of the host epithelium by the bacteria *Salmonella* and to assist its dissemination in the host by reaching of the blood stream (Rescigno et al. 2001).

Escherichia coli-Mode of Infection

E. coli is a most important constituent of the normal intestinal microbial flora of human beings. Enteric pathogenic *E. coli* have been generally alienated into enterotoxigenic *E. coli* (ETEC) and enteropathogenic *E. coli* (EPEC), Shiga toxin producing *E. coli* (STEC), enteroaggregative *E. coli* (EAEC) enteroinvasive *E. coli* (EIEC) and diffusely adherent *E. coli* (DAEC).

EHEC strains of the O157:H7 serovar are the majority considerable pathogens but several further serotypes, mainly those of the O26 and O111 serotypes, be able cause disease and are more important than O157:H7 in numerous nations.

E. Coli (EHEC) Virulent factors and their functions

Virulent factors	Target	Effect
Shiga Toxin	rRNA	Depurinates rRNA, inhibit protein synthesis and induce programmed cell death (apoptosis)
Urease	Urea	Convert the Urea into ammonia and CO_2
Esp P	Auto transporter	Cleaves coagulation factor V ; Serine protease activity
Cycle inhibiting factor	Unknown	Inhibits mitosis G2/M Phase and inactivates Cyclin depedend kinase 1
Tir	Nck	Nucleation of cytoskeletal proteins, GAP like activity and loss of microvilli
Stc E	C1 Esterase inhibition	Cleaves C1 Esterase and disturbs the complement cascade.
Ehx	Erythrocyte and Leukocyte	Erythrocyte and Leukocyte lysis

E. Coli (EIEC) Virulent factors and their functions

Virulent factors	Target	Effect
Ipa A	Vinculin	Actin depolymerization
Ipa B	Caspase 1	Apoptosis,Interleukin 1 release
Ipa C	Actin	Activation of cdc42 and Rac
Vir A	Tubulin	Membrane ruffling and Microtubule destabilization
Sep A	Unknown	Serine protease
Sig A	Unknown	Ion seceretion
Ipg D	Ptdlns	Membrane blebbing,Inositol 4 Phosphate

E. Coli (EPEC) Virulent factors and their Functions

Virulent factors	Target	Effect
Tir	Nck	Loss of microvilli, Nucleation of cytoskeletal proteins, GAP like activity
Esp C	Unknown	Ion secretion; Serine protease
Esp F	Unknown	Induce apoptosis
Esp H	Unknown	Modulates pedestal and filopodia formation
Map	Mitochondria	Disrupts mitochondrial membrane potential
Tir	Nck	GAP like activity, Nucleation of cytoskeletal proteins and loss of microvilli.
Cif	Unknown	Inactivation of cdk 1 and blocks the mitosis in G2/M phase.

Various other probable adherence components have been explained for O157:H7 and/or non-O157:H7 strains, one probable adhesin is a *Tox B*, large 362-kDa protein encoded by the 93kb plasmid, which is found in O157:H7 and other EHEC strains. This protein allocates sequence homology with *Clostridium* toxin lineage.

This pO157 plasmid also predetermines an RTX toxin that is analogous to haemolysin, a serine protease (Esp P) and the *Stc E* protein. *Stc E* cleaves the C1 esterase inhibitor (C1-

INH) of the harmonize pathway and might significantly cause thrombotic abnormalities, tissue injure and intestinal oedema of EHEC infections.

The genetic sequence of O157:H7 exposed several chromosomal islets that predetermine further impending virulence components (Uyeyama et al. 1982).

The key stature of Enterohemorragic *E. coli* pathogenicity is the progression of 'attaching and effacing' (A/E) lesions on epithelial cells of the intestine. 'Attaching and effacing' (A/E) lesions are distinguished by the localized obliteration of brush border microvilli and the cherished bond of *E. coli* to the membrane of the infected host cells. Formation of 'Attaching and Effacing' (A/E) lesions is intervened by the type 3 secretion systems (T3SS), which transfers virulence factors into host cells and the outer membrane protein, intimin is essential for attachment (Melton-Celsa and O'Brien 1998).

The principle virulence factor for Enterohemorragic *E. coli* (EHEC) is *stx*, which is also recognized as verocytotoxin (VT).

Toxin *stx* comprises of five alike B subunits that are conscientious for attaching the holotoxin units to the glycolipid globotriaosylceramide receptors (Gb3) on the target cell surface. The A subunit that split ribosomal RNA thereby leads to the termination of protein synthesis process. *Stx* provokes programmed cell death in epithelial cells of intestine which is synchronized by the Bcl 2 family.

Toxin *stx* was initially isolated and purified from *Shigella dysenteriae* and hemolytic uremic syndrome can in addition result from infection with the species *Shigella dysenteriae*, even though not with other *Shigella* species or enteroinvasive *E. coli*, do not generate *stx*.

Moreover toxin *stx* mediates injury in the colon which consequences in necrosis, haemorrhagic colitis, intestinal perforation and bloody diarrhoea.

The *stx* family contains subgroups *stx* 1 and *stx* 2 that share similarities of the amino acid sequence are not encoded by *E. coli* chromosome rather they are encoded by λ like bacteriophage. It has been adopted that during the evolution this λ bacteriophage participated in horizontal gene transfer of *stx* genes from *Shigella* to *E. coli*. The stx encoding toxin is produced in the colon and moves through the bloodstream to the kidney.

E. Coli (ETEC) Virulent factors and their functions

Virulent factors	Target	Effect
LT Heat labile enterotoxin	G_5	ADP ribosylates and activates the enzyme adenylate cyclase
ST Heat stable entero toxin a	Guanylate cyclase	Activates the guanylate cyclase
ST Heat stable entero toxin b	Unknown	Increase intra cellular calcium results in ion secretion
ShET2 (*Shigella* enterotoxin 2)	Unknown	Ion secretion

Shigella Pathogenesis-Entry and Dissemination

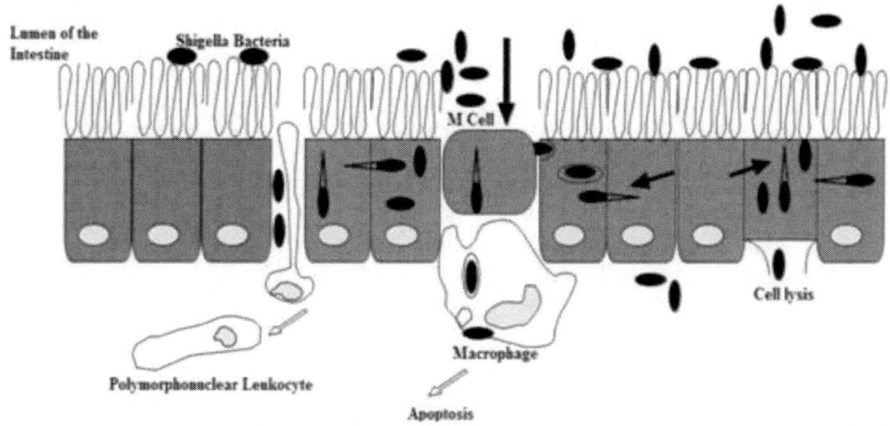

1 *Shigella* enters into the Micro fold cells through the process of endocytosis and escape from the endocytic vacuole,then the bacteria invade the epithelial cells and macrophage as well.

2 *Shigella* invasion induces apoptosis in macrophages which triggers the initial stages of inflammatory response.

3 *Shigella* multiplication takes place in the cytoplasm causes consequent epithelial cell death

Enterohemorrhagic E. coli (EHEC) Pathogenesis

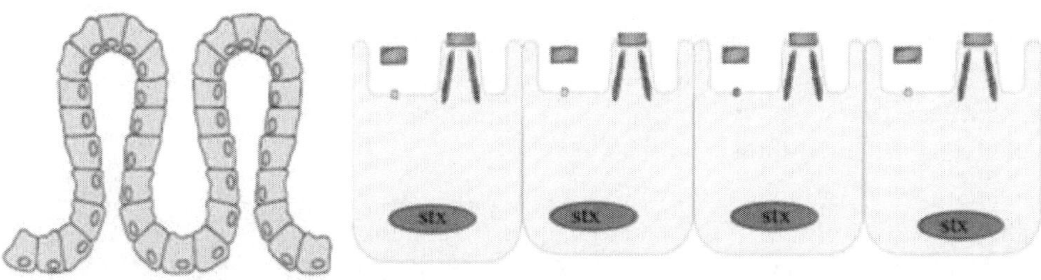

1 Enterohemorrhagic E.coli(EHEC) also induce the attaching and effacing lesion in the colon. The distinctive feature of EHEC is the expansion of Shiga toxin (Stx), systemic absorption of which leads to potentially life-threatening impediment.

2 Stx produced in Colon,and enters into the blood stream reaches kidney results in endothelial cell damage. This eventually consequences in Hemolytic Uremic Syndrome (HUS)

It results in damage of renal endothelial cells and stimulation of cytokine and chemokine assembly which ultimately leads to renal inflammation. In comparable to these mechanisms of bacterial adhesion, the EPEC (Enteropathogenic *E. coli*) and EHEC (Enterohemorragic *E. coli*) pathogens, which are responsible correspondingly for diarrheal disease in children and severe foodborne infections, use a extremely meticulous mechanism to make a close contact with host cells: they insert an effector called, *Tir* that inserts into the host cell plasma membrane and provides as an exogenous receptor for the bacterial exterior protein intimin (Lai et al. 2013).

Tir is delivered into the host cell cytoplasm through EPEC or EHEC type 3 secretion systems (T3SS), a multifarious protein forming a needle like construction that pass through the bacterial cell wall and the host cell plasma membrane. *Tir* thus tethers the bacteria to the host epithelial cell surface and gives an association between the bacteria and the host's cytoskeleton. Adhesion of bacteria to host surfaces is at last a key element in the development of bio film. The bio film development composes a limited mode of growth that allows bacteria to endure in antagonistic surroundings.

In the milieu of infectious diseases, bio film may be important as matrix embedded bacterial aggregates are more divergent to host defences or antibiotic treatments. Hence, adhesion represents a critical step for extracellular bacteria that helps their persistence in the host. For intracellular bacteria, it is an initial step that leads their internalization within host cells (Crepin et al. 2010). For numerous bacterial adhesins, the prospect of bond contravention increases with the tensile force derived from shear stress. This counter intuitive phenomenon can be explained by the existence of specific force strengthened bonds. Catch bonds can be observed for example with the *E. coli* Fim H adhesin, which exhibits a shear-enhanced binding to mannose glycoprotein molecule.

Helicobacter Pylori-Mode of Infection

Helicobacter pylori are curved Gram-negative organism that colonized the stomach. Infection may furthermore results in more severe clinical manifestations; such gastric mucosa associated lymphoid tissue (MALT) lymphoma, as peptic ulcer disease and gastric carcinoma for which the assortment in virulence of *H. pylori* strains is a significant factor. Polar flagella are essential virulence feature for *Helicobacter pylori*, a cause of gastric ulcers, as motility allows the bacteria to contact the gastric epithelium, adhere to it with some adhesins, and colonize the intestinal epithelium (Ogura et al. 2009).

The majority vital variations in virulence among *H. pylori* organism is the existence of the *Cag* pathogenicity island, which encodes type 4 secretion systems (T4SS) that permits migration of the bacterial effector molecule *Cag A* into host cells. T4SS mediated *Cag A* translocation occurs through the host beta1 integrin receptor situated at the epithelial cell baso-lateral surface. Inside the host cell, *Cag A* might endure tyrosine phosphorylation by host kinases and together non-phosphorylated and phosphorylated *Cag A* can trigger a range of signaling pathways directing to cytoskeletal reorganizations and disturbance of cell-cell junctions and cell proliferation (Frank et al. 2006).

Persons infected with H. pylori Cag A positive strains have rigorous inflammation and epithelial cell injury in the stomach and improved menace for peptic ulcer disease and gastric cancer than persons infected with Cag A negative variant of H. pylori. The threat for gastric carcinoma is elevated particularly in individuals infected with H. pylori strains harboring augmented tyrosine phosphorylation sites in Cag A. In addition, Cag A interacts with JAM-A and ZO-1 and employs these proteins to the sites of bacterial adhesion, changing the arrangements and role of the rigid junctional complex.

H. Pylori Pathogenesis

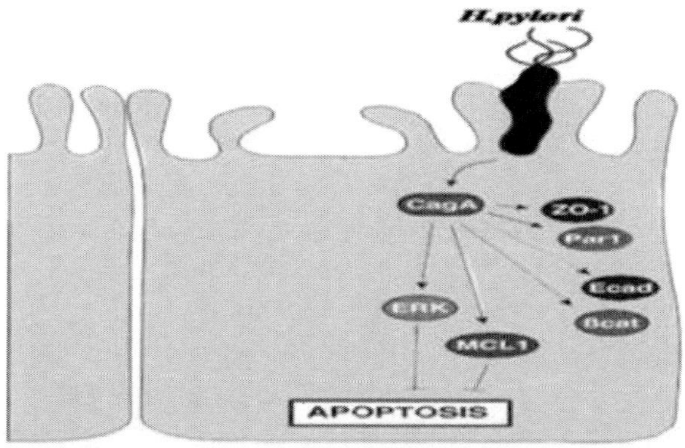

1 Bacterial virulence factors aiming host proteins concerned both in epithelial cell-cell junctions or in cell death and turnover.

2 CagA, an effector of *Helicobacter pylori*, interacts with ZO-1, a factor of tight junctions and Par1 a monitor of cell polarity, and activates distraction of epithelial rigid junctions.

3 This virulence factor also interrupts adherens junctions by targeting E-cadherin (Ecad) and promoting the discharge of b-catenin (bcat) from the adherence multipart.

It has also been scrutinized that H. pylori attains the intercellular spaces in the tight junctions.

It penetrates the epithelium in the direction of the lamina propria on the basolateral part of the cells, showing that H. pylori is capable to interrupt the adherens junctions. H. pylori targets E cadherin by numerous methods and methylation of Promoter CDH1 gene encoding *E cadherin* is often distinguished in *H. pylori* infected persons (Frank et al. 2006).

Additionally to epigenetic silencing, *H. pylori* has been related with further system of annoyance of *E cadherin* functions for instance proteolytic cleavage of its extracellular domain and protein delocalization from the cell membrane. This pathogen also makes *E cadherin* translocated to the cytoplasm from the cell membrane.

While E cadherin alterations intervened by H. pylori are self-determining of Cag A, physical relations among these proteins. Additionally, and in similar with Cag A/E cadherin interaction, communications involving p120 and Cag A and among c-Met and Cag A were also considered. Indeed, silencing of c-Met in these cells eliminated the communications among Cag A and p120 and Cag A and E cadherin signifying that Cag A interface with constituents of the adherens junctions is intervened by c-Met (Frank et al. 2006).

B Catenin and p120 Catenin Role in *H. Pylori* Infection

The binding of catenins *E cadherin* has a significant functional responsibility in the stabilization of adherens junctional complex, cell signaling and association to the cell cytoskeleton. While not joined at the membrane in the adherens junction, axin, adenomatous polyposis coli (APC), β catenin is phosphorylated by the serine/threonine kinase, glycogen synthase kinase 3b (GSK3b) and casein kinase1a (Ck1a) multipart and besieged to degradation through the ubiquitin/proteasome pathway. This deprivation process is offseted when the Wnt signalling pathway is dynamic resulting in stabilization of β catenin in the cytoplasm. Cytoplasmic stabilized β catenin could possibly be moved into the nucleus and it forms a multipart with the transcriptional factor of the T cell factor (TCF)/lymphoid enhancer binding factor (LEF), endorsing the switching -on of several genes (Nina et al. 2013).

Numerous researches have revealed the consequence of *H. pylori* infection in β catenin signaling and exposed *H. pylori* infection directs to the delocalization of *β* catenin from the membrane of the cell. *H. pylorus* phosphorylates GSK3b and by suppressing GSK3b activity, directs to quiet of β catenin phosphorylation and ubiquitin dependent deficiency. *H. pylori* intervened GSK3b suppression via phosphatidylinositol 3-kinase/protein kinase B (PI3K/Akt) enzyme activation (Nina et al. 2013). p120 catenin is an additional significant constituent in adherens junctions consistency and signaling. The p120 catenin binds to the membrane province of *E cadherin* and mutations in this area abolish *E cadherin* umpired cell–cell adhesion. Additionally to *E cadherin* stabilization, p120 could interrelate with the transcription factor. Several researches exposed that *H. pylori* changes the cellular localization and the phosphorylation condition of p120 however not entire p120 protein level (Nina et al. 2013).

Conclusion

There are numerous researcher groups globally that are working at deciphering the combined genome of the human microbiota. Intestinal microbiota is the community of live microbes existing in the gastrointestinal tract. The microbiota is requisite for exact body growth, the improvement of immunity, and nutrition. Establishment of bacterial infection is strongly dependent on host susceptibility. Genetic polymorphism in the particular population accounts for an vast variability in the type or amount of responses triggered against the come across pathogen. Identical bacterium can thus cause a huge spectrum of clinical consequences from asymptomatic infection to lethal disease, based on host genetic variability. Genetic determined host susceptibility, it is well recognized that the microbiota is playing a significant function to limit colonization and invasion by enteric microorganisms. Additionally, there is an immense need of consideration how precisely the pathogen survives under the condition and the pathways unique to the intracellular environment that could help us for the development of new drug candidate.

References

Crepin, Girard, Schuller, Phillips, Mousnier, Frankel. Dissecting the role of the Tir:Nck and Tir: IRTKS/IRS p53 signalling pathways *in vivo*. *Mol. Microbiol.*, 2010; 75: 308-23.

Cossart P., Helenius A. Endocytosis of viruses and bacteria. *Cold Spring Harb Perspect. Biol.,* 2014; 6.

Frank I. Tovey, Michael Hobsley, John Holton. *Helicobacter pylori* virulence factors in duodenal ulceration: A primary cause or a secondary infection causing chronicity. *World J. Gastroenterol.*, 2006; 7, 12(1): 6-9.

Johanna Haiko and Benita Westerlund-Wikström. The Role of the Bacterial Flagellum in Adhesion and Virulence, *Biology,* 2013; (2),1242-1267.

Johansson, Phillipson, Petersson, Velcich, Holm L., Hansson. The inner of the two Muc2 mucin-dependent mucus layers in colon is devoid of bacteria. *Proc. Natl. Acad. Sci. USA*, 2008; 105: 15064-9.

Lai, Rosenshine, Leong, Frankel. Intimate host attachment: enteropathogenic and enterohaemorrhagic Escherichia coli. *Cell Microbiol.*, 2013; 15: 1796-808.

Lai, Rosenshine, Leon, Franke., Intimate host attachment: enteropathogenic and enterohaemorrhagic *Escherichia coli. Cell Microbiol.*, 2013; 15: 1796-808.

Linden, Sheng, Every, Miles, Skoog, Florin, *et al.* MUC1 limits Helicobacter pylori infection both by steric hindrance and by acting as a releasable decoy. *PLoS Pathog.,* 2009; 5:e1000617.

Ma B., Forney L. J., Ravel J. Vaginal microbiome: rethinking health and disease. *Annu. Rev. Microbiol.*, 2012; 66:371-89.

McGuckin, Linden, Sutton, Florin. Mucin dynamics and enteric pathogens. *Nat. Rev. Microbiol.*, 2011; 9: 265e78.

Melton-Celsa, A. R., and A. D. O'Brien. 1998. Structure, biology, and relative toxicity of Shiga toxin family members for cells and animals.,p. 121-128. In J. B. K. a. A. D. O'Brien (ed.), *Escherichia coli* O157:H7 and other Shiga toxin-producing *E. coli*. American Society for Microbiology, Washington, D.C.

Melville S., Craig L. Type IV pili in Gram-positive bacteria. *Microbiol. Mol. Biol. Rev.*, 2013; 77:323-41.

Melville and Craig. Type IV pili in Gram-positive bacteria. *Microbiol. Mol. Biol. Rev.*, 2013; 77:323-41.

Nina., Salama, Mara., Hartung and Anne Müller. Life in the human stomach: persistence strategies of the bacterial pathogen Helicobacter pylori. *Nature Reviews, Microbiology,* 2013; 11(393), 385-399.

Ogura., Ooka., Iguchi., Toh., Asadulghani., Oshima., Kodama., Abe., Nakayama., Kurokawa, Tobe, Hattori, Hayashi. Comparative genomics reveal the mechanism of the parallel evolution of O157 and non-O157 enterohemorrhagic *Escherichia coli*. Proceedings of the National Academy of Science, USA, 2009; 106, 17939–17944.

Pedron, Sansonetti. Commensals, bacterial pathogens and intestinal inflammation: an intriguing menage a trois. *Cell Host Microbe*, 2008; 3:344e-7.

Roberts, Marklund, Ilver, Haslam, Kaack, Baskin, *et al.* The Gal (alpha 1-4)Gal-specific tip adhesin of Escherichia coli P-fimbriae is needed for pyelonephritis to occur in the normal urinary tract. *Proc. Natl. Acad. Sci. USA,* 1994; 91: 11889-93.

Rescigno, Urbano, Valzasina, Francolini, Rotta, Bonasio *et al.*, Dendritic cells express tight junction proteins and penetrate gut epithelial monolayers to sample bacteria. *Nat. Immunol.*, 2001; 2:361-7.

Stecher B., Hardt W. D. Mechanism's controlling pathogen colonization of the gut. *Curr. Opin. Microbiol.*, 2011; 14:82-91.

Stecher, Barthel, Schlumberger, Haberli, Rabsch, Kremer, *et al.* Motility allows *Sal. typhimurium* to benefit from the mucosal defence. *Cell Microbiol.*, 2008; 10: 1166-80.

Schommer N. N., Gallo R. L. Structure and function of the human skin microbiome. *Trends Microbiol.*, 2013; 21:660-8.

Uyeyama, Werner, Chin S., Pearce S. F., Kollip C. L., Williams L. P., Googins J. A.,. Isolation of *E. coli* O157:H7 from sporadic cases of hemorrhagic colitis: United States. *MMWR,* 1982; 31, 580–585.

Winter, Thiennimitr, Winter, Butler, Huseby, Crawford, *et al*. Gut inflammation provides a respiratory electron acceptor for *Salmonella*. *Nature,* 2010; 467:426-9.

In: Disorders of Gastrointestinal Systems … ISBN: 978-1-63485-366-8
Editors:S. Rajagopal, S. Murugan and S. Ramachandran ©2016 Nova Science Publishers, Inc.

Chapter 10

ROLE OF CORIANDRUM ESSENTIAL OIL AGAINST *CALLOSOBRUCHUS CHINENSIS* IN THE GASTRO INTESTINAL SYSTEM DISORDERS

M. Madhavi*[*], *PhD
Department of Zoology, Nizam College,
Osmania University, Hyderabad, Andhra Pradesh, India

ABSTRACT

Cereals and pulses form an important component in the diet of inhabitants of the world. After harvest, these goods are usually stored for long periods to provide a food reserve. Although stored grains can be destroyed by insects, fungi, and vertebrates pest, insect pests are often the most important because of the favorable climatic conditions for their development. The estimated global post-harvest losses caused by insects are huge. Synthetic chemical pesticides have been used to protect grains but their wide spread usage has led to the development of pest resistance. When properly used; synthetic insecticides may continue to play an important role in reducing storage losses due to insect pest activities. However, these insecticides have serious drawbacks such as development of genetic resistance in the treated pests, toxic residue problems, toxicity to consumers in the gastro intestinal system and hence causing disorders. It is therefore necessary to reduce such losses by controlling pests on stored grains. Alternative to synthetic chemical insecticides are highly desirable. Research on the use of natural pesticides for storage is increasing because of their low toxicity to human beings. Plant essential oils are often environmentally safe with rapid biodegradation and are non-toxic to humans. These facts may help in the Integrated Pest Management (IPM) programs and pest control strategies, including using plant derivatives against economic insect-pests. Essential oil isolated from coriander (*Coriandrum sativum*) was tested for their larvicidal and ovicidal activity aganist the important stored grain pest, the *Callosobruchus chinensis*. Hence, this chapter will discuss role of Coriander Essential oil against *Callosobruchus chinensis* in the gastro intestinal system disorders.

---

[*] Corresponding author: M. Madhavi, PhD., Assistant Professor; E-mail: prsmadhavi@gmail.com, Mo: +919848569309.

Keywords: coriander, *Callosobruchus chinensis*, gastro intestinal system disorders, genetic resistance, pesticides

1. Introduction

An imperative among the cultivation and harvesting strategies is the assessment of damage caused by insects in cereal crops, either by farmers themselves, or by traders, and technicians in animal farms in which grain feeds remain stored (Adams and Sculten 1976; Rajendran and Parveen 2005). Damage may be prevented by shortening storage time of adequate treatments financially and practically accessible to poor communities (Farrell et al. 1996; Stathers et al. 2002, Cox 2004; Epidi and Odili 2009). Effective pest control is no longer a matter of heavy application of pesticides, partly because of the rising cost of petroleum derived products but largely because excessive pesticides use promotes speedier evolution of resistance in insects pests, destroys natural enemies, turns formally innocuous species into pests, harms other non target species, and contaminates food (Anon 1980; Shukla et al. 2000). However because of the increasing problems associated with the use of toxic synthetic pesticides, such as loss of efficacy, development of pest resistance, regulatory restrictions as a result of adverse effects on non-target organisms, and ecotoxicity (Daglish 2004; Lorini et al. 2007; Sausa et al. 2009; Umoetok et al. 2009) there has been a pressing need for the development of safer, alternative crop protectants such as botanical insecticides, repellants and anti feedants (Isman 2006; Rajendran and Sriranjini 2008; Ukeh et al. 2011). Bioactivity of essential oils is related to their chemical composition, part of the plant extracted, phonological state of the plant, environmental conditions and the method of extraction (Isman 2000; Angioni et al. 2006; Zapata and Smagghe 2010; Nerio et al. 2010).

One of the major consequential benefits of improvements in drying and cooling processes for stored products is for the control of arthropod pests, particularly in an environment where chemical treatments are coming under greater and greater pressure. There are indeed growing market and regulatory constraints on the use of chemicals for pest control and serious insect resistance problems, especially with the major fumigant, Phosphate (Beckett 2011; Nayak et al. 2010; Lorini et al. 2007; Collins et al. 2002).

Plant products and their components have been known to exhibit biological activities (Barris et al. 2006). During the middle ages powdered mint leaves were used to whiten teeth (Hajlaoui et al. 2008). Even today about 80% of the world population relies predominantly on plants and plant extracts for health care (Peeyush et al. 2011; Werka et al. 2007). Particularly, in the recent years, plant extracts and their components are gaining increasing interests due to being relatively safe for the environment as well as the human health, their wide acceptance by consumers, and their exploitation for potential multi-purpose functional use. Plant insecticides have been used to fight pests for centuries (Isman 2006). More than 1500 species of plants have been reported to have insecticidal value, and many more exists. Although compared with modern synthetics the plant substances are relatively less effective, their relatively safer nature has resulted in the opening up of a new vista in plant insecticides research (Peeyush et al. 2011). Aqueous solutions are crude plant extracts obtained by using water as a solvent. Aqueous solutions are employed more frequently in the spraying of growing crops, and their use as protectants of stored products is rather restricted. This is probably their application increases the moisture content of the stored products.

Yalamanchilli et al., (2000) and Anand (2008) found that the oil isolated from turmeric leaves at 2% concentration (w/w) could effectively protect pulses from the attack of *Callosobruchus chinensis*. Chand et al., (2001) reported that oral administration of *Artemisia calamus* extract affected larval and adult forms of *Tribolium castaneum*. Rahman et al., (2003) evaluated the botanical products viz. leaf powder and extract of *Vitex negundo,* eucalyptus (*Eucalyptus globulous* Labill.), balkalmi (*Ipomoea* sp.), ash of babla wood (*Acacia arabica*), oil of neem, and sesame and saff flower against the attack of grain weevil *(Sitophilus granarious*) on wheat. The results showed that the higher concentration of oil (0.25-1.0%) indicated the lower infestation, less emergence of adults, less seed damage, less weight loss and higher inhibition rate.

Rahman and Talukder (2006) studied the bio-efficacy of extract, powder, ash and oil of *Vitex negundo*, eucalyptus (*Eucalyptus globules* Labill.), balkalmi (*Ipomoea sepiaria*), saf flower (*Carthamus tintorious* L.) sesame (*Sesame Indicum*. L) and bablah (*Acacia arabica* L.) against *Callosobruchus maculates* F. fed on vigna mungo seeds, for oviposition inhibition. Rajendran and Sriranjini (2008) reviewed plant essential oils and thin constituents as fumigants that are compounds acting on target insects in the vapour or gaseous phase against stored product insects such as *Tribolium. castaneum*, *Rhyzopertha dominicam*, and *Sitophilus Zeamais* but little or no attention has been paid towards moths such as *Corcyra cephalonica and Sitotroga cerealella*. Plant products therefore have the potential for small scale treatments, space fumigations and as adjuvant for conventional fumigants.

Coriander (*coriandrum sativum L.*) is an important plant in medicine, food production as well as in cosmetics and perfume industry. The components of coriander essential oil inhibit the growth of microorganisms. Corinder essential oil in particular linalool contained in it, is responsible for proper intestinal peristalsis. In fixed combinations, coriander oil is used in digestion difficulties, abdominal distension and excessive intestinal fermentation. Coriander essential oil shows antioxidant and antibacterial properties. The pulse beetle *Callosobruchus chinensis* is a major pest of economically important leguminous grains, such as cowpeas, lentils, green gram and black gram. The larvae bore into the pulse grain which becomes unsuitable for human consumption, variability for replanting, or production of sprouts. They are important pests of pulses crops in tropics under storage conditions.

Among Callsobruchus species, C. chinensis is frequently infesting different pulses in different parts of India. These are polyphagous pest larvae bore within the cotyledons and eventually hollow out the seed within the testa, typically three larvae bore per seed. Essential oil isolated from coriander (*Coriandrum sativum*) was tested for their larvicidal and ovicidal activity against the important stored grain pest, the *Callosobruchus chinensis*.

Serious problems of genetic resistance by insect species, pest resurgence, residual toxicity, and vertebrate toxicity, wide spread environmental hazards and increasing costs of application of presently used synthetic pesticides have directed the need for effective, biodegradable pesticides. The essential oil of *coriandrum sativum* was reported to have insect growth regulating activity, antibacterial activity and abortifacient properties. Irritable bowel syndrome is a common functional gastrointestinal disorder, which may result from alteration of the gastrointestinal microbiota following gastrointestinal infection, or with intestinal dysbiosis or small intestinal bacterial overgrowth. This may be treated with antibiotics, but there is concern that widespread antibiotic use might lead to antibiotic resistance. Some herbal medicines have been shown to be beneficial, but their mechanism of action remains incompletely understood. Essentialoils of coriander was tested for their activity on stored pests Callosobruchus chinensis which causes gastrointestinal disorder (Thompson et al. 2013). Hence, this chapter will discuss role of Coriander Essential oil against *Callosobruchus chinensis* in the gastro intestinal system disorders.

2. Experimental Insect -- Callosobruchus Chinensis

2.1. Classification

Kingdom - Animalia
Phylum - Arthropoda
Class - Insecta
Order - Coleoptera
Family - Bruchidae
Genus - Callosobruchus
Species - chinensis

Callosobruchus species, are commonly known as Pulse Bruchids/cowpea bruchids is of Asian origin, where it is still the dominant species, among others and now widely distributed throughout the warmer parts of the world. These are serious pests of pulse crops, intially in the field and later in produce stores, throughout the warmer parts of the world.

The species of family Bruchidae are small, oval, hard, covered by setae or scales with short elytra and abdominal tip exposed. Abdomen contains atleast five free sternites. Larvae undergo metamorphosis. The first instars is caraboid with well developed legs, toothed thoracic plates to help entry into the seed of plants on which the egg is laid. After the first moult the larva, becomes cruciform and often more or less apodous, blind pale grub. These beetles feed exclusively on seeds of leguminaceae. A number of species are of considerable economic importance. *Callosobruchus chinnensis* is the cosmopolitan pest of legumes.

The most valuable feature in the recognition of bruchid species is the arrangement of teeth and ridges on the hind femur. The commonest species of *Callosobruchus chinensis* were described and differentiated by Southgate and Pope (1957) and Sothgate (1958). *Callosobruhus chinensis* ia a serious pest on stored pulses, these are polyphagous insects and infest variety of pulses like chickpea, cowpea, lentils, greengram, blackgram, and redgram and cause severe damage in storage conditions.

3. Life Cycle of Callosobruchus Chinnensis

C. chinensis lifecycle takes 36 days at the 25°C and 70% RH. Usually, six to seven generations occur in a year. The period of lifecycle may vary according to the change of temperature, Relative humidity and type of pulses. *C. chinensis* is a major pest of *Cajanus cajan* (Red gram), *Cicer arietinum* (chick peas), Lens culinaris (lentils), Vigna radiate (green gram), *Vigna unguiculata* (cowpeas) in various tropical regions. It also attacks other pulses on occasions, but appears to be incapable of developing on *Phaseolus vulgaris* (common beans).

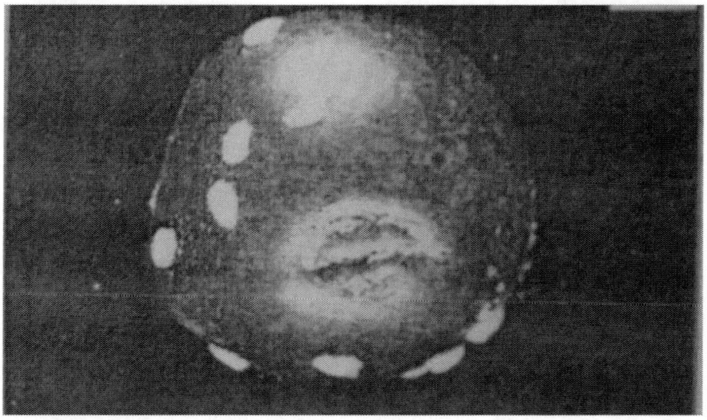

Figure 1. Eggs Laid By Control Insects on Red Gram.

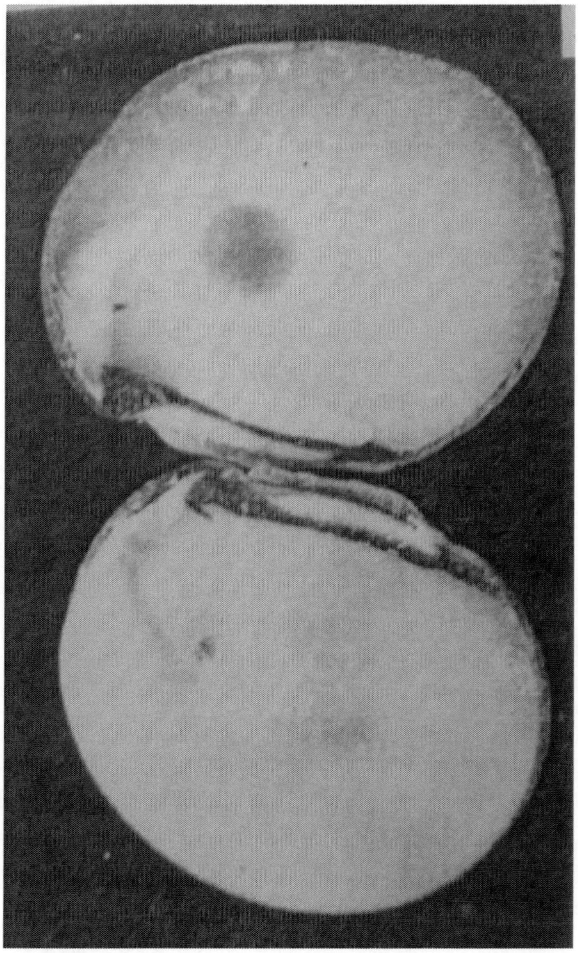

Figure 2. Damaged Red Gram Cup Open to Show the II Instar Lava.

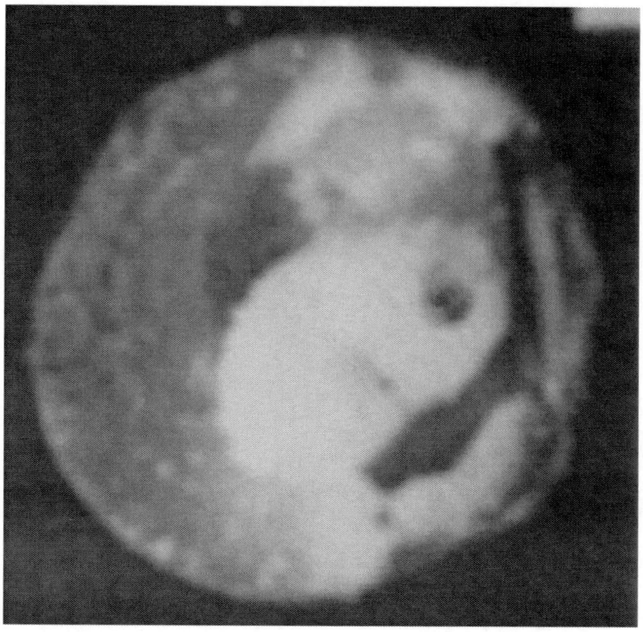

Figure 3. Damaged Red Gram Cup Open to Show the III Instar Larva.

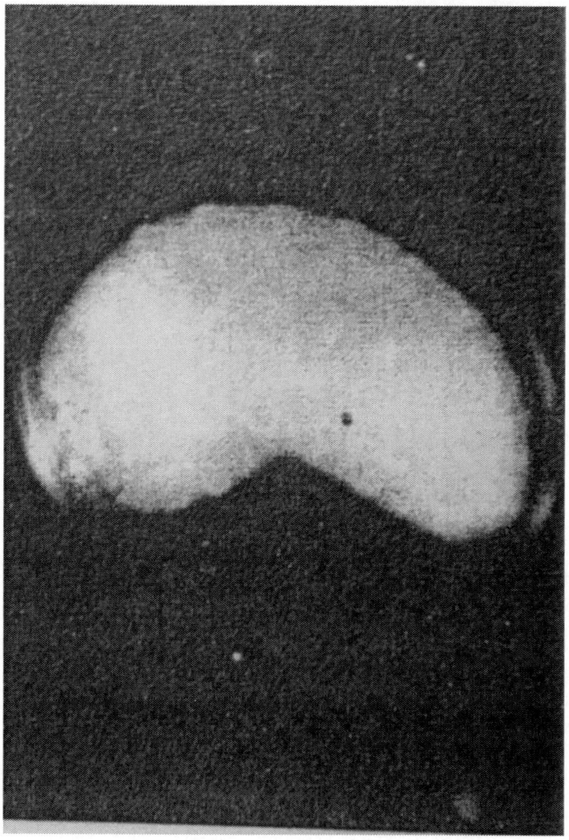

Figure 4. IV Instar Larva.

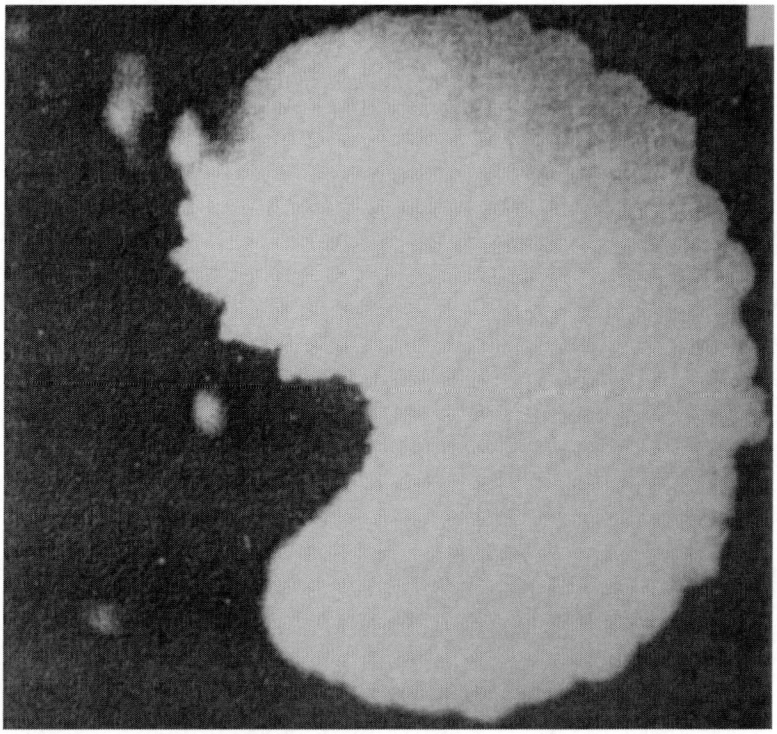

Figure 5. V Instar Larva.

EGG

The adult beetles, which do not feed on stored products, are very short lived (usually not more than 12 days under optimum conditions) and during this time the females lay many eggs (85-100). The optimum temperature for oviposition is low about23°C. The eggs are laid, they are firmly glued to the surface of the host seed, and smooth seeded varieties being more suitable rather than rough seeded varieties. The eggs are domed structures with oval, flat bases. When newly laid they are small, translucent grey and inconspicuous. Eggs hatch within 5-6 days of oviposition.

Larva (1-24 Days)

The developing feed entirely witin a single seed, excavating achamber within the cotyledons as it grows. The hatching larvae bit through the base of the egg, directly through the testa and into the cotyledons.

The larva is scarabaeiform and under gone 4 moults (5 instars) in about22-24 days at 25°C and 70% RH.

The whole time of the larvae is spent within a single seed. Larval stages are the main feeding stages. Larvae are fleshy, curved, white, and creamy in color with black mouth parts; the last instars larva before pupation stops feeding and contracts and this called pre- paul stage."

Pupal Stage (25-30days)

During this period the tissues are broken down and changed for preparation of adult. Pupation takes place inside the seed.

Adults

Adults have a very active period of reproduction. Adults fly quite well, but they do not feed on stored products and are usually short lived. Infestation commonly begins in the field, where eggs are laid on maturing pods. As the pods dry, the pest's ability to infest them decreases. Thus, dry seeds stored in their pods are quite resistant to attack, whereas the threshold seeds are susceptible to attack throughout storage.

4. Plant Material-Coriander Essential Oil Extraction

Essential oil was extracted from the seed of coriander, coriander sativum L. of the family Apiaceae. The essential oil was extracted by steam distillation for 4-6 hours using a Clevenger type apparatus where 250g of seeds in 250 ml of water is subjected to hydrodistillation (Marcus and Lichtenstein 1979; Weaver et al. 1994).

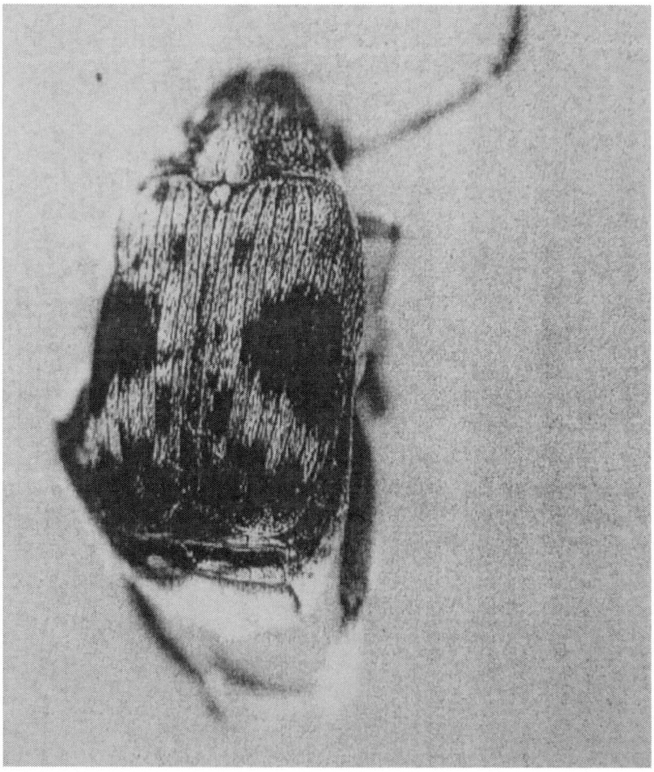

Figure 6. Adult Female.

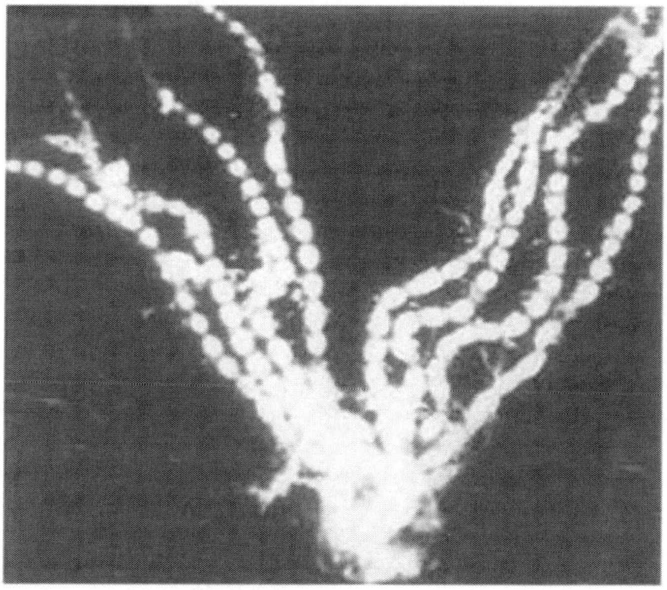

Figure 7. Ovary with Ovarioles.

The oil was separated dried over anhydrous sodium sulfate and stored in dark glass bottles at 4°C in the refrigerator until used. The isolated oil is a colorless or pale yellow liquid with a characteristic odor and taste of coriander. The larvae and adults were treated with the coriander essential oils prepared using ethyl alcohol (95%) as solvent. After suitable gap of time the insects were transformed into the diet. The treated larvae were observed daily to note the changes and the resulting abnormal intermediates were collected from the diet media.

4.1. Effect of Coriander Essential Oil on the IV And V Instar Grubs

The larvae were treated with coriander essential oil and the resultants exhibited the following results:

- ✓ 30% of the treated larvae died during moulting. If any insects survived initially, they also died during the process of treatment. The rate of mortality increased with increased dosage.
- ✓ 10% of the larvae remained as "over-aged" larvae for an extended period of time without moulting. These over-aged larvae were called as permanent larvae in which stage they continue for several days and eventually died.
- ✓ 20% of the V instar larvae were resulted as larval-pupal intermediates. In the resultant larval-pupal intermediates, larval exuvium was seen attached with the pupal case and the abdominal region was undifferentiated when compared with the control pupae.
- ✓ 8% of the treated resultant V instar larvae pupated normally but to enclose into adults and resulted as pupal –adult intermediates
- ✓ 10% of the V instar treated resultants metamorphosed into adults and these adults the body was shruken with deformed wings.

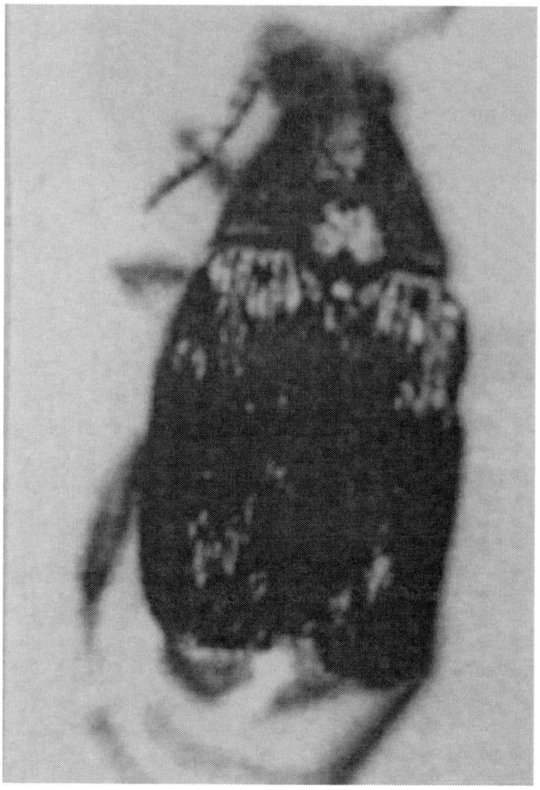

Figure 8. Pupal Adult Intermediate.

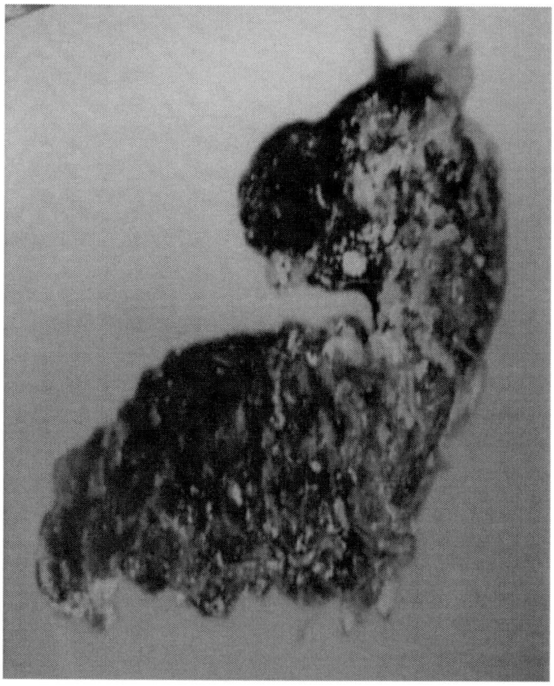

Figure 9. Abnormal Adult with Deformed Wings and Appendages.

- ✓ 22% of the v instar treated resultants metamorphosed into morphologically normal adults. However; the fecundity was reduced when compared with the normal control adults.

Pupal Treatment

The pupae were treated with coriander essential oil and the resultants exhibited the following results:

- ✓ 26% of the treated resultant pupae failed to eclose into adults and eventually died in the pupal case. These pupae were unable to metamorphose into adults and died within the pupal case.
- ✓ 34% of the treated resultant pupae were formed as the pupal –adult intermediates. The resultant pupal-adult intermediates were characterized by specimens which were developed within the pupal case but were unable to eclose. In some cases the mouth parts and legs were freed to a limited extent so that they were able to move up to a limited extent. These forms survived for a short period and eventually died.

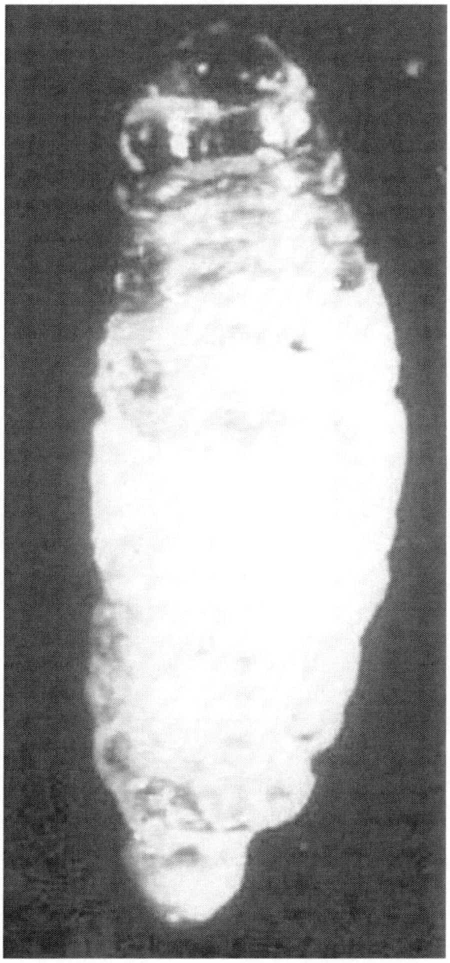

Figure 10. Larval – Pupal intermediate with larval head.

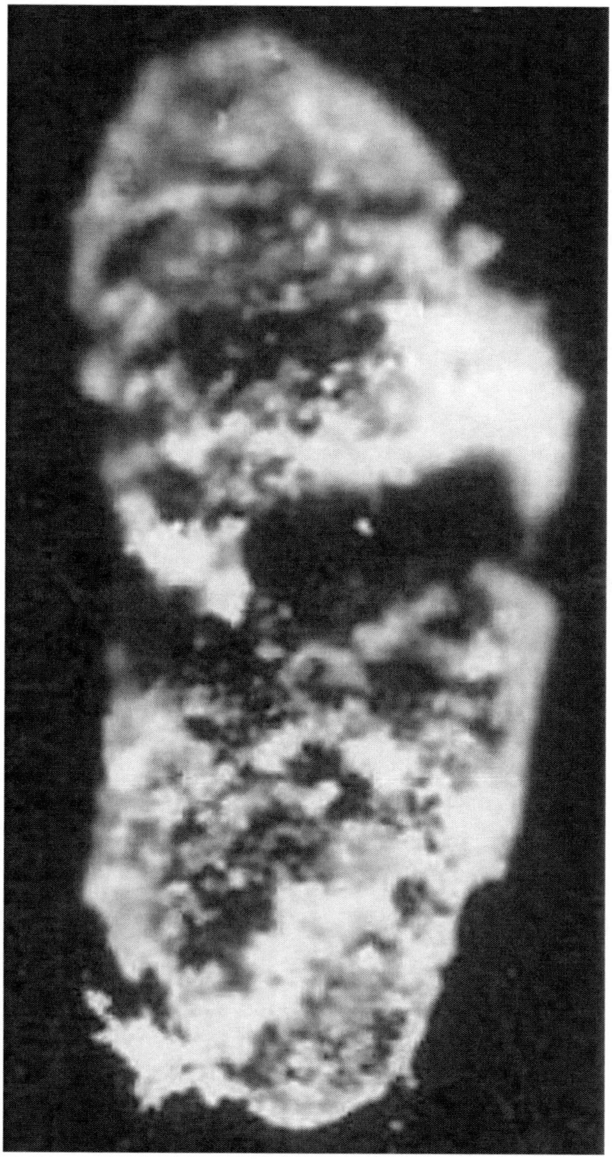

Figure 11. Larval Pupal Intermediates with Cuticular Patches on the Posterior Region.

Ovaries

In the control *C. chinensis* there are two distinct ovaries, each with six ovarioles. each telotrophic ovariole is clearly demarcated into germarium and vitellarium (plate-3).

- ✓ The ovaries of the treated resultant aduklts showed severe disorders in the development. There was a variation in the number of ovarioles and deformities were observed in the ovaries when compared with the ovaries from the control adults.
- ✓ In certain cases the terminal oocytes were abnormally large and unable to ovulate due to dislodging of their linear position. The abnormal terminal large oocytes block the ovulation.

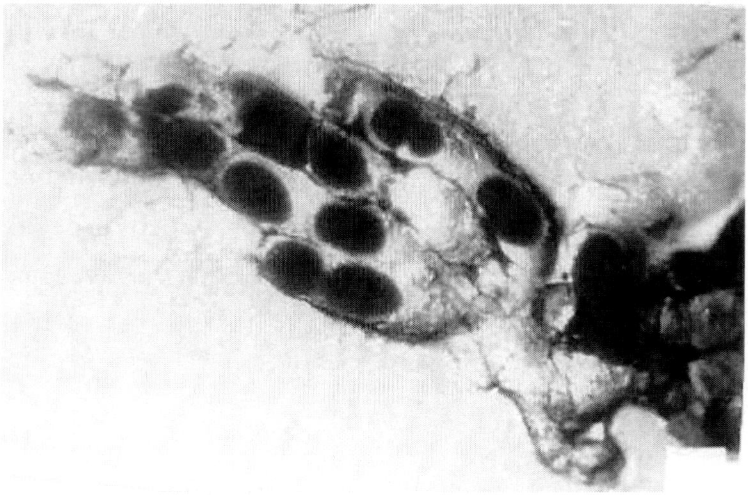

Figure 12. Ovarioles with Unequal Size of Oocytes in Abnormal Adult.

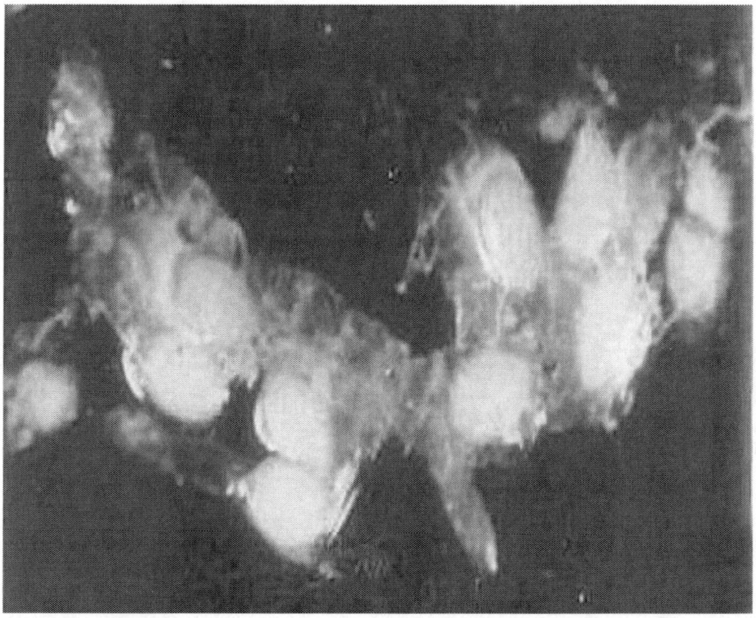

Figure 13. Deformed Ovary with Less Number of Ovarioles, Large Oocytes Unovulated in Abnormal Adult.

- ✓ In the ovaries of the treated resultant adults ovarioles were varying in length with abnormal sized oocytes when compared with the oocytes of the control insect
- ✓ In some cases deformed ovarioles were showing large un-ovulated chorionated oocytes
- ✓ In the ovaries of the treated resultant adults few ovarioles showed well developed oocytes while in the rest of the ovarioles oocytes were underdeveloped
- ✓ In some cases the two ovaries were with large terminal oocytes and malformed small oocytes.

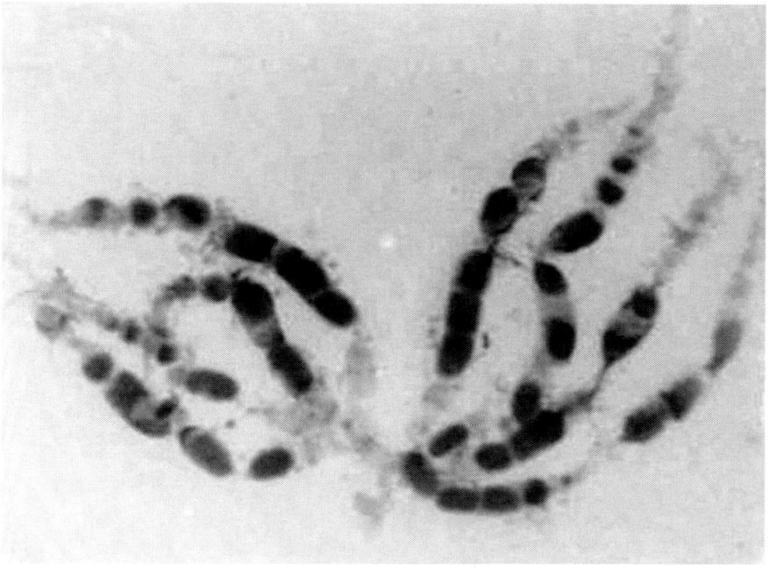

Figure 14. Ovaries with Ovarioles Reduced in Size – Malformed Adults.

CONCLUSION

The essential oil of coriander sativum was reported to have insect growth regulating activity and abortifacient properties. In the present study the effects of administering coriander sativum essential oil topically have detrimental effects on the development of larvae and pupae of *C. chinensis* which led to eclosion of abnormal adults. The treated insects could not moult normally due to which flight and reproduction were hindered. The prolongation of larval periods was observed. The treated ones resulted in malformed pupae and larval-pupal intermediates. The feeding activity was reduced in the treated resultant grubs with corinder essential oil which indicates the antifeedant activity. The similar effects were observed on other pests.

In *C. chinensis* coriander essential oil induced abnormal development of ovaries showing the variation in the development of ovarioles. The abnormally large sized and chlorinated oocytes hindered ovulation. In the ovaries, certain ovarioles remained underdeveloped. So, these abnormalities in the treated resultants drastically decreased the fecundity of the pest which led to the control of population of the pest. The results show that the considerable physiological effects on the pulse beetles, such as ovipositional activity, growth inhibition and adult mortality.

The main action of the coriander essential oil is prevention of molting. The effects on the endocrinal mechanisms of the insect such as molting and metamorphosis without causing any direct toxicity to the insect. Essential oil has affected the cuticle of soft-bodied insect.

The *C. chinensis* was unable to cast their exuviate. For both reasons, the individuals are not viable because they were prevented from feeding or defecation. It is interesting to note that if molting was achieved despite treatment, disruption becomes apparent in the next stage, when a new molting-endocrinological cycle occurs, so a very specific and long term and irreversible action occurs.

The ovaries of the treated resultant *C. chinensis* pupal-adult intermediates and abnormal adults showed oocytes degeneration and resorption and one or two bulky deposited chlorinated eggs blocks the oviducts. The reduced amounts of proteins in the ovaries of treated females of insect clearly indicate that the Essential oil of *Coriander sativum* caused a lower uptake of proteins by the ovary. Hence, the treated resultant adults exhibited inhibition of vitellogenesis and reduced fecundity.

Thus, it is evident that coriander essential oil acts as insect growth regulator and it influences the metamorphosis in the treated resultant larvae and pupae metamorphosed into larval-pupal intermediates, pupal-adult intermediates and malformed adults. Ovaries also exhibited the deformities like large oocytes, chlorinated oocytes which blocked the ovarioles and reduced fecundity. The protein levels also were variable with that of control insects.

The decreased protein levels indicate the effect of Coriander essential oil on protein synthesis and uptake during larval pupal transformation and vitellogenesis. This also inhibited the growth and development of the stored grain pest *C. chinensis* suggesting its use as a cheap, safe and eco-friendly pesticide.

REFERENCES

Adams, J. M. and Sculten, G. G. M. (1976). Losses caused by insects, mites and microorganisms. In: K. L., Linblad, C. J. (Eds), Postharvest Grain Loss Assessment Methods. American Association of Cereal Chemists, Slough, England, pp.83-89.

Anon. (1980). World Conservation Stratergy. International Union of Conservation of Nature and Natural Resources.

Angioni, A., Barra, A., Coroneo, V., Dessi, S. and Cabras, P. (2006). Chemical composition, seasonal variability, and antifungal activity of *Lavandula stoechas* L. ssp. stoechas essential oils from stem/leaves and flowers. *J. Agri. Food Chem.*, 54, 4364-4370.

Beckett, S. J. (2011). Insect and mite control by manipulating temperature and moisture before and during chemical-free storage. *J. Stored Product Research*, 1-9.

Barris, O., Gulluce, M., Sahin, F., Ozer, H. and Ozbek, T. (2006). Biological activities of essential oil and methanol extract of *Achillea biebersteini* Afan. (Asteraceae), *Turkish J. Biol.*, 30, 65-73.

Chand, S., Basu, P. and Maheshwari, N. (2001) Effect of *Artemisia calamus* extract on the development of *Tribolium castaneum*. *J. Stored Products Research,* 3:53-54.

Collins, P. J., Daglish, G. J., Bengston, M., Lambkin, T. M. and Pavic, H. (2002). Genetics of resistance to phosphine in *Rhizoppertha dominica* (Coleoptera: Bostrichidae). *J. of Economic Entomology*, 95, 862-869.

Cox, P. D. (2004). Potential for using semiochemicals to protect stored products from insect infestation. *Journal of stored Product Research*, 40.1-25.

Daglish, G. J. (2004). Effect of exposure period on degree of dominance of phosphine resistance in adults of *Rhyzopthera dominica* (Coleoptera: Bostrychidae) and *Sitophilus oryzae* (Coleoptera: Curculionidae). *Pest. Mang. Sci.,* 60, 822-826.

Epidi, T. T. and Odili, E. O. (2009). Biocidal activity of selected plant powders against *Tribolium castaneum* Herbst in stored groundnut (Arachys hypogaeak L.) *African Journal of Environmental Science and Technology*, 3, 1-5.

Farrell, F., Hill, M. G., Nang, F. L. O. and Stabrawa, A., (1996). A review of investigations to improve pest management of stored maize in smallholder farms in Kenya. *Integrated Pest Management Reviews*, 1, 251-263.

Hajlaoui, H., Snoussi, M., Jannet, H. B., Mighri, Z. and Bakhrough, A. (2008). Comparison of chemical composition and antimicrobial activities of *Mentha lobgifolia L. ssp*. From two Tunisian localities (Gabes and Sidi Bouzid). *Ann. Microbiol.*, 58,103-110.

Isman, M. B. (2000). Plant essential oils for pest and disease management. *Crop Prot.*, 19. 603-608.

Isman, M. B. (2006). Botanical insecticides, deterrents, and repellents in modern agriculture and an increasingly regulated world. *Annu. Rev. Entmol.*, 51, 45-66.

Lorini, I., Collins, P. J., Daglish, G. J., Nayak, M. K. and Pavic, H. (2007). Detection and charecterization of strong resistance to phosphine in Brazilian *Ryzopertha dominica (F)* (Coleoptera: Bostrychidae), *Pest Mang. Sci.*, 63, 358-364.

Nayak, M., Holloway, J., Pavic, H., Head, M., Reid, R. and Collins, P. J. (2010). Developing stratergies to manage highly phosphine resistant populations of flat grain beetles in large bulk storages in Australia. Proceed. Of the 10th International Working Conference on Stored Product Protection 27 June to 2 July 2010, Estoril, Portugal. pp. 396-401.

Nerio, L. S., Olivero-Verbel, J. and Stashenko, E. (2010). *Repellent activity of essential oils: a review Bioresource Technol.*, 101, 372-378.

Peeyush kumar, Sapna Mishra. (2011). Insecticidal properties of *Mentha species*– A Review. *J. Industrial crops and products*, 34.802817.

Rahman, M. A., Jaleb, M. A. and Biswas, M. M. (2003). Evalution of botanical product as grain protectant against grain weevil, *Sitophilus granaries* L. on wheat, *Asian J. Plant Sci.*, 2(6): 501-504.

Rahman, A. and Talukdar, F. A. (2006). Bioefficacy of some plant derivatives that protect grains against puls beetle, *callosobruchus maculates* F. (coleopteran: Bruchidae) *J. Insect Sci.*, 6:03.

Rajendran, S. and Sriranjini, V. (2008). Plant products as fumigants for stored product insect control. *J. Std. Prod. Res.*, 44(1); 126-135.

Sausa, A., Faroni, L., Pimentel, M., Guedes, R. (2009). Developmental and population growth rates of phosphine-resistant and susceptible populations of stored-product insect pests. *J. Stored Prod. Res.*, 45,241-246.

Shukla, A. C., Shahi, S. K., Dikshit, A. and Saksena, V. C. (2000). Plant products as a Fumigant for the Management of Stored-Product Pests. Proc. Int. Conf. Controlled Atmosphere and Fumigation in Stored Products, pp 125-132.

Stathers, T. E., Chigariro, J., Mudiwa, M., Mvumi, B. M., Golob, P. (2002). Small-scale farmer perceptions of diatomaceous earth products as potential stored grain protectants in Zimbabwe. *Crop Protection*, 21, 1049-1060.

Southgate, B. J. and Pope R. D. (1957), The groundnut seed beetle,a study of its identity and taxonomic position. *Annals and Magazine of Natural History, Series 12,* 10,669-672.

Southgate, B. J. (1958) Systemics notes on the species of Callosobruchus of economic importance. *Bulletein of Entomological research*, 49(3), 591-599.

Thompson A., Meah D., Ahmed N. (2013). Comparision of antibacterrial activity of essential oils and extracts of medicinal and culinary herbs to investigate potential new treatments for irritable bowel syndrome. *J. Stored Pests,* 10.1186/1472-6882-13-338.

Umoetok, S. B. A. Osuagwu, A. N., Udo, I. A., Idiongette, M. I., Ukeh, D. A. (2009). Effects of *Azadirachta indica* produces on the management of Ootheca mutabilis on *Telfaria occidentalis* in Calabar, Southeast Nigeria. *Crop Prot.,* 28, 583-587.

Werka, J. S., Boehme, A. K., Setzer, W. N. (2007). Biological activities of essential oils from *Monteverde, Costa Rica. Nat. Prod. Commun*., 2, 1215-1219.

Yalamanchilli, R. P., Punukollu, B., Kumar, S., Kukreja, A. K., Dwivedi, S. and Singh, A. K. (2000). Bioefficacy studies on leaf oil of *curcuma domestica valeton*, grain protectant activity. *J. med., Aroma. Plant sci.,* 22(1B):715-716.

Zapata, N. and Smagghe, G. (2010). Repellency and toxicity of essential oils from the leaves and bark of *Laurelia sempervirens* and *Drimys winteri* against *Tribolium castaneum, Indus. Crop. Prod*., 32, 405-410.000.

In: Disorders of Gastrointestinal Systems … ISBN: 978-1-63485-366-8
Editors:S. Rajagopal, S. Murugan and S. Ramachandran ©2016 Nova Science Publishers, Inc.

Chapter 11

CHRONIC KIDNEY DISEASES AND GASTROINTESTINAL DISORDERS

Murugavel Ponnusamy**, PhD
Centre for Developmental Cardiology, Institute for Translational Medicine,
College of Medicine, Qingdao University, Qingdao, China

ABSTRACT

Chronic kidney disease (CKD) is the major health problem worldwide. Global burden of CKD is increasing continuously at the rate of 6-8% per annum. Every year millions of adults die prematurely due to complications associated with CKD. The gastrointestinal (GI) disorder is one of the major complications associated with CKD and more than 50% of patients with end-stage renal disease (ESRD) have GI problems. Uremia and dialysis procedure increases the risk of GI tract and accessory organs related problems. The most common GI disorders in CKD patients are gastroparesis, gastroesophageal reflux disease, ulcerative esophagitis, peptic ulcer disease, irritable bowel syndrome, watermelon stomach, angiodysplasia, stercoral ulcer, and its associated GI bleeding. In this chapter, the unique features of GI complications associated with CKD and pathophysiological mechanism of GI complications in those patients are discussed. The clinical manifestations, diagnosis, and management of GI disorders in CKD patients is also demonstrated.

Keywords: chronic kidney disease, end stage renal disease, dialysis, gastrointestinal disorders

---

* Corresponding author: Murugavel Ponnusamy, PhD., Center for Developmental Cardiology, Institute of Translational Medicine, College of Medicine, Qingdao University, Qingdao 266021, China, Email: spmvel@gmail.com.

1. INTRODUCTION

Chronic kidney disease (CKD) is a condition characterized by gradual loss of kidney function that emerges from both non-communicable and infectious diseases. In recent years, CKD is gaining attention as more than 10% of global population is affected by this disorder, and millions die every year due to this problem. The global burden of CKD continuously increases at an annual growth of 6 to 8%. This is mainly due to the growing number of elder population and a dramatic increase in patients with diabetes and hypertension, which are closely associated with CKD development. The incidence of CKD is even higher in developing countries due to lifestyle modifications and food-habits (Stenvinkel, 2010; Thomas et al., 2008).

CKD is defined as the presence of renal tissue damage and progressive loss of renal function, which is manifested by a persistent proteinuria (albumin excretion) and a decrease in estimated glomerular function (blood creatinine concentration) for more than 3 months (Thomas et al., 2008). Clinically, a persistent fall in glomerular filtration rate (GFR) below 60 ml/min/1.73 m^2 even without any kidney damage is a hallmark of CKD. Unlike acute kidney injury, CKD is asymptomatic until it reaches advanced stages. CKD is unpreventable in advanced stages, but it is possible to slow down the progression if it is recognized and treated in the early stages. Severity of CKD is determined based on the GFR rate and albumin in urine, and is classified into 5 stages (Thomas et al., 2008) as showed in Table 1. Regardless of GFR, the high amount of albumin in urine increases the risk of quick progression to ESRD.

Table 1. Stages of chronic kidney diseases

Stage of CKD	GFR (ml/min/1.73m^2)	Albuminuria (UACR level in mg/mmol)	Description and Action Plan
1	≥ 90	LOW RISK Less than 3 mg/mmol	Kidney damage with normal GFR or increased GFR. Treatment for prevention and slow down of CKD progression. Reduce the risk of comorbid conditions especially CVD.
2	60-89	MODERATE RISK 3-29 mg/mmol (Microalbuminuria)	Kidney damage with slight decrease of GFR. Estimate progression and diagnosis for complications.
3	30-59	HIGH RISK $\geq$30 mg/mmol (Macroalbuminuria)	Moderate decrease of GFR. Evaluate and treat complications.
4	16-29		Severe decrease of GFR. Required dialysis and preparation for transplantation
5	<15 (End Stage Renal Disease)		Renal Failure. Required dialysis and immediate transplantation

CKD - Chronic Kidney Disease; GFR - Glomerular Filtration rate; UACR - Urinary albumin-creatinine ratio; Normal albumin level - less than 2 mg albumin/mmol of creatinine.

In the early stages (stage 1 and 2) of CKD, the kidney function (GFR) is almost normal (90-120 ml/min/1.73 m^2) but there is a stable increase of proteinuria (albumin in the urine). Although patients at this stage have normal kidney function, it silently increases the risk of hypertension, cardiovascular disease (CVD) and diabetes. As the CKD progresses to advanced stages, the GFR decreases below 30 ml/min/1.73 m^2 along with a very high level of proteins in urine, which raises several other complications as well as worsen preexisting extra-renal disorders. A complete failure of the kidney is indicated by the GFR level below 15 ml/min/1.73 m^2, which is defined as end stage of renal disease (ESRD). These patients required regular dialysis for maintenance until they get a kidney replacement (Levey et al., 2005; Weiner, 2007).

CKD is associated with the development of various disorders. The primary route cause for the development of non-renal complications in CKD patients is the drastic changes in circulatory compositions since kidney is the key regulator of volume and composition of blood. Of many irregularities, uremia and imbalance in electrolytes causes a variety of damage to different systems. As the CKD progresses, it also augments the prevalence and severity of co-morbidities such as cardiovascular diseases, diabetes, hypertension, anemia, and gastrointestinal (GI) complications. In fact, most of the CKD patients do not reach ESRD rather they prematurely die due to worsening of one or more of these complications (Thomas et al., 2008).

Among various complications, GI disorder is the most commonly observed non-renal complication in CKD patients. A different form of GI lesions always accompany advanced stages of CKD. The CKD patients with a very high urea level and patients under dialysis are more prone to the development of GI disorders. The overall incidence of GI complication in CKD patients is about 70% and it is higher in patients on maintenance dialysis (Dong et al., 2014). In CKD patients, GI disorders can be seen in all segments of the GI tract, however, most of the problems occur in the upper GI (Nand et al., 2014; Thomas et al., 2013). As the number of patients with CKD increases steadily, the nephrologists confront with the management of complex medical problems associated with CKD, including GI complications, until the patients requires/undergoes renal replacement therapy. In this background, this chapter focuses on the functional abnormalities of the GI tract in CKD patients. In addition, this chapter briefly illustrates pathological changes that occur in the GI tract and practical approaches to manage them in CKD patients.

2. Causes of CKD

CKD is characterized by the relentless progression of renal tubular injury and irreversible structural modification of renal tissue. The formation and abundance of fibrotic proteins (tubulointerstitial fibrosis) and tubular atrophy is the final common pathway of CKD regardless of the underlying causes and contributing factors (Boor et al., 2007; Hodgkins and Schnaper, 2012). The primary route cause of tubulointerstitial damage and fibrosis is the alterations in glomerular function, which is due to misdirected glomerular ultrafiltration, proteinuria, obstruction of filtration, chronic hypoxia or toxic insults. The major pathological mechanisms involved in the development of tubulointerstitial injury and activation of fibrotic processes are oxidative stress, increased production of proinflammatory cytokines, microvascular injury, overproduction of connective tissue growth factors and profibrotic growth factors (Boor et al., 2007; Hodgkins and Schnaper, 2012).

Metabolic syndrome is the leading cause of CKD. There is a close relationship between the incidence of CKD and metabolic disorders such as hyperglycemia, hypertension, dyslipidemia, and obesity. Among various metabolic diseases, diabetes and hypertension are the prominent causes of CKD. Nearly two-third of patients with CKD is having pre-existing diabetes and/or high blood pressure. The uncontrolled high blood pressure increases intraglomerular pressure and damages the blood vessels in renal tissue, which consequently impairs filtration function of glomeruli resulting in abnormally increased levels of protein in the urine. A small amount of albumin in the urine (microalbuminuria) is the first sign of CKD despite normal levels of creatinine and urea. As the CKD progresses, macroalbuminuria is developed, which is the warning sign for the decline of kidney function.

Numerous cross-sectional and observational studies found that diabetes, hypertension, and hyperlipidemia also emerges in patients with established CKD. This indicates the casual bi-directional relationship between these two conditions (Nashar and Egan, 2014; Prasad, 2014; Shiba and Shimokawa, 2011). The other conditions such as repeated infections (pyelonephritis), inflammatory diseases of kidney (interstitial nephritis and glomerulonephritis), inherited disorders of kidney (polycystic kidney disease), autoimmune disorders (lupus nephritis caused by systemic lupus erythematosus), long-term use of non-steroidal inflammatory drugs (Ibuprofen, aspirin), renal blockage such as kidney stones and prostate diseases also causes CKD (Weiner, 2007).

3. Gastrointestinal Complications in CKD Patients

GI complication is one of the major contributors to early morbidity and mortality among CKD patients. The signs and symptoms of GI complications appear in CKD patients are non-specific. In most cases, the symptoms of GI complications are seen in stage 3 of CKD during which there is a drastic change in the circulatory composition (Dong et al., 2014; Salamon et al., 2013). The GI associated early symptoms include weakness, nausea, vomiting, fatigue, anorexia, constipation, and loss of appetite. Some of these symptoms can also be seen in early stages of CKD (stage 1 and 2). As the CKD progresses to advanced stages, the patients acquire some common digestive tract discomforts like glossitis (inflammation of the tongue), diarrhea and ulcer. With further worsening of CKD (stage 4 and ESRD), eating dysfunction, gastritis, angiodysplasia, diverticular diseases, and bleeding in the lower and upper GI tract are more prominent. In most instances, these complications are reported in patients undergoing dialysis (Dong et al., 2014; Salamon et al., 2013). Among dialysis patients, the prevalence, diversity, and severity of GI symptoms are different depending on the dialysis procedures (hemodialysis or peritoneal dialysis). For instance, the incidence of constipation, abdominal pain and diarrhea are very high in hemodialysis patients when compared to patients under peritoneal dialysis. At the same time, peritoneal patients experience more frequent and severe gastric reflux problems, gastroparesis and eating dysfunction (Dong et al., 2014; Salamon et al., 2013).

Most of the GI lesions occurring in CKD patients leads to GI bleeding (hemorrhage), which accounts for mortality up to 7% of CKD patients and about 20% of ESRD patients receiving renal transplantation (Shah, 1993). The incidence of GI bleeding is very high in patients with advanced stages of CKD as well as dialysis patients. The upper GI bleeding is predominant in CKD patients, and the mortality risk due to upper GI bleeding is about 3 fold higher than all other causes of hospital death in CKD patients (Liang et al., 2014b; Sood et al., 2012).

The most important causes of hemorrhage in CKD patients are angiodysplasia (vascular malformations), peptic ulcers (gastric and duodenal), watermelon stomach, ischemic bowel disease, colonic and rectal ulcers, and diverticular disease (Figure 1). The frequent use of heparin and other anticoagulants and uremic platelet dysfunction are implicated to the increased bleeding diathesis in CKD patients. The bleeding in CKD patients contributes to a quick loss of red blood cells (RBC) and acute anemia. As the circulating RBC helps platelets to contact with subendothelium at the site of wall injury, anemia itself can promote bleeding diathesis (Saeed et al., 2011). In addition, vascular calcification and volume overload also lead to spontaneous bleeding in patients with advanced stages of CKD. In clinical settings, the blood vomiting (hematemesis), dark coloured sticky faeces with partially digested blood (melena), the passage of fresh blood from anus (hematochezia), and/or unexplained decrease in the hemoglobin level (>2 g/dL) are indicators of GI bleeding in CKD patients (Song et al., 2015).

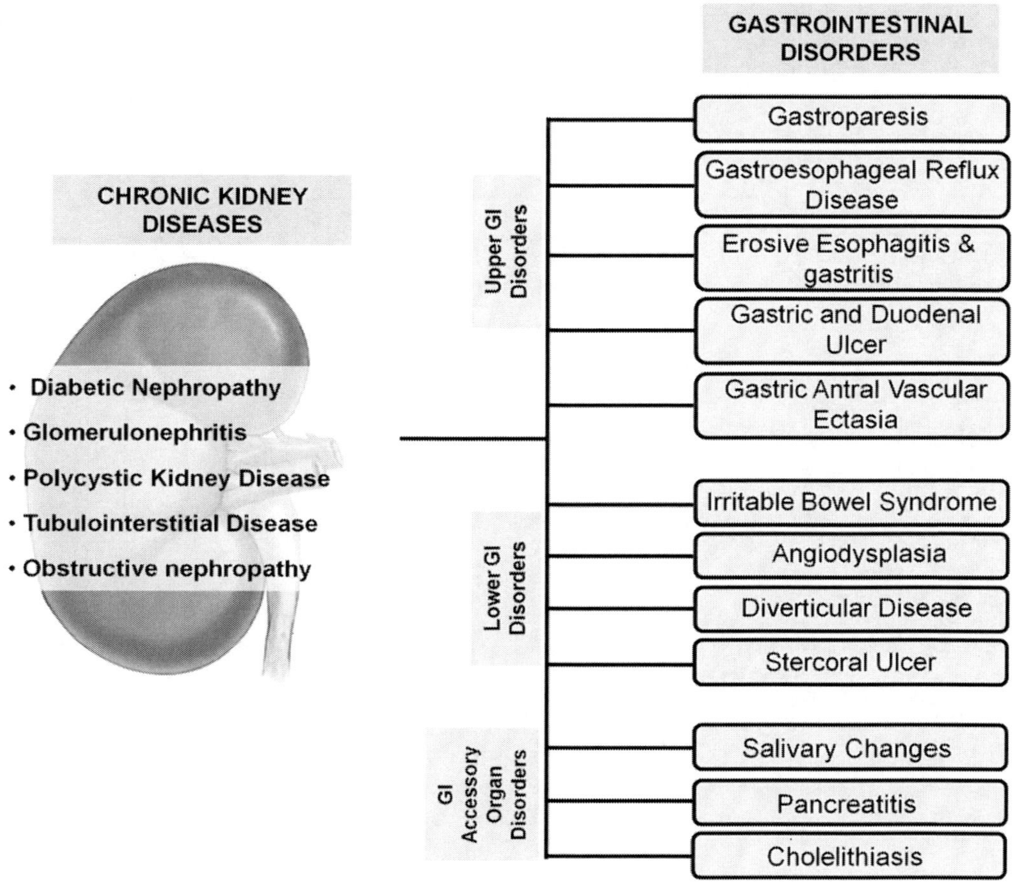

Figure 1. Most common GI disorders in CKD patients.

3.1 Factors Associated with GI Complications in CKD Patients

The occurrence of GI disorders in CKD patients is largely attributed to the underlying conditions, increased level of blood urea, imbalance of hormones regulating GI function, effects of dialysis, and medications used in treatments (Figure 2).

3.1.1. Metabolic Neuropathy

About 60% of ESRD patients are experiencing neuropathy symptoms due to uremia, hyperkalemia, and hyperphosphatemia (Krishnan and Kiernan, 2007; Ogura et al., 2001). The uremic neuropathy has been observed in ESRD patients and it is associated with functional disorders of GI systems. In addition, the metabolic disturbance caused by diabetes is also implicated in polyneuropathy in CKD patients. A molecular insight found that a very high urea and potassium depolarizes nerves membrane potential and resulting in the nerve dysfunction (Krishnan and Kiernan, 2007). A clinical study found that the dialysis patients exhibit impaired gastric myoelectric activity, which is indicated by abnormal waves of cutaneously recorded electrogastrograph (EGG) (Furgala et al., 2012). In this context, CKD-induced metabolic polyneuropathy can affect esophagus and gastric motor function, thereby impairing the upper GI function. Moreover, the regular use of calcium-channel blockers and nitrites are also important contributors to the development of GI disorders in CKD patients (Kawaguchi et al., 2009; Promberger et al., 2013).

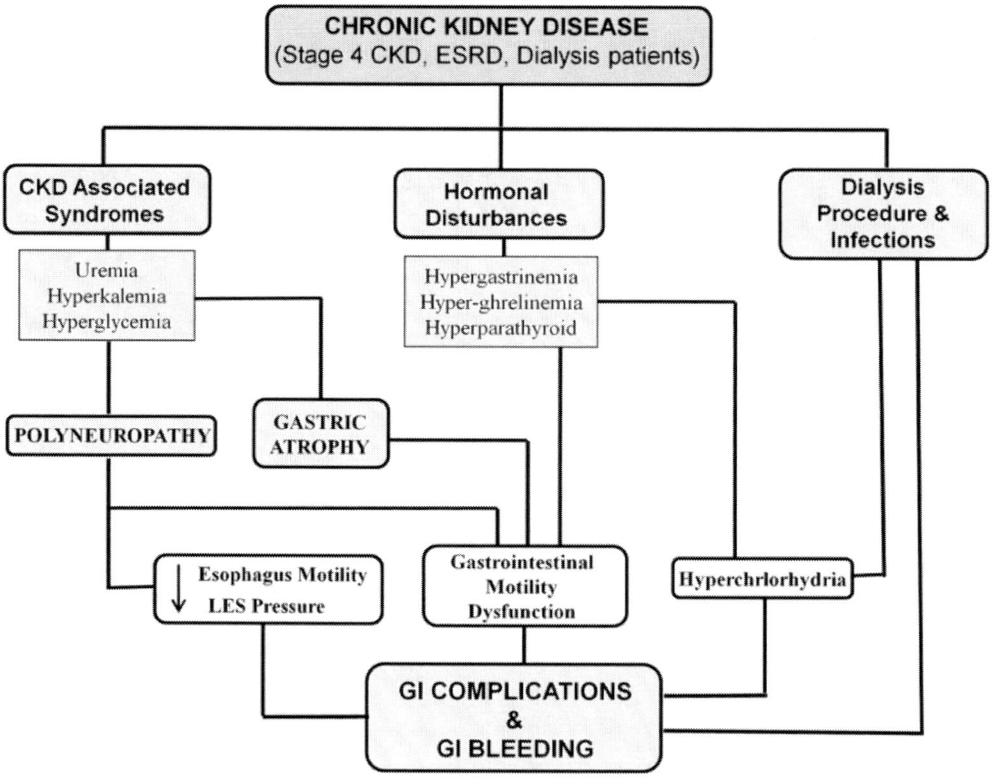

Figure 2. Factors associated with the development of GI disorders in CKD patients.

3.1.2. Hypergastrinemia

Gastrin is a key regulator of stomach acid production and secretion from parietal cells. Gastrin positively controls the lower esophageal sphincter (LES) pressure and relaxation. It also regulates gastric contraction, antrum muscle mobility, and pyloric sphincter. Given the fact that the kidney plays a central role in the elimination of gastrin, a very low GFR in CKD patients reduces the clearance of gastrin from circulation and resulting in hypergastrinemia. However, this may be secondary to overproduction of gastrin due to increased density of gastrin producing G-cells in CKD patients, which apparently results in hypergastrinemia. This increase is a vital aggressive factor for CKD associated gastroesophageal reflux disease (GERD) and other GI lesions (Fallone and Mayrand, 2001; Straathof et al., 1997).

An infection could also partly contribute to hypergastrinemia in ESRD patients. Clinical studies found that *Helicobacter pylori* (*H. pylori*) infection is common in patients under dialysis. The eradication of this infection reduced fasting gastrin concentration, and also restored gastric juice pH by decreasing ammonia in gastric juice, as it is already known that *H. pylori* produces ammonia from urea (Khedmat and Taheri, 2009; Tokushima et al., 1998). Further, ammonia production is detrimental to mucosal layer and GI tract epithelial cells due to its toxic nature, which might be responsible for GI bleeding in CKD patients with *H. pylori* infection (Megraud et al., 1992). In CKD and ESRD patients with *H. pylori* infection, a combination of proton pump inhibitor (PPI) with antibiotics (amoxicillin and clarithromycin) for 1 week, is more effective for the early eradication of *H pylori* and to avoid recurrent peptic ulcer diseases (Chang and Hu, 2015).

3.1.3. Hyper-Ghrelinemia

Ghrelin is an appetite stimulating peptide hormone, which is also an important contributor in the regulation of gastric and intestinal motility. This hormone also promotes intestinal cell proliferation and inhibits intestinal epithelial cell apoptosis caused by inflammation. Ghrelin exists in different forms such as acyl-ghrelin (active form), desacyl-ghrelin (non-active form) and C-ghrelin. These three forms have independent functions. The desacyl-ghrelin antagonizes the effects of acyl-ghrelin and ghrelin. Normally, about 80-90% of circulatory ghrelin is in the form of desacyl-ghrelin. Given the fact that ghrelin is primarily secreted by stomach and small intestine and degraded by the kidney, the metabolism and homeostasis of ghrelin is affected by renal dysfunction (Cheung and Mak, 2010; Delporte, 2013). Earlier studies suggest that the abnormal level of ghrelin primarily leads to the development of anorexia (loss of appetite) and cachexia (weight loss and muscle wastling) in CKD patients. In addition, severe gastroparesis and GERD are also correlated with the elevated level of circulatory ghrelin. But in all these studies, the assay method detected only total ghrelin (total of acyl-ghrelin, desacyl-ghrelin and ghrelin fragments) (Barros Ade et al., 2013).

Recent advancement in detection of ghrelin fractions revealed that the acyl-ghrelin level is low in CKD patients especially in hemodialysis patients. At the same time, the level of desacyl-ghrelin, an inactive form of ghrelin, is high in CKD patients due to poor clearance of this molecule by the kidney (Barros Ade et al., 2013). As the desacyl-ghrelin has an antagonistic effect on acyl-ghrelin and unacylated ghrelin, the increased concentration of desacyl-ghrelin contributes to GERD and gastric dysmotility related disorders in CKD patients. In support of this, recent findings revealed that acyl-ghrelin and ghrelin exert a stimulatory effect on motility of the antrum and duodenum, and the afferent pathway of vagus nerves is implicated in this response. In contrast, desacyl-ghrelin inhibits the motility of antrum. The vagal nervous response does not take part in this effect, but desacyl-ghrelin directly activates corticotropin-releasing factor (CRF) type 2 receptor (Fujimiya et al., 2010; Fujimiya et al., 2012). In this background, the impairment of ghrelin signaling due to uremia and metabolic disturbances mediated neural dysfunction is attributed to the functional disorders of the GI tract in CKD patients (Krishnan and Kiernan, 2007; Nahata et al., 2012; Ogura et al., 2001).

3.1.4. Hyperchlorhydria

The gastric acidity state varies (ranging from low to high) among the CKD patients. But in majority of CKD patients, gastric hypersecretory state has been found (Cervelli et al., 2012). Given the fact that the parathyroid hormone and the level of potassium are important regulators of gastric acid secretion, the hyperparathyroid and hyperkalemia state in CKD patients tend to increase gastric acid secretion by parietal cells (hydrochloric acid producing cells of stomach), resulting in hyperchlorhydria in these patients. However, a decrease in the secretion of gastric acid (hypochlorhydria) is observed in some ESRD patients especially in hyperuremic terminal ESRD patients as well as in patients on chronic maintenance dialysis. This is mainly due to gastric atrophy caused by chronic uremia and infections (Fallone and Mayrand, 2001). Although *H. pylori* infection primarily shows an increasing tendency of gastric acidity, the chronic uremia and persistent *H. pylori* infection causes atrophic gastritis, which leads to the insensitivity and dysfunction of parietal cells to gastrin resulting in hypoacidity state. In addition, the neutralization of stomach acid by ammonia produced from urea by *H. pylori* and other enterogenic microbes also leads to hypoacidity (Moustafa et al., 1997; Muto et al., 1985). Apart from this, the reduced sensitivity of gastric mucosal cells also leads to impairment of the negative feedback mechanism of gastrin production, and this could also be responsible for hypergastrinemia (Muto et al., 1985). Regardless of acid secretory state in the stomach, the CKD patients experience indigestion, delaying of stomach emptying, and peptic ulcer diseases.

3.2. Upper GI Disorders in CKD Patients

3.2.1. GERD and Gastroparesis in CKD Patients

GERD is one of the upper GI tract related digestive disorders, which is characterized by frequent reflux of gastric contents into the esophagus. As CKD is associated with increased incidence of digestion related disorders, these patients frequently encounter acid reflux diseases (Fallone and Mayrand, 2001). Gastroparesis is a condition of delaying in emptying of the stomach, which is often associated with dysmotility of the stomach and intestine (Hirata et al., 2012; Van Vlem et al., 2000). The incidence esophageal motility disorder, dyspepsia, gastroparesis, and GERD are relatively high in chronic kidney failure patients compared to the general population. A high proportion of this disorder is observed in uremia patients and patients under dialysis. In particular, peritoneal dialysis patients are easily susceptible to GERD due to intraperitoneal pressure. A frequent heartburn, regurgitation of acid and stomach content, and feeling fullness are most commonly observed in these patients (Hirata et al., 2012; Kawaguchi et al., 2009; Van Vlem et al., 2000).

3.2.1.1. Pathophysiology of GERD and Gastroparesis in CKD patients

The pathophysiology of gastroparesis, dyspepsia, and GERD in CKD patients are multifactorial. In CKD patients, this condition is mainly due to increased relaxation of LES, a ring of muscle between the esophagus and stomach. In addition, decreased clearance of esophageal contents due to impaired peristalsis (a wave-like contraction of GI tract muscle) also contributes to GERD (Fallone and Mayrand, 2001). The hormonal disturbances, electrolyte imbalance and uremic toxins are are important contributors in the functional disorders of the esophagus and stomach. The uremic polyneuropathy and abnormal levels of GI motility regulating hormones such as gastrin and ghrelin plays a vital role in the development of gastroparesis and GERD in CKD patients (Fallone and Mayrand, 2001).

3.2.1.2. Treatment and Management of Gastroparesis and GERD

The general symptoms of GERD and gastroparesis do not accurately predict these disorders in CKD patients because of overlap of multiple disorders in those patients. In most instances, recurrent nausea, anorexia and vomiting are indicators of these disorders. The improvement of esophageal and gastric motility and emptying of the stomach is the primary target for the treatment of GERD in CKD patients. The suppression of uremic neuropathy is the best effective therapy for functional disturbances of the GI tract and its associated disorders including GERD and gastroparesis. Given the fact that potassium (K^+) has a vital role in the development of uremic neuropathy, a dietary restriction of K^+ could help to prevent the neuropathy in the early stage of CKD (Krishnan et al., 2006). Although hemodialysis reduces blood urea, it does not improve the gastric emptying time, hence, symptom based therapy provides relief from these disorders (Van Vlem et al., 2000). The *H. pylori* based GERD in CKD patients can be treated with a short-course (1 week) of triple based eradication therapy, which consists of proton pump inhibitor (lansoprazole or omeprazole) along with antibiotics such as amoxicillin (750 mg a day) and clarithromycin (400 mg a day) (Itatsu et al., 2007; Liang et al., 2011). However, the long-term use of PPI can worsen CKD.

Currently, metoclopramide and erythromycin are considered as gastroprokinetic drugs to increase gastric emptying in hemodialysis patients. These drugs promote gastric and intestinal motility thereby improves gastroparesis and consequently attenuates GERD. A clinical study found that long-term use of these drugs at lower and safest dose can improve the serum albumin level within 3 months, which indicates the improvement in gastric motility and nutritional status in dialysis patients (Silang et al., 2001). Recently, ghrelin mimetics are developed and they are providing great relief from gastroparesis by increasing gastric emptying. In addition, ghrelin mimetics potentially reduces nausea and vomiting (Sanger and Furness, 2016). The administration of exogenous ghrelin and ghrelin receptor agonists also increases appetite, reduces muscle wastling, improves malnutrition conditions (Deboer et al., 2008). Although there are multiple treatment options for uremic and hyperkalemic neuropathy related GI disorders, renal transplantation is the only effective treatment to prevent neurological disturbance induced disorders, including GERD and gastroparesis (Krishnan et al., 2006; Ramírez and Gómez, 2012).

3.2.2. Peptic Ulcer Disease (PUD)

Peptic ulcer disease (PUD) is the most common upper GI problem in advanced stages of CKD (Parasa et al., 2013). In general, PUD is predominantly due to erosion of gastric mucosa by hyperacidity, which occurs mainly in stage 4 and 5 of CKD during which elevated level of positive regulators (parathyroid hormone, calcium and potassium) of gastric acid secretion has been observed (Fallone and Mayrand, 2001). In ESRD patients, diabetes, congestive heart failure, hypoalbuminemia, and peritoneal dialysis are important risk factor for PUD (Chen et al., 2010). The incidence of PUD substantially increased in elder and non-steroidal anti-inflammatory drug (NSAID) receiving CKD patients. The *H. pylori* infection is common in ESRD patients and this colonization can also cause chronic superficial gastritis, which ultimately leads to peptic ulcer.

Clinical studies disclosed that the recurrent rate of PUD is high in hemodialysis patients even without *H. pylori* infection (Liang et al., 2014a). This indicates that CKD itself is an independent risk factor for PUD. The influence of hemodialysis on the occurrence of PUD remains largely unknown. However, the intradialytic hypotension and hemodynamic changes might contribute to PUD in patients on maintenance dialysis. Given that hypotension is more frequent in hemodialysis patients, the hypotension induces gastrointestinal ischemia by splanchnic hypoperfusion resulting in a stress induced ulcer like gastric mucosal lesions in these patients (Liang et al., 2014a). The chronic and severe PUD leads to bleeding in CKD patients. The patients with ESRD and a moderate degree of CKD who are suffering from peptic ulcer bleeding, frequently encounters rebleeding related mortality (Lin et al., 2012).

3.2.2.1. Diagnosis and Treatment of PUD in CKD Patients

The endoscopic findings of active bleeding, visible vessels, blood in the stomach, adherent clot are indicators of PUD associated bleeding in the upper GI tract. In the case of *H. pylori* induced PUD, the determination of ratio of urea to ammonium in the intragastric sample is a reliable method to confirm infection related PUD in CKD patients (Neithercut et al., 1993). In ESRD patients with recurrent PUD-related gastric and duodenal bleeding, an early endoscopic procedure for initial hemostasis and a short course of high intravenous dose of PPI can reduce the rebleeding incidence (Lin et al., 2012). A clinical study suggests that omeprazole is effective in reducing the incidence of PUD in hemodialysis patients (Liang et al., 2011). In NSAID drug (aspirin) related PUD, early treatment with lower doses of PPI can prevent non-variceal bleeding in the upper GI tract of CKD patients (Lim et al., 2015). However, some PPI can interfere with CKD management therapeutics. For example, the acid suppressing drugs such as pantoprazole and ranitidine interacts with calcium carbonate ($CaCO_3$), which is a phosphate binder used to control hyperphosphatemia in CKD patients but omeprazole does not influence the activity of phosphate binders (Cervelli et al., 2012; Sechet et al., 1999). Since the gastric acid suppression therapy is regularly used in dialysis patients, physicians should be aware of the potential influence of acid suppression on the efficacy of phosphate binders.

3.2.3. Gastric Antral Vascular Ectasia

The gastric antral vascular ectasia (GAVE) is currently recognized as one of the important causes of the occult and obscure gastric bleeding in CKD patients especially in patients under maintenance dialysis (Iguchi et al., 2011). This pathological condition is commonly called as 'watermelon stomach' due to its unique appearance in the gastric antrum as like stripes on watermelon. GAVE is endoscopically characterized by multiple long stripes of red blood vessels (watermelon stomach) or a diffused pattern of red vessels (diffuse antral vascular ectasia) from the pylorus to antrum, along with dilatation of the gastric capillaries and hemorrhage. The histological assessment revealed that capillary ectasia with thrombosis, superficial hyperplastic antral mucosa, fibromuscular hyperplasia in the lamina propria, and abnormal submucosal vasculature are common features of GAVE (Iguchi et al., 2011; Ohira et al., 2013).

The pathogenesis of GAVE in CKD patients remains largely unknown. However, uremia-induced failure of gastric emptying increases mechanical stress on the antrum, which is believed to contribute to the development of GAVE in CKD patients. In these patients, the platelet dysfunction due to uremia is the primary risk factor for antrum bleeding (Iguchi et al., 2011). Apart from this, liver cirrhosis and portal hypertension are often associated with the development of GAVE (Iguchi et al., 2011). So the co-existence of CKD and chronic liver disease leads to the development of GAVE in renal patients.

3.2.3.1. Diagnosis and Treatment

The capsule endoscopy is a more reliable method for the detection of GAVE, which does not need gastric inflation and sequent compression of the vasculature as like in conventional endoscopy (Iguchi et al., 2011). Given the fact that severe erosive gastritis shares many of the endoscopic features of watermelon stomach (Saadah, 2011), a careful examination should be carried out to avoid diagnostic misconception. A clinical study suggests that GAVE in ESRD patients under hemodialysis can be improved by switching to continuous ambulatory peritoneal dialysis (Yorioka et al., 1996). This study also indicates that volume overload does not engage in GAVE development. The pharmacological treatment with tranexamic acid or estrogen-progesterone is efficacious in CKD patients with GAVE (Lata et al., 2012). The argon plasma coagulation (APC) is a standard endoscopic therapy used to treat GAVE with bleeding, which is safer and easier to use, but the patients is required to undergo this therapy multiple times to achieve the efficient benefit (Iguchi et al., 2011). The endoscopic bipolar electrocoagulation with gold probe also provides a significant endoscopic and hematologic improvement from GAVE related GI bleeding in ESRD patients (Stefanidis et al., 2006). The blood transfusion is required in the case of bleeding, which helps to improve severe anemia due to blood loss.

3.3. Lower GI Disorders in CKD Patients

3.3.1. Angiodysplasia of the Colon

Angiodysplasia is a malformation of small vessels of the GI tract, which is characterized by colon swelling and fragile blood vessels in the colon. Angiodysplasia is a degenerative lesion, which is primarily due to chronic and repeated damage to the walls of vessels. In CKD patients, this is mainly due to the intestinal dysmotility, constipation, vascular stenosis due to hyperphosphatemia and hyperkalemia, and punctures in the muscular layers of the colon. This leads to deformation of vessels and eventually causes hypoxemia and hypoxia in the colon wall, which can further extend the intestinal vessel damage, especially in older CKD patients (Galanopoulos, 2012). It is the most common cause of bleeding in the lower part of GI mainly in the cecum and ascending colon, however, angiodysplasia can also occur in other sections of the GI tract of CKD patients. Multiple hemorrhagic episodes are common and are mostly occult and intermittent in nature. This vascular lesion accounts for 19-32% recurrent bleeding in the lower GI tract of patients with chronic renal failure, and this incidence is even high in patients under maintenance dialysis (Galanopoulos, 2012; Saeed et al., 2011).

Diagnosis and Treatment: A computerized tomographic angiography (CT angiography) can reveal the early signs of angiodysplasia. This technique helps in localizing the hemorrhage site in patients with prolonged and active draining vessels. This procedure requires intravenous administration of contrasting agent and the sensitivity of detection is low in the case of intermittent bleeding. These are major limitations in using the CT angiography method in CKD patients (Galanopoulos, 2012). The colonoscopy is a sensitive method to detect the angiodysplasia in the colon. Endoscopically, lesions are flat or raised above the mucosal layer. However, a false positive can occur by minor trauma during endoscopy. Similarly, a false negative could also occur in volume depleted as well as in severe anemic patients. So repeated endoscopy helps to refine the specificity of this problem in CKD patients (Galanopoulos, 2012; Kaaroud et al., 2008). In recent years, colon capsule endoscopy (CCE), a minimal invasive procedure, is the best option for diagnosis of the colon angiodysplasia, which offers a higher possibility to reveal the hemorrhage sites in the intestine when other types of endoscopy fails to detect this lesion (Kaaroud et al., 2008).

In general, the angiodysplasia bleeding stops spontaneously in more than 90% cases. The endoscopic hemostatic therapy is the initial form of treatment for the patients with active hemorrhagic angiodysplasia (Thomas et al., 2008). APC and bipolar coagulation treatment with endoscopic procedure have been successfully used to treat angiodysplasia in the colon as well as in the small intestine. However, surgical resection should be carried out in patients with persistent or recurrent hemorrhage (Galanopoulos, 2012; Kaaroud et al., 2008).

3.3.2. Diverticular Disease and Bleeding

Diverticulosis is one of the common causes of lower GI bleeding in ESRD patients. The incidence of lower GI bleeding due to this disorder in CKD is same as in general population (about 30-50%). The patients on maintenance dialysis for adult polycystic kidney disease have a high incidence (60-80%) of diverticular bleeding (Kumar et al., 2006; Saeed et al., 2011). Diverticuli is a outpouching of intestinal mucosa in the weakened area of muscle layers. Constipation is the major cause of diverticulosis and it is also associated with overt or occult bleeding from diverticula in ESRD patients. The usage of phosphate and calcium binders (to reduce the circulatory level of these two elements) in ESRD patients under dialysis, is also associated with the development of diverticulitis (inflammation of diverticula) by increasing constipation (Saeed et al., 2011). Atherosclerosis, visceral fat, and adipose tissue accumulation lead to arteriolar changes in the larger intestine and diverticulum, and this contributes to colonic diverticular hemorrhage in CKD patients (Nagata et al., 2015).

Diagnosis and Treatment of diverticular disease in CKD patients: Colonoscopy is the initial choice for the examination when the presence of diverticulosis is suspected. This procedure is used to diagnosis and treat if bleeding of diverticula is identified in CKD patients but this procedure is not always useful as some patients have intermittent bleeding. A contrast-enhanced magnetic resonance angiography (MRA) is a more reliable technique to detect intermittent bleeding diverticula. The volume resuscitation is useful for the management of diverticular bleeding in the colon. In peritoneal dialysis patients, the presence of more than 10 diverticulum in a size of >10mm in the colon increases the risk for acute peritonitis (Saeed et al., 2011). A prompt laparotomy is necessary to avoid severe complications such as peritonitis and death.

3.3.3. Stercoral Ulcer of the Colon

The hard and larger fecal mass induces necrosis and ulceration of the mucosal layer of the colon, which is called as stercoral ulcer. As the prolonged constipation is quite common in advanced stages of CKD and in elder chronic dialysis patients, the stercoral ulcer is mostly developed in the sigmoid colon and rectum of CKD patients. The use of phosphate binders (sevelamer), fluid restriction, and slower bowel movement are important contributors of chronic constipation in CKD patients (Saeed et al., 2012). The patients with long-term stercoral ulcer are at risk for life threatening perforation in this segment of the colon, which is due to secondary infections, fibrosis and fecal material induced granulomatous inflammation in the ulcer. The stercoral perforation leads to acute peritonitis and is associated with high mortality (more than 50%) caused by stercoral ulcer (Saeed et al., 2011).

Diagnosis and Treatment: Stercoral ulcer also causes hemorrhage from the lower intestine and it can be identified by endoscopic procedures. The fecal masses on imaging along with colonoscopy and histological examination of biopsy can help to identify the factors associated with this problem in CKD patients. Endoscopically, the lesions are irregular in shape, vary in depth (mucosal ulceration to perforation) and sharply protrude from the mucosal layer. The bleeding stercoral ulcer can be treated with endoscopic multipolar electrocoagulation or APC therapy with prophylactic antibiotics. However, surgical intervention is required in patients with perforation and massive/uncontrolled bleeding (Saeed et al., 2011; Saeed et al., 2012).

3.3.4. Irritable Bowel Syndrome

Irritable bowel syndrome (IBS) is one of the functional disorders of the large intestine. This complication is also frequently observed in CKD patients under dialysis (Kahvecioglu et al., 2005). The pathophysiology of IBS in CKD patients is multifactorial with an unknown etiology. The altered intestinal activity (motility and secretion), visceral hypersensitivity, and impairment of the brain-gut axis are thought to play a central role in the emergence of IBS in CKD patients (Fiderkiewicz et al., 2011). In addition, anxiety and generalized mood depression are common in dialysis patients, and these psychological stress also leads to IBS in ESRD patients under maintenance dialysis (Kahvecioglu et al., 2005). The symptoms of IBS are epigastric pain associated with defecation or changes in bowel habit with disorders in defecation along with diarrhea or constipation (Fiderkiewicz et al., 2011).

Diagnosis and Management of IBS in CKD patients: As the IBS is not a single disorder entity, a definitive therapeutics has not been outlined for this GI problem in the general population and ESRD patients. In the general population, the treatment is preceded based on symptoms. Various symptomatic therapeutics include laxatives, dopamine antagonists, histamine antagonists, sedatives, and/or antibiotics. For IBS patients with diarrhea, probiotics along with antidiarrheal agents (loperamide and diphenoxylate) are required. The pharmacological agents such as linaclotide and lubiprostone are promising for the relief of multiple symptoms in IBS patients suffering from constipation (Lazaraki et al., 2014). But in CKD patients, these drugs should be used cautiously to avoid detrimental effects. Recently, rifaximin, an antibiotic, is approved by FDA for the treatment of IBS with diarrhea. This drug also improves systemic hemodynamics and renal function in patients with advanced liver cirrhosis (Kalambokis et al., 2012).

4. Complications in Accessory Digestive Organs

The organs such as salivary glands, liver, gallbladder and pancreas play a crucial role in the process of digestion although they are not part of the GI tract. CKD apparently causes an alteration in the functions of these organs. In CKD patients, the metabolic disturbances, endocrinological abnormalities, and imbalance in electrolytes lead to several systemic complications in extra-renal organs including salivary glands, gallbladder, and pancreas.

4.1. Oral and Salivary Changes in CKD Patients

Saliva is a unique fluid, which initiates the digestion of food. In patients with chronic renal diseases, the salivary composition, flow and concentration is drastically changed. A high level of urea in ESRD patients adversely affects salivary gland function and saliva composition (Anuradha et al., 2015). In ESRD patients, the discharge of urea into saliva not only affects the digestion but also has a detrimental effect on oral and GI tract health. Several clinical studies have observed a very high rate of oral pathology in dialysis patients. The most common oral symptoms in CKD patients are taste disturbances, uremic odor in the mouth, dysphagia, mucosal inflammation, oral mucosal ecchymosis/erythematous, oral ulceration, and/or enamel hypoplasia. A typical ammoniacal odor is often observed in CKD patients, which is due to the breakdown of urea in saliva and formation of ammonia. In addition, a persistent level of urea and ammonia in saliva alters taste sensation in CKD patients, and some patients have unpleasant and/or metallic taste in the mouth. The sweet and sour tastes are most seriously affected in ESRD patients (Akar et al., 2011; Kaushik et al., 2013). In addition, these patients are easily susceptible to dental calculus due to a very high level of salivary urea and phosphate (Anuradha et al., 2015).

Gingival bleeding and periodontitis are well documented oral manifestations in ESRD patients. The accumulation of ammonia in the mouth can result in gingival mucosal inflammation (gingivitis) and irritation. A decrease in salivary mucin prone to infections and ammonia-induced inflammation and tissue damage, which consequently leads to gingival bleeding, mucosal and tongue pain in ESRD patients. However, we cannot exclude the oral bleeding due to uremia-induced platelet dysfunction, and repeated use of anticoagulants during dialysis (Kaushik et al., 2013). The gingival bleeding facilitates the opportunity for the colonization of pathogenic organisms (bacteria, candida albican, and herpes simplex virus) due to compromised salivary defense and humoral defense system in ESRD patients. The sustained infection may cause life threading sepsis in CKD patients. The presence of plaque and calculus in CKD patients indicates insufficient oral care. The oral hygiene measures such as flossing, tooth brushing, and mouthwashes can reduce gingivitis. The mechanical debridement and prophylaxis with antibiotics can effectively prevent the development of periodontal diseases (Akar et al., 2011).

4.2. Pancreatitis in CKD Patients

Pancreatic disorders are most commonly reported in ESRD patients receiving chronic dialysis. The frequency of pancreatic abnormalities are very high (up to 60%) in both hemodialysis and peritoneal dialysis patients (Hou et al., 2013; Quraishi et al., 2005). Pancreatitis, an inflammation of the pancreas, is found in the majority of ESRD patients undergoing chronic dialysis (Quraishi et al., 2005). The mortality due to acute pancreatitis in CKD patients is up to 56%. The etiology of pancreatitis in renal failure patient is multifactorial. The dialysis induced hypotension, ischemia events during dialysis, underlying co-morbidity mainly hyperinsulinemia are important contributors in the generation of acute pancreatitis in chronic hemodialysis patients (Kishino et al., 2005). The autopsy study from patients died due to chronic renal failure disclosed the diffused pattern of histological changes in the pancreas including duct ectasia, periductal fibrosis, atrophy, calcification, amyloidosis, and necrosis of peripancreatic fat.

The serum amylase activity higher than 3 fold together with acute abdominal pain is an indicator of pancreatitis. However, the diagnosis of pancreatitis in dialysis patients by using routine biochemical assay is difficult due to the fact that plasma amylase activity is always elevated in uremic and CKD patients under chronic dialysis (Villacorta et al., 2010). In peritoneal dialysis patients, the use of icodextrin (a colloid osmotic agent derived from maltodextrin used for peritoneal dialysis) interferes with serum amylase assay, which shows a falsely low serum activity of α-amylase in PD patients with pancreatitis. In this case, the serum lipase concentration along with dialysate concentration of amylase at least 100 IU/L confirms the presence of acute pancreatitis (Villacorta et al., 2010). These patients require clinical screening to evaluate the nature and severity of pancreatitis. The conventional methods such as bowel rest and nasogastric suction help to manage pancreatitis in CKD patients. To reduce the risk of pancreatic hemorrhage, the use of heparin during dialysis should be minimized.

4.3. Gallbladder Stone in CKD Patients

Gallbladder disorders are due to the formation of solid calculi in the gallbladder (cholelithiasis) or bile duct (choledocholithiasis). The gallstones are classified depending on the concentration of cholesterol as follows: cholesterol stone (>70% cholesterol content), black pigment stone (<30% cholesterol content) and mixed stone (cholesterol content between 30-70%). The incidence of gallstone diseases is high in advanced stages of chronic renal insufficiency (Genctoy et al., 2014). Chronic uremia and hyperthyroidism are important contributors in gallstone formation in CKD patients (Cariati, 2013). The metabolic changes in the kidney disease along with high phosphorus and calcium access may initiate a series of alterations in bile composition and consequently leads to choledocholithiasis (Li Vecchi et al., 2003). The pathogenesis of gallstone in these patients is linked to decreased gallbladder motility, changes in bile composition and increased tendency to nucleation (Bektas et al., 2005). The autonomic neuropathy due to uremia could partly contribute to gallbladder stone formation and its associated disorders in hemodialysis patients (Genctoy et al., 2014).

The real-time ultrasound is reliable to detect gallstones in CKD patients. The asymptomatic lithiasis usually does not require surgical treatment. But patients presenting with acute abdominal pain or gallstone associated complications such as cholecystitis, cholangitis, jaundice or pancreatitis, are required immediate surgical interventions to avoid mortality. The laparoscopic cholecystectomy (LC) is a gold standard therapy for patients with symptomatic uncomplicated cholelithiasis (Brito et al., 2010). Endoscopic papillary balloon dilation (EPBD) is also an effective and safe method to remove bile duct stones in CKD patients. However, EPBD should be carefully performed in ESRD patients taking anticoagulants at the time of dialysis, which increases bleeding risk in these patients (Takahara et al., 2012).

Conclusion

The chronic renal disease frequently leads to the development of different GI lesions. The GI associated symptoms in CKD patients are ranging from salivary changes to GI bleeding. The GI disorders in renal patients depend on the severity and nature of CKD, therapeutics and renal maintenance procedures (hemodialysis or peritoneal dialysis), and comorbidities (CVD, hypertension, diabetes, etc.). The most frequent GI complications in CKD patients are gastroparesis, GERD, peptic ulcer disease, watermelon stomach, irritable bowel syndrome, angiodysplasia, diverticular bleeding, stercoral ulcer, and pancreatitis. The pathophysiology of GI disorders in CKD patients is multifactorial and complicated. However, the metabolic disturbances (uremia, diabetes, hypertension), endocrinological abnormalities (hyperparathyroidism, hypergastrinemia, hyper-ghrelinemia), and imbalance in electrolytes (hyperkalemia, hyperphosphatemia, hypercalcemia) are important contributors in the emergence of functional disorders of GI in CKD patients. Many of the CKD patients experience bleeding from upper and lower GI lesions due to vascular anomalies and coagulation abnormalities. Endoscopic procedures are useful in diagnosis and therapy of GI abnormalities with bleeding in ESRD patients. Sometimes therapeutic attempt for GI disorder in CKD patients may be hindered by overlapping of many complications. Hence, the awareness and adequate knowledge of caregivers about CKD associated GI disorders can offer prompt recognition and appropriate therapy.

References

Akar H, Akar GC, Carrero JJ, Stenvinkel P, Lindholm B, Systemic consequences of poor oral health in chronic kidney disease patients. *Clin J Am Soc Nephrol,* 2011; 6: 218-26.

Anuradha BR, Katta S, Kode VS, Praveena C, Sathe N, Sandeep N, Penumarty S, Oral and salivary changes in patients with chronic kidney disease: A clinical and biochemical study. *J Indian Soc Periodontol,* 2015; 19: 297-301.

Barros Ade F, Moraes C, Pinto MB, Lobo JC, Mafra D, Is there association between acyl-ghrelin and inflammation in hemodialysis patients? *J Bras Nefrol,* 2013; 35: 120-6.

Bektas A, Belet U, Kelkitli E, Bakir T, Acikgoz A, Akpolat T, Ultrasonic gallbladder function in chronic kidney disease: does predialysis, hemodialysis, or CAPD affect it? *Ren Fail,* 2005; 27: 677-81.

Boor P, Sebekova K, Ostendorf T, Floege J, Treatment targets in renal fibrosis. *Nephrol Dial Transplant,* 2007; 22: 3391-407.

Brito AT, Azevedo LS, Nahas WC, Matheus AS, Jukemura J, Cholelithiasis in patients on the kidney transplant waiting list. *Clinics* (Sao Paulo), 2010; 65: 389-91.

Cariati A, Blackberry pigment (whitlockite) gallstones in uremic patient. *Clin Res Hepatol Gastroenterol,* 2013; 37: e69-72.

Cervelli MJ, Shaman A, Meade A, Carroll R, Mcdonald SP, Effect of gastric acid suppression with pantoprazole on the efficacy of calcium carbonate as a phosphate binder in haemodialysis patients. *Nephrology* (Carlton), 2012; 17: 458-65.

Chang SS, Hu HY, Helicobacter pylori: Effect of coexisting diseases and update on treatment regimens. *World J Gastrointest Pharmacol Ther,* 2015; 6: 127-36.

Chen YT, Yang WC, Lin CC, Ng YY, Chen JY, Li SY, Comparison of peptic ulcer disease risk between peritoneal and hemodialysis patients. *Am J Nephrol,* 2010; 32: 212-8.

Cheung WW, Mak RH, Ghrelin in chronic kidney disease. *Int J Pept,* 2010; 2010.

Deboer MD, Zhu X, Levasseur PR, Inui A, Hu Z, Han G, Mitch WE, Taylor JE, Halem HA, Dong JZ, Datta R, Culler MD, Marks DL, Ghrelin treatment of chronic kidney disease: improvements in lean body mass and cytokine profile. *Endocrinology,* 2008; 149: 827-35.

Delporte C, Structure and physiological actions of ghrelin. Scientifica (Cairo), 2013; 2013: 518909.

Dong R, Guo ZY, Ding JR, Zhou YY, Wu H, Gastrointestinal symptoms: a comparison between patients undergoing peritoneal dialysis and hemodialysis. *World J Gastroenterol,* 2014; 20: 11370-5.

Fallone CA, Mayrand S, Gastroesophageal reflux and hyperacidity in chronic renal failure. *Perit Dial Int,* 2001; 21 Suppl 3: S295-9.

Fiderkiewicz B, Rydzewska-Rosolowska A, Mysliwiec M, Birecka M, Kaczanowska B, Rydzewska G, Rydzewski A, Factors associated with irritable bowel syndrome symptoms in hemodialysis patients. *World J Gastroenterol,* 2011; 17: 1976-81.

Fujimiya M, Asakawa A, Ataka K, Chen CY, Kato I, Inui A, Ghrelin, des-acyl ghrelin, and obestatin: regulatory roles on the gastrointestinal motility. *Int J Pept,* 2010; 2010.

Fujimiya M, Ataka K, Asakawa A, Chen CY, Kato I, Inui A, Regulation of gastroduodenal motility: acyl ghrelin, des-acyl ghrelin and obestatin and hypothalamic peptides. *Digestion,* 2012; 85: 90-4.

Furgala A, Blaut-Kadzielska U, Stojakowska M, Dobrek L, Mazur M, Machowska A, Thor PJ, Gastric dysfunction in dialysed patients with chronic renal failure. *Folia Med Cracov,* 2012; 52: 39-55.

Galanopoulos G, Angiodysplastic lesions as a cause of colonic bleeding in patients with chronic renal disease: is there an association? *Saudi J Kidney Dis Transpl,* 2012; 23: 925-8.

Genctoy G, Ayidaga S, Ergun T, Lakadamyali H, Erbayrak M, Sezer S, Increased frequency of gallbladder stone and related parameters in hemodialysis patients. *Turk J Gastroenterol,* 2014; 25: 54-8.

Hirata ES, Mesquita MA, Alves Filho G, Camargo EE, Gastric emptying study by scintigraphy in patients with chronic renal failure. *Rev Bras Anestesiol,* 2012; 62: 39-47.

Hodgkins KS, Schnaper HW, Tubulointerstitial injury and the progression of chronic kidney disease. *Pediatr Nephrol,* 2012; 27: 901-9.

Hou SW, Lee YK, Hsu CY, Lee CC, Su YC, Increased risk of acute pancreatitis in patients with chronic hemodialysis: a 4-year follow-up study. *PLoS One,* 2013; 8: e71801.

Iguchi A, James Kazama J, Komatsu M, Kaneko Y, Iino N, Goto S, Narita I, Three cases of gastric antral vascular ectasia in chronic renal failure. *Case Rep Nephrol Urol,* 2011; 1: 15-9.

Itatsu T, Miwa H, Nagahara A, Kubota M, Miyazaki A, Sato N, Hayashida Y, Eradication of Helicobacter pylori in hemodialysis patients. *Ren Fail,* 2007; 29: 97-102.

Kaaroud H, Fatma LB, Beji S, Boubaker K, Hedri H, Hamida FB, El Younsi F, Abdallah TB, Maiz HB, Kheder A, Gastrointestinal angiodysplasia in chronic renal failure. *Saudi J Kidney Dis Transpl,* 2008; 19: 809-12.

Kahvecioglu S, Akdag I, Kiyici M, Gullulu M, Yavuz M, Ersoy A, Dilek K, Yurtkuran M, High prevalence of irritable bowel syndrome and upper gastrointestinal symptoms in patients with chronic renal failure. *J Nephrol,* 2005; 18: 61-6.

Kalambokis GN, Mouzaki A, Rodi M, Pappas K, Fotopoulos A, Xourgia X, Tsianos EV, Rifaximin improves systemic hemodynamics and renal function in patients with alcohol-related cirrhosis and ascites. *Clin Gastroenterol Hepatol,* 2012; 10: 815-8.

Kaushik A, Reddy SS, Umesh L, Devi BK, Santana N, Rakesh N, Oral and salivary changes among renal patients undergoing hemodialysis: A cross-sectional study. *Indian J Nephrol,* 2013; 23: 125-9.

Kawaguchi Y, Mine T, Kawana I, Yasuzaki H, Kokuho T, Toya Y, Ohnishi T, Umemura S, Gastroesophageal reflux disease in chronic renal failure patients: evaluation by endoscopic examination. *Tokai J Exp Clin Med,* 2009; 34: 80-3.

Khedmat H, Taheri S, Current knowledge on helicobacter pylori infection in end stage renal disease patients. *Saudi J Kidney Dis Transpl,* 2009; 20: 969-74.

Kishino T, Nakamura K, Mori H, Yamaguchi Y, Takahashi S, Ishida H, Saito S, Watanabe T, Acute pancreatitis during haemodialysis. *Nephrol Dial Transplant,* 2005; 20: 2012-3.

Krishnan AV, Kiernan MC, Uremic neuropathy: clinical features and new pathophysiological insights. *Muscle Nerve,* 2007; 35: 273-90.

Krishnan AV, Phoon RK, Pussell BA, Charlesworth JA, Bostock H, Kiernan MC, Neuropathy, axonal Na^+/K^+ pump function and activity-dependent excitability changes in end-stage kidney disease. *Clin Neurophysiol,* 2006; 117: 992-9.

Kumar S, Adeva M, King BF, Kamath PS, Torres VE, Duodenal diverticulosis in autosomal dominant polycystic kidney disease. *Nephrol Dial Transplant,* 2006; 21: 3576-8.

Lata S, Gupta V, Nandwani A, Sharma P, Watermelon stomach in end-stage renal disease patient. *Indian J Nephrol,* 2012; 22: 477-9.

Lazaraki G, Chatzimavroudis G, Katsinelos P, Recent advances in pharmacological treatment of irritable bowel syndrome. *World J Gastroenterol,* 2014; 20: 8867-85.

Levey AS, Eckardt KU, Tsukamoto Y, Levin A, Coresh J, Rossert J, De Zeeuw D, Hostetter TH, Lameire N, Eknoyan G, Definition and classification of chronic kidney disease: a position statement from Kidney Disease: Improving Global Outcomes (KDIGO). *Kidney Int,* 2005; 67: 2089-100.

Li Vecchi M, Soresi M, Cusimano R, Carroccio A, Corrado C, Gioe A, Montalto G, Prevalence of biliary lithiasis in a Sicilian population of chronic renal failure patients. *Nephrol Dial Transplant,* 2003; 18: 2321-4.

Liang CC, Muo CH, Wang IK, Chang CT, Chou CY, Liu JH, Yen TH, Huang CC, Chung CJ, Peptic ulcer disease risk in chronic kidney disease: ten-year incidence, ulcer location, and ulcerogenic effect of medications. *PLoS One,* 2014a; 9: e87952.

Liang CC, Wang IK, Lin HH, Yeh HC, Liu JH, Kuo HL, Hsu WM, Huang CC, Chang CT, Prophylactic use of omeprazole associated with a reduced risk of peptic ulcer disease among maintenance hemodialysis patients. *Ren Fail,* 2011; 33: 323-8.

Liang CC, Wang SM, Kuo HL, Chang CT, Liu JH, Lin HH, Wang IK, Yang YF, Lu YJ, Chou CY, Huang CC, Upper gastrointestinal bleeding in patients with CKD. *Clin J Am Soc Nephrol,* 2014b; 9: 1354-9.

Lim H, Kim JH, Baik GH, Park JW, Kang HS, Moon SH, Park CK, Effect of low-dose proton pump inhibitor on preventing upper gastrointestinal bleeding in chronic kidney disease patients receiving aspirin. *J Gastroenterol Hepatol, 2015*; 30: 478-84.

Lin SC, Wu KL, Chiu KW, Lee CT, Chiu YC, Chou YP, Hu ML, Tai WC, Chiou SS, Hu TH, Changchien CS, Chuah SK, Risk factors influencing the outcome of peptic ulcer bleeding in end stage renal diseases after initial endoscopic haemostasis. *Int J Clin Pract,* 2012; 66: 774-781.

Megraud F, Neman-Simha V, Brugmann D, Further evidence of the toxic effect of ammonia produced by Helicobacter pylori urease on human epithelial cells. *Infect Immun,* 1992; 60: 1858-63.

Moustafa FE, Khalil A, Abdel Wahab M, Sobh MA, Helicobacter pylori and uremic gastritis: a histopathologic study and a correlation with endoscopic and bacteriologic findings. *Am J Nephrol,* 1997; 17: 165-71.

Muto S, Murayama N, Asano Y, Hosoda S, Miyata M, Hypergastrinemia and achlorhydria in chronic renal failure. *Nephron,* 1985; 40: 143-8.

Nagata N, Sakamoto K, Arai T, Niikura R, Shimbo T, Shinozaki M, Aoki T, Sekine K, Okubo H, Watanabe K, Sakurai T, Yokoi C, Yanase M, Akiyama J, Noda M, Uemura N, Visceral fat accumulation affects risk of colonic diverticular hemorrhage. *Int J Colorectal Dis,* 2015; 30: 1399-406.

Nahata M, Muto S, Oridate N, Ohnishi S, Nakagawa K, Sadakane C, Saegusa Y, Hattori T, Asaka M, Takeda H, Impaired ghrelin signaling is associated with gastrointestinal dysmotility in rats with gastroesophageal reflux disease. *Am J Physiol Gastrointest Liver Physiol,* 2012; 303: G42-53.

Nand N, Malhotra P, Bala R, Evaluation of upper gastrointestinal symptoms and effect of different modalities of treatment in patients of chronic kidney disease. *JIACM,* 2014; 15: 182-187.

Nashar K, Egan BM, Relationship between chronic kidney disease and metabolic syndrome: current perspectives. *Diabetes Metab Syndr Obes,* 2014; 7: 421-35.

Neithercut WD, Rowe PA, El Nujumi AM, Dahill S, Mccoll KE, Effect of Helicobacter pylori infection on intragastric urea and ammonium concentrations in patients with chronic renal failure. *J Clin Pathol,* 1993; 46: 544-7.

Ogura T, Makinodan A, Kubo T, Hayashida T, Hirasawa Y, Electrophysiological course of uraemic neuropathy in haemodialysis patients. *Postgrad Med J,* 2001; 77: 451-4.

Ohira T, Hokama A, Kinjo N, Nakamoto M, Kobashigawa C, Kise Y, Yamashiro S, Kinjo F, Kuniyoshi Y, Fujita J, Detection of active bleeding from gastric antral vascular ectasia by capsule endoscopy. *World J Gastrointest Endosc,* 2013; 5: 138-40.

Parasa S, Navaneethan U, Sridhar AR, Venkatesh PG, Olden K, End-stage renal disease is associated with worse outcomes in hospitalized patients with peptic ulcer bleeding. *Gastrointest Endosc,* 2013; 77: 609-16.

Prasad GV, Metabolic syndrome and chronic kidney disease: Current status and future directions. *World J Nephrol,* 2014; 3: 210-9.

Promberger R, Lenglinger J, Riedl O, Seebacher G, Eilenberg W, Ott J, Riegler F, Gadenstatter M, Neumayer C, Gastro-oesophageal reflux disease in type 2 diabetics: symptom load and pathophysiologic aspects - a retro-pro study. *BMC Gastroenterol,* 2013; 13: 132.

Quraishi ER, Goel S, Gupta M, Catanzaro A, Zasuwa G, Divine G, Acute pancreatitis in patients on chronic peritoneal dialysis: an increased risk? *Am J Gastroenterol,* 2005; 100: 2288-93.

Ramírez BV, Gómez PaB, Uraemic neuropathy: A review. *Int J Genet Mol Biol,* 2012; 3: 155-160.

Saadah OI, Erosive gastritis mimicking watermelon stomach in a child. *Arab J Gastroenterol,* 2011; 12: 201-2.

Saeed F, Agrawal N, Greenberg E, Holley JL, Lower gastrointestinal bleeding in chronic hemodialysis patients. *Int J Nephrol,* 2011; 2011: 272535.

Saeed F, Kalra A, Kousar N, Pace LA, Holley JL, Stercoral ulcer as a cause of lower gastrointestinal (LGI) bleeding in chronic hemodialysis patients. *Clin Nephrol,* 2012; 77: 75-8.

Salamon K, Woods J, Paul E, Huggins C, Peritoneal dialysis patients have higher prevalence of gastrointestinal symptoms than hemodialysis patients. *J Ren Nutr,* 2013; 23: 114-8.

Sanger GJ, Furness JB, Ghrelin and motilin receptors as drug targets for gastrointestinal disorders. *Nat Rev Gastroenterol Hepatol,* 2016; 13: 38-48.

Sechet A, Abighanem O, Said S, Rasombololona M, Moriniere P, Brazier M, Fournier A, [Inhibition of gastric secretion by omeprazole and efficacy of calcium carbonate in the control of hyperphosphatemia in patients on maintenance hemodialysis]. *Nephrologie,* 1999; 20: 213-6.

Shah SH, Upper gastrointestinal bleeding in chronic renal failure. *J Pak Med* Assoc, 1993; 43: 85.

Shiba N, Shimokawa H, Chronic kidney disease and heart failure--Bidirectional close link and common therapeutic goal. *J Cardiol,* 2011; 57: 8-17.

Silang R, Regalado M, Cheng TH, Wesson DE, Prokinetic agents increase plasma albumin in hypoalbuminemic chronic dialysis patients with delayed gastric emptying. *Am J Kidney Dis,* 2001; 37: 287-93.

Song YR, Kim HJ, Kim JK, Kim SG, Kim SE, Proton-pump inhibitors for prevention of upper gastrointestinal bleeding in patients undergoing dialysis. *World J Gastroenterol,* 2015; 21: 4919-24.

Sood P, Kumar G, Nanchal R, Sakhuja A, Ahmad S, Ali M, Kumar N, Ross EA, Chronic kidney disease and end-stage renal disease predict higher risk of mortality in patients with primary upper gastrointestinal bleeding. *Am J Nephrol,* 2012; 35: 216-24.

Stefanidis I, Liakopoulos V, Kapsoritakis AN, Ioannidis I, Eleftheriadis T, Mertens PR, Winograd R, Vamvaka E, Psychos AK, Potamianos SP, Gastric antral vascular ectasia (watermelon stomach) in patients with ESRD. *Am J Kidney Dis,* 2006; 47: e77-82.

Stenvinkel P, Chronic kidney disease: a public health priority and harbinger of premature cardiovascular disease. *J Intern Med,* 2010; 268: 456-67.

Straathof JW, Lamers CB, Masclee AA, Effect of gastrin-17 on lower esophageal sphincter characteristics in man. *Dig Dis Sci,* 1997; 42: 2547-51.

Takahara N, Isayama H, Sasaki T, Tsujino T, Toda N, Sasahira N, Mizuno S, Kawakubo K, Kogure H, Yamamoto N, Nakai Y, Hirano K, Tada M, Omata M, Koike K, Endoscopic papillary balloon dilation for bile duct stones in patients on hemodialysis. *J Gastroenterol,* 2012; 47: 918-23.

Thomas R, Kanso A, Sedor JR, Chronic kidney disease and its complications. *Prim Care,* 2008; 35: 329-44, vii.

Thomas R, Panackal C, John M, Joshi H, Mathai S, Kattickaran J, Iqbal M, Gastrointestinal complications in patients with chronic kidney disease--a 5-year retrospective study from a tertiary referral center. *Ren Fail,* 2013; 35: 49-55.

Tokushima H, Tamura H, Murakawa M, Matsumura O, Itakura Y, Itoyama S, Mitarai T, Isoda K, Eradication of Helicobacter pylori restores elevation of serum gastrin concentrations in patients with end-stage renal disease. *Intern Med,* 1998; 37: 435-9.

Van Vlem B, Schoonjans R, Vanholder R, De Vos M, Vandamme W, Van Laecke S, Lameire N, Delayed gastric emptying in dyspeptic chronic hemodialysis patients. *Am J Kidney Dis,* 2000; 36: 962-8.

Villacorta J, Rivera M, Alvaro SJ, Palomares JR, Ortuno J, Acute pancreatitis in peritoneal dialysis patients: diagnosis in the icodextrin era. *Perit Dial* Int, 2010; 30: 374-8.

Weiner DE, Causes and consequences of chronic kidney disease: implications for managed health care. *J Manag Care Pharm,* 2007; 13: S1-9.

Yorioka N, Hamaguchi N, Taniguchi Y, Asakimori Y, Nishiki T, Oda H, Yamakido M, Gastric antral vascular ectasia in a patient on hemodialysis improved with CAPD. *Perit Dial Int,* 1996; 16: 177-8.

In: Disorders of Gastrointestinal Systems ... ISBN: 978-1-63485-366-8
Editors:S. Rajagopal, S. Murugan and S. Ramachandran ©2016 Nova Science Publishers, Inc.

Chapter 12

Gastrointestinal Complications in Solid Organ Transplant Recipients

Murugavel Ponnusamy[1,*], PhD, Senthilkumar Rajagopal[2], PhD and Amarnathsatheesh Maruthamuthu[3], PhD

[1]Center for Developmental Cardiology, Institute for Translational Medicine, College of Medicine, Qingdao University, Qingdao, China
[2]Department of Biotechnology, Rayalaseema University, Kurnool, AP, India
[3]Department of Cellular and Molecular Biology, Bio Medical Research, University of Texas Health Science Center, Tyler, Texas, US

Abstract

Organ transplantation has made major progress and it is the successful form of treatment saving life of thousands of patients who have been doomed to death due to vital organ failure. Among various complications, gastrointestinal (GI) complications are common and unavoidable after transplantation of solid organs such as kidney, liver, pancreas, heart, and lung. GI complications have a significant impact on the quality of life and survival of the transplant recipients. The origin of GI complications in solid organ transplant (SOT) recipients is multifactorial, including preexisting disorders, surgical stress on the abdomen, use of non-steroidal anti-inflammatory drugs, impairment of gastric and intestinal system due to immunosuppressive drug toxicity. The post-transplant GI complications are fall into one of the following main categories: infections, ulceration, biliary tract disorders and malignancy. This chapter illustrates clinical features of most frequently occurring GI complications in transplant recipients and also describes pathogenesis, clinical diagnosis and management of GI disorders during post-transplant period.

Keywords: clinical management, drug toxicity, gastrointestinal problems, solid organ transplantation

---

* Corresponding author: Murugavel Ponnusamy, PhD. Center for Developmental Cardiology, Institute for Translational Medicine, College of Medicine, Qingdao University, Qingdao 266021, China. Email: spmvel @gmail.com.

1. Introduction

Organ transplantation is one of the greatest achievements in medical therapy that restores life and health of thousands of people from failure of vital organs. The first success of human kidney allograft resulted in the development of transplantation of other essential organs such as liver, heart, lungs, pancreas, etc. (Modi et al., 2014). In recent years, dual organ transplantation such as kidney-pancreas, heart-lung, and liver-kidney is also carried out under certain circumstances. Every year, more than 1, 00,000 people are receiving lifesaving organ transplantation worldwide. The recent advancement of medical science increased the number of organ replacement therapy by receiving organs from deceased donors in addition to live donors (Kellar, 2015).

In the past two decades, modern medical techniques have made more progress in organ transplantation to improve post-transplant life quality after transplantation, which is complicated in the early period of transplant era. This field has advanced to a robot-assisted transplant surgery, which is providing minimal invasive procedures, quick healing and a lower rate of complications when compared to traditional transplant surgery (Modi et al., 2014; Tzvetanov et al., 2013). The standard of care, development of preventive and prophylaxis strategies, refinement of antimicrobial and immunosuppressive regimens, and enhancement in monitoring methods significantly improved the success rate of solid organ transplantation (Kellar, 2015). A good indicator of the transplantation success in recent years is the dramatic increase of one-year graft and patient survival rates (Fortunato et al., 2008; Kim and Marks, 2014; Mathis, 2015). However, there is a least improvement in the long-term survival rate, which is due to the emergence of several other internal complications during the post-transplant period.

The post-transplantation period is critical and several complications has been observed during the early and long term period after grafting the organ (Torricelli et al., 2014). Most of the complications are mild or transient. They can be managed or cured under medical surveillance in this modern era. The complication depends upon the organ to be transplanted, the magnitude of ischemic injury, surgical procedure, and use of anti-rejection drugs and antimicrobials. The risk factor for complications is age, medical condition of the patient, bleeding, genetic polymorphism, immunosuppressive and therapeutic drug related toxicities, malignant disease, and development of graft-versus-host-disease (GVHD).

Within a week after transplantation, the most frequently observed complications are associated with surgery that includes surgical wound infections, vascular compromise, and anastomatic disruption and leak. During this period, infection is the predominant cause of death (>30%) due to high usage of immunosuppressive agents. The infection causes fever and more than 80% fever incidence occurs in transplanted ICU patients (Bouza et al., 2007). The incidence of other organ dysfunction and malignancy has also been considerably observed in later period after transplantation. The central nervous system damage and neurological lesions are also found in transplant recipients, but it is a rare event nowadays (Chung et al., 2014).

One of the major challenges in transplant community is gastrointestinal (GI) complications. GI tract problems considerably account for morbidity and mortality associated with transplantation (Gautam, 2006). Some patients have pre-existing GI complications and that can be exacerbated after transplantation. However, the prevalence of post-transplant GI problems exceeds more than 50% in solid organs such as liver, kidney and lungs recipient

(Bravo et al., 2007; Gil-Vernet et al., 2007; Herrero et al., 2007; Ryan et al., 2004). The unnoticed and persistent GI problems in transplant recipients can also lead to other disorders within the first year of organ replacement and it may become life threatening. In this chapter, we focus most commonly seen GI related complications developing during post-transplant period of solid organs such as kidney, liver, lung, heart, and pancreas. This chapter also illustrates the pathogenesis, differential diagnosis and management of post-transplant GI complications.

2. Major Factors Associated with GI Complications in Transplant Recipients

A multifactorial etiology often related to post-transplant GI disorders. However, infections (bacterial, viral and fungi) and immunosuppressive regimens (immunosuppressive agents and other medications) are major factors associated with the development of GI complications (Helderman and Goral, 2002). Some of these medications directly cause damage to different sections of the GI tract and lead to discomfort in transplant recipients.

2.1. Infections

Infection is the major problem in transplant recipients. Although patients are under antibiotic prophylaxis, infection is unavoidable and more than half of solid organ transplant (SOT) recipients are suffering from infections. It is not only occurring in GI tract, but also in other systems, which is due to suppression of the body immune system during organ transplantation (Danziger-Isakov, 2014). In renal and liver transplant, the infectious etiology is more than 70%, as these patients are under high doses of immunosuppression for the preservation of grafted organ. Early after transplantation (1-6 months), GI infections are resulting from pre-existing infectious microbes in patients, transmitted from donors or from surgical wound sites. The patients who are repeatedly hospitalized after transplant surgery or with marginal graft function and taking additional immunosuppressants are having a high risk for opportunistic infections. But patients with well functioning graft have a risk of infections from community acquired enteric pathogenic microbes (Danziger-Isakov, 2014; Gautam, 2006; Snydman, 2001).

Bacterial infection related GI complications are predominantly found in most cases of transplant recipients. *Clostridium difficile*, a gram positive anaerobic bacteria, associated diseases have been frequently observed in the majority of SOT patients. *C. difficile* also accounts for nosocomial and infectious diarrhea in early times after transplantation (Honda and Dubberke, 2014). The other bacterial species like *Shigella, Campylobacter*, nontyphoidal *Salmonella spp.*, and *Shiga* toxin producing *E. coli* are also responsible for GI complications (Gautam, 2006).

The viral infections caused by organisms such as cytomegalovirus (CMV), Herpes simplex virus (HSV), Epstein-Barr virus (EBV), BK polyomavirus type BK (BKV) and norovirus also significantly contribute to GI complications during the post-transplant period (Danziger-Isakov, 2014). CMV infection usually occurs within the first month after transplantation. In patients receiving cyclosporine A (CsA) or tacrolimus (TAC), the incidence of CMV infected enteritis is high and this organism can affect any segment of the GI tract. Infection with this organism also increases the risk for co-infection with bacterial and fungal infections (Helderman and Goral, 2002; Snydman, 2001). HSV infection is another common opportunistic viral infection found in transplant recipients. This viral agent causes ulcer like mucocutaneous lesions in the oral cavity and pharynx, in addition to esophagitis. The post-transplant HSV infection usually presents with dysphagia or odynophagia. Since the esophagus is the predominant site of HSV infection, the untreated patients susceptible to hemorrhage and fatal esophageal perforation (Helderman and Goral, 2002). EBV also an important organism, which is the major contributor in late onset of post-transplant malignancy, chiefly post-transplant lymph proliferative disorder (PTLD) (Wasson et al., 2006). In addition, BKV associated viremia and viruria is asymptomatic and this can be seen in more than 30% of renal patients after transplantation (Garces, 2010).

The opportunistic fungal infections are also common within two months after transplant surgery due to several risk factors, including frequent use of antibiotics, steroids, and catheters. The Candida albicans induced candidiasis very commonly appears in patients who are receiving a high dose of steroids or broad spectrum antibiotics. Nowadays, infections with the antifungal resistant *C. glabrata, C. tropicalis,* and *C. parapsilosis* are also found in transplant patients (Hagerty et al., 2003; Munoz et al., 2012). The parasitic infections are rare, but it is an important threat to patients traveling to endemic areas for transplantation or visit after transplantation (Helderman and Goral, 2002; Munoz et al., 2012).

2.2. Immunosuppressive and Anti-Rejection Medications

The standard immunosuppressive regimen consists of induction therapy and maintenance therapy. The induction therapy is started immediately after transplantation to block acute rejections. The maintenance therapeutics are administered lifelong to preserve grafted organ function as well as to avoid chronic or delayed rejections. The immunosuppressive therapy is always targeting T-Cell activities. In detail, T-cells recognizes antigens from grafted organ and promotes antigen driven secretion of several cytokines, including IL-2, a molecule required for T-cell proliferation and differentiation as well as activation of B-cell. This cytokine stimulates B-Cell to produce antibodies against implanted organ, and it also increases cytotoxic T-Cell activity against the grafted organ. Hence, attenuation of T-Cell proliferation and activation can prevent rejection of implanted organ (Enderby and Keller, 2015).

The immunosuppression induction therapy starts with immediate administration of antibodies such as anti-CD25-receptor antibodies (basiliximab, daclizumab), anti-CD52 monoclonal antibody (alemtuzumab), or depleting polyclonal antibodies (thymoglobulin or ATG), which specifically targeting cell surface epitope of B and T Cells. Usually, these antibodies are used immediately after renal, liver and pancreas transplant surgery, in which there is a need for delaying calcineurin inhibitors or decreased use of steroids (Mahmud et al., 2010; Saidi, 2012). The maintenance therapeutic regimen is generally a combination of medication with different actions. This includes a calcineurin inhibitor (CsA, TAC, etc.), an antiproliferative agent (mycophenolate, azathioprine, etc.), a corticosteroid, or a mammalian-target-of-rapamycin (mTOR) inhibitor (rapamycin or sirolimus) (Enderby and Keller, 2015).

The selection of these medications depends on the transplanted organ and preexisting condition of patients. The most commonly used transplant drugs and their mechanism of action are listed in Table 1.

Table 1. Commonly Using Drugs and Medicines Solid Organ Recipients and Their Mechanism of Action

Drugs/Medicine	Mechanism of action
Medications used in immunosuppression induction therapy	
Anti-Lymphocyte Antibodies	
Thymoglobulin/ATGAM	A Polyclonal antibody depletes T-lymphocytes concentration through complement dependent cytolysis (Administered 7-14 days after Transplant surgery).
Muromonab-CD3 (OKT3)	A Monoclonal antibody targeting circulating T-lymphocytes and induces apoptosis in T-lymphocytes (Administered 5-10 days after Transplant surgery)
Basiliximab/Daclizumab	Monoclonal antibody against α-subunit (CD25) of IL-2 receptor. Specifically targets MHC-antigen stimulus activated T-cells (Basiliximab - 2 hrs prior to transplant surgery and another 4 days after surgery; Daclizumab - 24 hrs prior to transplant surgery and additional 4 doses in 14 days intervals)
Antimicrobials	
Amphicillin/Sulbactum (For liver transplantation)	Antibacterial (1 dose prior to surgery and for another 3 days in 6 hrs intervals)
Vancomycin (For patients Allergic to Amphicillin)	Antibacterial (1 dose prior to surgery and for another 1-3 days in 8 hrs intervals)
Cefazolin/Cefoxitin (For kidney/ pancreas/heart transplantation)	Antibacterial (1 dose prior to surgery and for another 1-3 days in 12 hrs intervals)
Immunosuppressants Used In Induction/Maintanance Therapy	
Calcineurin Inhibitors	
Cyclosporine A	Binds with cyclophilin and inhibits the phosphatase activity of calcineurin, a key enzyme in T cell activation
Tacrolimus	Binds with cytoplasmic protein FK506-binding protein 12 (FKBP12) and inhibits phosphatase activity of calcineurin
Antiproliferatives	
Mycophenolate Mofetil (MMF)/ Mycophenolate Sodium (MPS)	Inhibits inosine monophosphate dehydrogenase, a key enzyme in denovo purine sythesis in T and B lymphocytes
Azathioprine	Blocks denovo purine synthesis in lymphocytes and halt DNA replications
Targets of Rapamycin Inhibitors (mTORs) Sirolimus/Everolimus	Binds the intracellular immunophilin (FKB12) and inhibits mTOR receptor. This leads to cell cycle halt at G1-S phase and results in blockage of T-cell activation
Corticosteroids Prednisone/Methylprednisolone	Down regulate transcription and expression of inflammatory cytokines (interleukins) by lymphocytes, antagonize macrophage differentiation, inhibit neutrophil adhesion to endothelial cells (anti-inflammatory effect), decreases circulating eosinophil and basophil.

CsA and TAC are blockers of calcineurin, a calmodulin dependent serine/threonine phosphatase enzyme, which is a key regulatory molecule in T-cell activation and IL-2 production. Thereby these drugs inhibit T-cell activation and rejection process. The antiproliferative agents are blockers of T and B cell proliferation by targeting cell cycle proteins. The most conventional antiproliferative drugs such as mycophenolate mofetil (MMF) and mycophenolate sodium (MPS) inhibits T cell proliferation by blocking the inosine monophosphate dehydrogenase (IMPDH), a key enzyme in the *de novo* synthesis of purine base. Since lymphocytes are only depending *de novo* pathway of purine synthesis during cell division, their blockage reduces those cell proliferation (Enderby and Keller, 2015). Another drug azathioprine (AZA) is an analog of purine, which incorporates into DNA and blocks DNA replication thereby it inhibits cell proliferation. AZA is used as alone or in combination with corticosteroids to prevent rejection of liver and kidney allograft (Maltzman and Koretzky, 2003).

mTOR inhibitors (Sirolimus and Everolimus) are used as an alternative or replacement for calcineurin and T-cell proliferation inhibitors. In some cases, mTOR inhibitors are used along with small doses of calcineurin inhibitors. mTOR inhibitors targets IL-2 driven T-Cell growth and proliferation by forming complex with FKBP12 and inhibiting mTOR pathway, a major pathway of ILs signaling (Enderby and Keller, 2015). This class of drugs is a better immunosuppressant for transplant recipients with pre-existing carcinoma (Bhat and Watt, 2015). Corticosteroids are used for maintenance of immunosuppression as well as for the treatment of acute rejections due to their anti-inflammatory properties. As a transplant medicine, they have a wide range of responses, including inhibition of cytokine production, suppression of inflammatory cell activation, and induction of lymphocyte apoptosis (Enderby and Keller, 2015). Due to their side effects upon long term use, these agents are mostly avoided in maintenance therapy. In addition to immunosuppressive drugs, the antimicrobial agents are required as a surgical prophylaxis before and immediately after transplant surgery. Some of them are continued for first 3-6 months after transplantation. The penicillin is used primarily for clean operative procedures and they administered during first 3 days of the post-operative period. If patients are allergic to penicillin, clindamycin is used as an alternative. In addition to this, cephalosporin also used to prevent gram-negative bacterial infections (Watson and Dark, 2012). Most of these medications are withdrawn after the infection is cleared or risk is decreased.

3. GI System Associated Complications in Transplant Recipients

The discomfort is frequently found in all the level of the GI tract after solid organ transplantation. The GI complications may be different depending upon the organ being affected and transplanted. In general, GI associated symptoms like diarrhea, a decrease in appetite; nausea, vomiting, and weight loss are most commonly seen in transplant recipients. Other symptoms of GI problems include changes in bowel movements, bloating, difficulties in swallowing, cramp in the abdominal area, constipation, and bloody or mucousy stool but these symptoms arise depending on the section of GI tract affected. The post-transplant associated GI complications mainly come under one of the following categories: infections, ulceration, mucosal injury, biliary tract disorders, pancreatitis, and rarely malignancy (Helderman and Goral, 2002; Ponticelli and Passerini, 2005).

3.1. Diarrhea in Transplant Recipients

Diarrhea is defined as three or more watery or loose stool per day. Diarrhea is the most frequently found complication in early time after transplantation, and that affects the outcome of transplantation. In fact, diarrhea is the warning sign of GI problems. In the majority of cases, diarrhea is mild or transient. Most of them can be relieved from diarrhea by proper diet, symptomatic therapy and careful adjustment of the dose of immunosuppressive agents. But severe diarrhea in these patients becomes life threatening (Arslan et al., 2007; Rice et al., 2009). Diarrhea can cause malabsorption, dehydration and electrolyte imbalance thereby increase the weakness in very young and old patients. Nevertheless, severe diarrhea leads to decline in the level of immunosuppressant agents in the body by reducing the absorption of them, which may result in rejection of implants (Arslan et al., 2007; Aulagnon et al., 2014; Gil-Vernet et al., 2007; Lee and Ison, 2014). In addition, severe diarrhea results in the reduction of intestinal multidrug resistance 1 (a p-glycoprotein) enzyme activity, which is required for CsA and TAC metabolism. This destruction leads to the elevation of level of un-metabolized immunosuppressive agents such as CsA and TAC in circulation and subsequently results in GI toxicity (Leroy et al., 2010).

3.1.1. Etiology and Pathogenesis

The etiology of diarrhea in transplant recipients is different from people having a normal immune system. In transplant patients, diarrhea is due to changes in normal intestine flora or infections in the intestinal system. The suppression of the immune system by anti-rejection agents is responsible for infection in GI system and leads to diarrhea (Aulagnon et al., 2014; Ginsburg and Thuluvath, 2005). GVHD is one of the reasons for diarrhea after engraftment of solid organs. Diarrhea due to GVHD is green, watery, mucoid and in large volumes and that can be accompanied by gastrointestinal bleeding and severe abdominal pain and vomiting (Zhang and Ruiz, 2010).

The episode of infectious diarrhea is due to one or more microbes, including bacteria (*Campylobacter jejune*, non-typhoidal *Salmonella* spp., *C. difficile, Enteropathogenic E. coli*), parasites and viruses (CMV and norovirus) (Echenique et al., 2015; Lee and Ison, 2014). In more than 90% cases of transplant recipients, *C. difficile, Helicobacter pylori, Enteropathogenic E. coli,* CMV and/or norovirus infection is a reason for diarrhea (Angarone and Ison, 2015; Echenique et al., 2015). In recent years, the incidence of antibiotic associated diarrhea is increasing worldwide in solid organ transplant patients as well as in generally hospitalized patients. In most cases, it is due to antibiotic resistant and hypervirulent strains of bacteria. Clinical studies reveal that the conventional antibiotic prophylaxis, such as ampicillin, cephalosporin and clindamycin are frequently associated with *C. difficile* infection. These antibiotics suppresses normal colon microbial growth and increase colonization of *C. difficile*, an organism that causes inflammatory diarrhea and colonic mucosal injury by producing endotoxins (Toxin A and B) (Honda and Dubberke, 2014).

Among various viral infections, the norovirus related diarrhea is frequently seen in transplant recipients, particularly in renal recipients. The norovirus infection causes gastroenteritis, nonspecific inflammation, and intestinal villi blunting and these pathological lesions lead to diarrhea in those patients. This viral infection is responsible for more weight loss than other causes of diarrhea. Diarrhea is also a common symptom in CMV infected patients, but it is the consequences of CMV-induced colitis and gastroenteritis. Molecular findings indicate that the usage of MMF critically involved in the persistence of this viral diarrhea, by preventing clearance of the virus as well as the repair of intestinal epithelial cells (Coste et al., 2013). So If patients are affected by virus related diarrhea, reduction of MMF and other immunosuppression agents and switch to inhibitors of mTOR based therapy is most the effective regimen to manage norovirus and other viral infection, since mTOR inhibitors have antiviral activities.

Regardless of microbes associated diarrhea, immunosuppressive medications can also cause non-infectious diarrhea, which increases the risk of graft rejection and patient death (Aulagnon et al., 2014; Ginsburg and Thuluvath, 2005). The incidence of non-infectious diarrhea is high in MMF (about 40%) and TAC. The villous atrophy is one of the frequent causes of chronic and persistent post-transplant diarrhea, and this incidence is high in renal transplant patients receiving MMF (Aiyangar et al., 2010; Hanif et al., 2015). In addition, the colonoscopy studies revealed that MMF grounds erosive enterocolitis, Crohn's disease-like changes in the colon, ulcerative esophagitis and GVHD like changes. These injuries to GI tract could also cause diarrhea in MMF receiving patients (Al-Absi et al., 2010; Parfitt et al., 2008). Generally, TAC has minimal side effects compared to CsA but mild diarrhea can increase trough level of TAC, which prone to toxic effects of this drug to gut and causes persistent diarrhea. This is attributed to the reduction of intestinal activity of cytochrome P450 3A4 (CYP3A4) and p-glycoprotein (PGP) during diarrhea, as these enzymes are determinants of bioavailability and clearance of TAC (Mayer et al., 1997).

3.1.2. Diagnosis and Clinical Management

The early and correct diagnosis is essential for the timely initiation of appropriate therapy and management of diarrhea in transplant recipients. In recent years, numerous diarrhea causing opportunistic infectious agents has been identified in transplant recipients and in the general population, which reveals the large unknown side of transplant diarrhea. For example, the microsporida is a protozoan parasite is responsible for un-explained chronic diarrhea in transplant recipients. This organism is low suspicion, and it cannot be detected by normal routine stool examination. This can be detectable only by modified trichome staining of stool samples (Gumbo et al., 1999; Hocevar et al., 2014). So un-identified post-transplant diarrhea should not be endorsed solely to the toxicity of immunosuppressive drugs, which could lead to diagnostic misconceptions and unsuitable treatments. Hence, the physicians should be familiar with the common etiologies and possible factors that resulting in post-transplant diarrhea.

A stepwise approach will help to the clinician to achieve a better diagnostic yield in post-transplant diarrhea (Figure 1). The routine post-transplant microbiological surveillance in blood, urine, and stool samples is helpful for identifying patients at high risk and also helps to evaluate whether the diarrhea is due to medications or infections. The routine microbiological tests also help to monitor the patient's response to therapy (Coste et al., 2013). Given the fact that the majority of diarrhea incidence in transplant recipients is due to infection by *C. difficile, Campylobacter spp.,* CMV and norovirus (Angarone and Ison, 2015; Echenique et al., 2015), the assessment for these microbes, at first, would help to quick finding of the causative factor. The molecular tools such as multiplex PCR assays become a useful tool for early detection and treatment of microbial infections. Nowadays, this molecular technique becomes a key element in the management of severe acute diarrhea in transplant recipients (Coste et al., 2013).

The histological and colonoscopic deteriorations are usually common in organ transplant recipients with diarrhea, but these findings rarely direct to changes in diagnosis or management. Hence, non-invasive testing for diarrhea along with a careful review and adjustment of medications should be performed before going for a colonoscopy and biopsy evaluations (Rice et al., 2009). The reduction in the degree of immunosuppression along with complement antiviral/antibiotic treatment could provide a better relief from infectious diarrhea in transplant patients (Arns, 2007).

In the cases of non-infectious diarrheal disease, diarrhea is obviously caused by drugs used for maintenance of graft. In these patients, the manipulation drug doses such as dose splitting (For example, changing doses to four times instead of two times daily), and/or reduction of dosage is effective strategy to manage GI toxicity and its associated diarrhea (Arns, 2007). Food safety is also important to decrease the incidence of diarrhea in transplant recipients. In patients with unidentified diarrhea even after extensive investigations, the management with antidiarrheal agents, probiotics and lactose-free diets could help to control diarrhea and its associated problems (Pant et al., 2013).

3.2. Ulcers in Transplant Recipients

Ulcers are a sore developed in the lining of soft tissues of the GI tract. The ulcer is resulting from disruption or rupture of the protective layer of the GI tract and imbalance in digestive fluid secreted by the stomach. As like in general populations, ulcer can develop in the esophagus (esophageal ulcer), stomach (gastric or peptic ulcer) and also formed in different sections of the intestine (duodenum, ileum, jejunum, and colon) of transplant recipients. Before the discovery of proton pump inhibitors and H2 antagonists, the incidence of ulcer (peptic ulcer and duodenal ulcer) was very high, and its related mortality was a major problem in transplant recipients, especially in renal transplant patients (Gautam, 2006).

3.2.1. Etiology and Pathogenesis

The infection and medications are major contributors in post-transplant associated ulcerative diseases (Figure 2). *H. pylori* is the key pathogenic bacterium, responsible for post-transplant ulcer development (Gautam, 2006). The opportunistic infections with CMV and EBV also present oral peptic ulcer in transplant recipients. These infectious agents weaken the mucous coating of the stomach and duodenum. When this protective barrier is ruptured, the epithelial lining of the stomach and intestine can be irritated by stomach acid and consequently causes ulcer (Helderman and Goral, 2002; Ponticelli and Passerini, 2005).

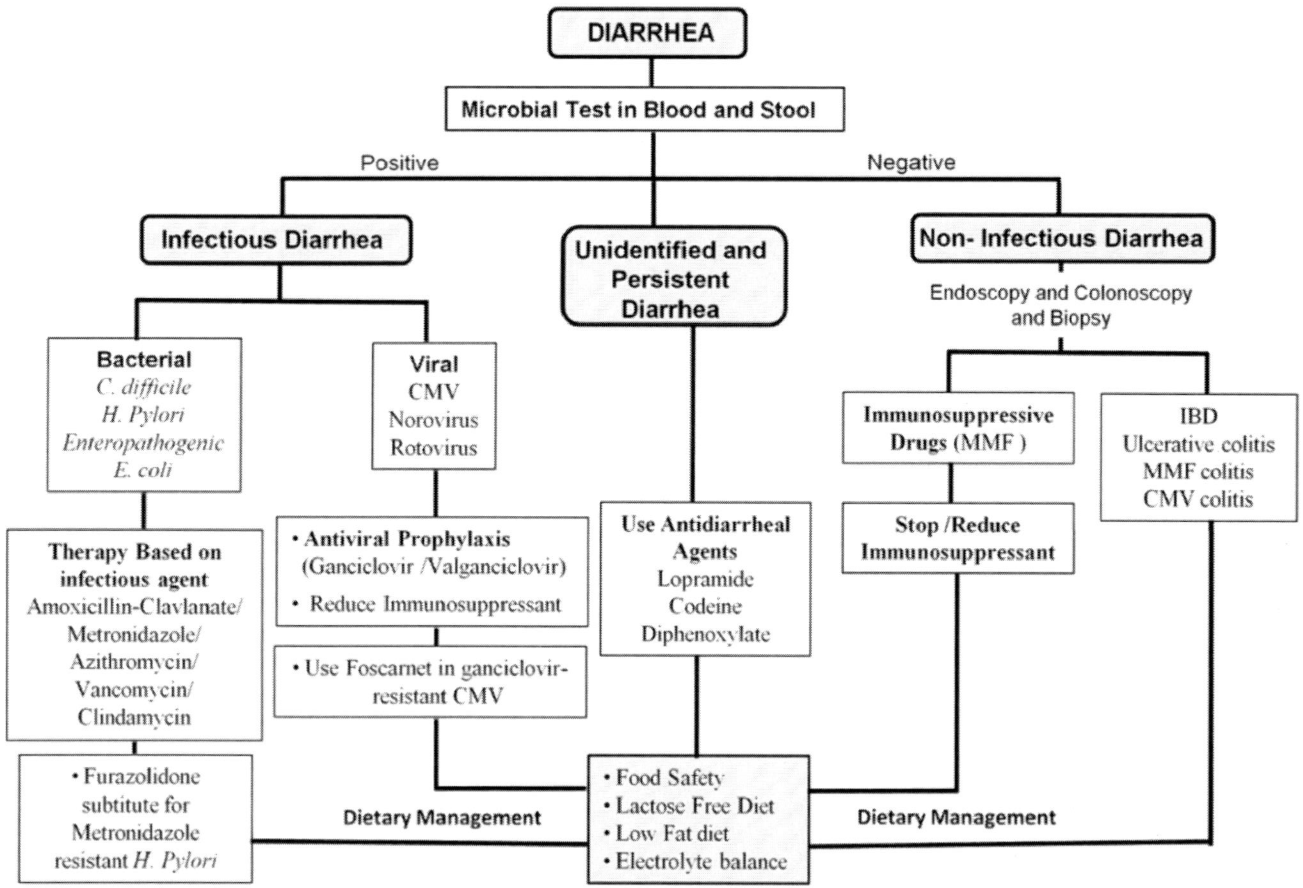

CMV - Cytomegalovirus; MMF - Mycophenolate Mofetil; IBD - Inflammatory Bowel Disease.

Figure 1. Etiology and Management of Diarrhea in Transplant Recipients.

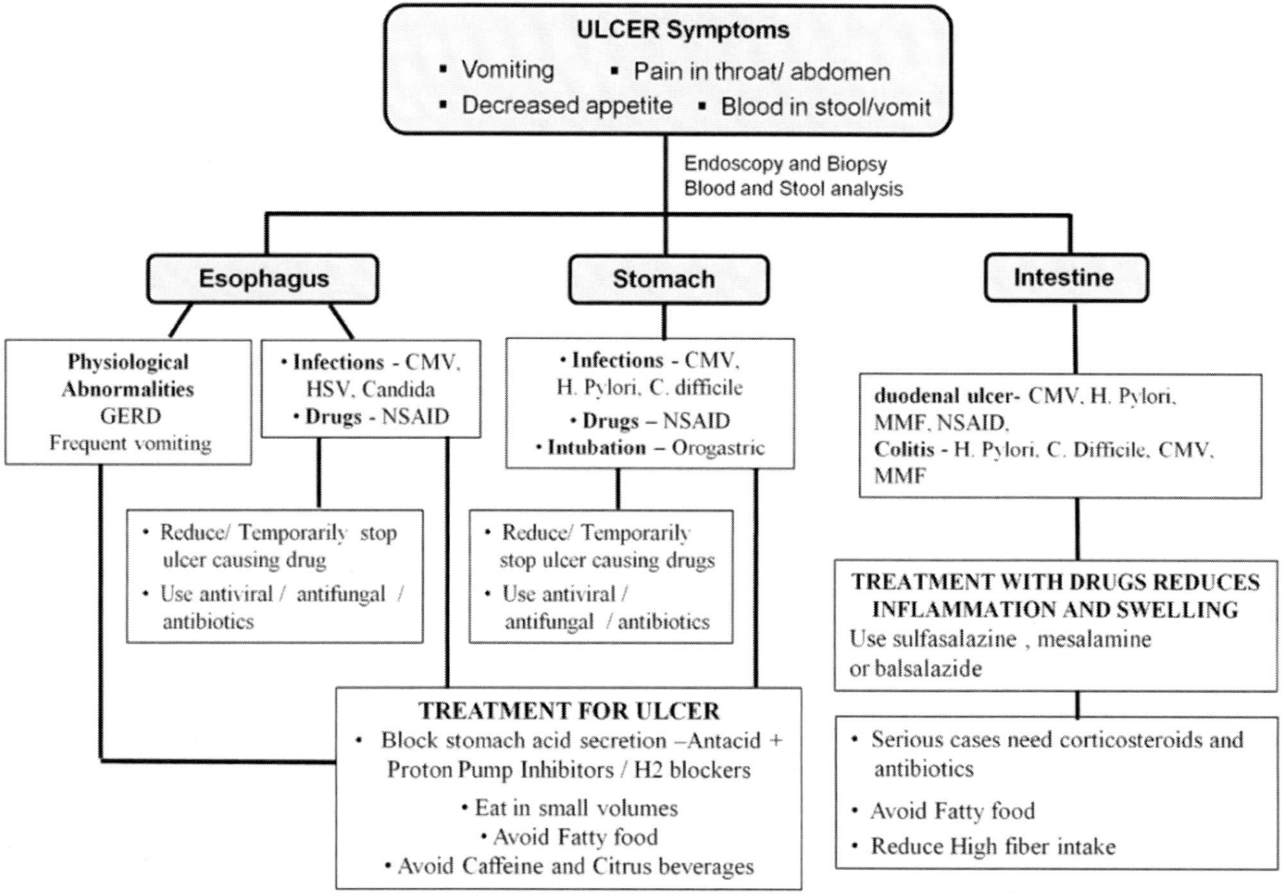

CMV - Cytomegalovirus; GERD - Gastresophageal Reflux Disease; HSV - Herpes Simplex Virus; H2 Blocker - Histamine Receptor 2 Blocker; MMF - Mycophenolate Mofetil; NSAID - Nonsteroidal Anti-inflammatory Drugs.

Figure 2. Etiology and Management of Ulcer in Solid Organ Transplant recipients.

In addition to infections, immunosuppressive agents and its conjugations with nonsteroidal anti-inflammatory drugs (NSAIDs) increase the risk for ulcer development in the stomach and intestine. The high dose of NSAID usage in bilateral lung transplantation predisposes ulcer, and it can be seen in both upper and lower GI tracts. The non-CMV enteritis in esophagus, stomach, duodenum and colon is also commonly seen in patients under NSAID regimen (Lipson et al., 1998). In fact, ulcers are completely asymptomatic in transplant recipients because of NSAID, which masks the clinical symptoms of various GI disorders, including ulcer (Helderman and Goral, 2002).

In patients under medications such as MMF and AZA are susceptible to ulcer development, since these drugs can reduce intestinal cell turnover and lead to GI tract damage. In particular, MMF associated irritation and damages leads to esophageal ulcer, duodenal ulcer, and also reactive gastrophathy. In the upper GI tract, MMF induced pathological changes resemble lesions of NSAID. In the lower GI tract, MMF induces the pathological changes including architectural changes, damaged and dilated crypts, and patchy inflammation in the colon and ileum, which is similar to the pattern of injury caused by GVHD (Davies et al., 2007; Parfitt et al., 2008). Unlike other organ recipients, the kidney transplant recipients have numerous additional factors that producing ulcers. For instance, heparin used during post-operative dialysis can increase secretion of gastric acids by elevation of histamine and gastrin levels (Steger et al., 1990).

3.2.2. Diagnosis and Clinical Management

The patients with ulcer are having one or more symptoms as follows: Nausea and vomiting after intake of food; Repeated burping; A decreased appetite. Some symptoms are also depends location of ulcers. The patients with esophageal ulcer have pain in throat when swallow the food. In the case of patients with ulcer in the stomach or intestine, a sharp and severe pain in the abdomen is observed. The gastric ulcer patients have a worse feeling of pain after eating food, but duodenal ulcer patients feel better after having food and the pain returns within one to two hours. In severe ulcer conditions, the stools of patients become bright red or black due to bleeding in the GI tract. A bloody vomiting or vomit like coffee grounds is also observed in patients with severe ulcer in the stomach.

As like in the general population, there are several examinations performed to diagnose factors involved in the development of ulcer in transplant recipients. In general, blood tests are performed to assess if there is any sign of infections especially for *H. pylori*. The stool sample is also checked for infectious agents. The endoscopic examination with sedations helps to examine the nature and degree of injury in the upper GI tract (esophagus, stomach and duodenum). The Tendoscopic procedure also visualizes the signs of irritation, swelling, any abnormalities in tissue and bleeding in the upper GI tract. Similarly, the colonoscopy examination helps to identify the ulceration in the large intestine.

The treatment for ulcer is mainly depends on the causative factor, severity and location (Figure 2). The primary target of ulcer treatment is blocking or reducing the production of excessive acid secretion by the stomach. The post-transplantation therapeutic strategy for ulcer includes both medications (one or more combinations) and avoiding the things that worsening the worse, which is proven to be effective in clinical settings. A histamine receptor 2 blocker (H2 blocker) or proton pump inhibitor (PPI) along with antacids is commonly prescribed for all kinds of transplant recipients with ulcerative disorders. The H2 blockers such as ranitidine, cimetidine, famotidine and nizatidine are usually prescribed to ulcer patients to block stomach acid production. The PPIs such as omeprazole, esomeprazole, pantoprozole, lansoprazole are also recommended to stop the secretion of acid into the stomach. Another approach is neutralizing stomach acid by using antacids such as bismuth subsalicylate. This antacid not only neutralizes stomach acid but also forms a coating on the stomach; thereby it protects the tissue from additional damage and promoting healing of ulcers (Cianciolo et al., 2007; Helderman and Goral, 2002).

The important concern of ulcer therapy in transplant recipient is their interference and interactions with immunosuppressive agents. This interaction may lift additional complications and also hurdles allograft survival. The H2 blockers such as cimetidine and ranitidine, and PPIs (omeprazole) can alter CsA trough level when they administered together. Similarly, sucralfate, a drug used for the treatment of gastric and duodenal ulcers, delays absorption of CsA (Helderman and Goral, 2002). The stomach acid environment is required for MMF cleavage and increased availability of mycophenolate acid (MPA). The co-administration of PPIs, in particular, pantoprazole with MMF can influence drug exposure and immunosuppressive potency of MMF by reducing stomach acid secretion, which increases the risk for acute rejections (Schaier et al., 2010). In addition, the long-term use of H2 blockers and PPIs for reduction of acid secretion increases the chance of colonization of various enteric infectious agents, including *C. difficile* by altering upper gut flora. So ulcer prophylaxis should be carefully carried out based on the immunosuppressive regimen. The physician should have the knowledge of certain drug interactions to avoid additional complications (Helderman and Goral, 2002; Reimer and Bytzer, 2012). To avoid complications caused by drug interactions, antacids and H2 blockers should be taken only two hours after calcineurin inhibitors (TAC or CsA) and/or antiproliferative agents (MMF). If the ulcer is caused by bacteria (*H. pylori*) or viruses (CMV or HSV-1), appropriate antibiotics or antiviral are included in the therapeutic regimen. The antiviral agents such as valganciclovir (VGCV) and ganciclovir (GCV) are most conventionally used in transplant patients. VGCV is a better agent for CMV associated disorder due to its greater bioavailability and less side effects (Vaziri et al., 2014).

3.3. Esophagitis and Gastro-Esophageal Reflux Disease (GERD) in Transplant Recipients

The esophagus is the muscular soft tissue that carries food from the mouth to stomach. The most frequently observed esophagus related disorders in post-transplant patients are gastro-esophageal reflux disease (GERD) and esophagitis (erosion or inflammation in the esophagus) (Davis et al., 2010; Mohammed and Neujahr, 2010). GERD primarily due to esophageal motility disorders (ineffective peristalsis or slow transit) and delaying in emptying of the stomach. The esophagitis and GERD are interlinked to each other that cause serious problems in transplant recipients. The lung and renal transplant recipients are more prone to these two esophageal related disorders. A considerable number of heart transplant recipients are also susceptible to GERD. In lung recipients, GERD is the crucial factor for acute and chronic lung transplant rejection (Abdulrahman and Al-Quorain, 2008; Davis et al., 2010; Mohammed and Neujahr, 2010).

3.3.1. Etiology and Pathogenesis

Clinical investigations suggest that delaying in emptying of the stomach (Gastroparesis) and ineffective peristalsis (abnormal motility of the esophagus) are important contributory in GERD development and its consequences in transplant patients, especially in lung and heart recipients. The primary pathogenic mechanism is interruption/transection of vagus nerves, which is unavoidable during lung and lung-heart transplant surgery (Basseri et al., 2010; Davis et al., 2010; Khan et al., 2013). In addition, the post-surgical esophageal tissue scarring also disturbs sympathetic (vagus) and parasympathetic nerves. The disturbance or complete dysfunction of these nerve systems imposes GERD and gastric disorder during the post-transplant period, as these nerve systems exert a regulatory function on lower esophageal sphincter (LES) and gastric motility. A severe GERD can be seen in patients with total dysfunction of vagus nerves, chiefly in bilateral lungs and heart-lung transplant patients (Basseri et al., 2010; Davis et al., 2010; Khan et al., 2013). In renal recipients, hyperuremia induced metabolic neuropathy prior to renal replacement is a route cause for gastroparesis and GERD in these patients.

The acid reflux or frequent vomiting causes severe inflammation and erosion, which results in esophagitis and esophageal ulcer. GERD contributes to these pathological lesions by increasing reflux of acidic gastric contents to upper esophageal sections. GERD also ultimately leads to dysphagia, odynophagia, and anemia. The patients with GERD and esophagitis have the following symptoms: A burning sensation or pain in the chest (heartburn), regurgitation highly specific after having fatty meal, sometimes sour taste in mouth, difficulties in swallowing (dysphagia) or feeling like something stuck in throat, nausea and vomiting (Basseri et al., 2010; Davis et al., 2010; Rosolowski and Kierzkiewicz, 2013).

In addition to physiological abnormalities, infection and immunosuppressive agents are major contributors to the development of esophageal disorder in transplant recipients. The yeast and viruses related esophagitis are frequently observed in transplant recipients. The fungus, Candida sp. responsible for oral thrush (oral candidiasis) in transplant recipients and its colonization causes esophagitis. This infection appears as a lining of white patches in the mouth (oral mucosa) and can spread to esophagus area and even further to stomach in patients received high doses of immunosuppressive agents. Candida esophagitis usually accompanied by difficulties in swallowing (dysphagia or odynophagia), heartburn, epigastric pain or sometimes GI bleeding. The early identification of lesions (superficial erosion and white plaques) caused by Candida is important because under severe condition, it may necrotizing esophagus and leads to the formation of perforation with tracheoesophageal fistula (Dongari-Bagtzoglou et al., 2009).

The infectious viruses such as HSV1 and CMV are also causing severe inflammation in the mouth and esophageal lining. The odynophagia and epigastralgia are symptoms appeared in virus esophagitis. The patients who have CMV and herpes esophagitis have severe pain while chewing and swallowing. They also have chills and joint pains (Albuquerque et al., 2012; Joo et al., 2013). The adverse effects of drugs also seem to be an important etiologic factor in the emergence of gastroparesis as well as non-infectious esophagitis. For example, the immunosuppressive drug MMF causes erosive esophagitis due its adverse effect on epithelial cell turnover (Kim et al., 2012).

3.3.2. Diagnosis and Management

The gastroparesis is characterized by postprandial nausea and vomiting. The electrogastrography (EGG) by using electrodes overlying on the stomach is the most convenient method to measure gastric slow-wave activity. In healthy persons, EGG records 3 cycles of uniform waves per minute, and it increases in amplitude after ingestion of food or water. EGG abnormalities indicate gastroparesis, especially the impairment of postprandial amplitude responses indicates delaying in stomach emptying (Hasler, 2008). The examination of walls of the esophagus by using endoscopy helps to find signs of inflammation, ulcers or bleeding in the esophagus. Based on this result, the gastroenterologist may collect biopsy samples for accurate diagnosis of the severity of esophageal tissue inflammation and its causative factor (Davis et al., 2010; Dongari-Bagtzoglou et al., 2009). This helps the physician to provide correct treatment for this complication in transplant recipients.

The patient suffers from esophagitis due to GERD or reflux of gastric contents, are advised to take stomach acid decreasing medications. Although the PPI inhibitors can provide great relief by controlling GERD and healing of gastritis, the inclusion of gastric motility stimulators is more efficient in post-transplant GERD and gastroparesis. The prokinetic drugs such as metocloprimide and domperidone are used to treat gastroparesis. The metocloprimide is a serotonin agonist and it also acts as a dopamine D2 antagonist thereby it accelerates stomach emptying by increasing lower esophageal and small bowel contractions. But domperidone only has a dopamine D2 antagonist effect. This drug increases LES pressure and enhances gastroduodenal co-ordination with stomach, thereby it facilitates acceleration of gastric emptying (Hasler, 2008).

In the case of infectious esophagitis, the source of infection can be identified by microbial testing and patients are prescribed antibiotics, antiviral or antifungal medications depending upon the infectious agent. Normally, the endoscopy shows the infections as a patchy colony of microbes in the different area of the esophagus and/or stomach. If the grafted organ is healthy and its functions are progressively improving, then the dose of immunosuppressive medication may have to be reduced to support the immune system fight against the infectious agents. The antifungal therapy for candida infection contains nystatin, clotrimazole, fluconazole or liposomal amphotericin B solution and their application depends on the segment of GI tract affected. Nystatin or clotrimazole is effective for upper GI tract fungal infection but fluconazole is only effective for oropharyngeal candidiasis (Gautam, 2006). Usually, 1-2 weeks therapy with fluconazole can clear candidiasis, but if there is no improvement and the symptoms are not resolved, esophagogastroduodenoscopy should be performed. In refractive cases, posaconazole, voriconazole or itraconazole are more useful (Rosolowski and Kierzkiewicz, 2013). In patients with viral esophagitis, a short course of oral acyclovir (200 mg five times a day or 400 mg three times a day) or valacyclovir (1 g three times a day) for 1 to 2 weeks helps to relief from CMV and HSV esophagitis (Rosolowski and Kierzkiewicz, 2013).

During the treatment for esophagitis and GERD, the transplant recipients are recommended to make changes in their diet and lifestyle as follows: Intake smaller and more frequent foods at certain intervals. Maintain a healthy weight and reduce fatty food. Avoid eating food at least 2 hours before going to bed. Avoid chocolate, caffeine, spicy foods, and citrus fruits. Raise the head about ten inches of the bed to avoid stomach acid reflux into the esophagus while sleeping. Avoid abdominal exercise and excessive bending which may increase pressure in the stomach and cause reflux (Frye and Peura, 2015).

3.4. Gastric Disorders in Transplant Recipient

The stomach is a major part of digestion, which encounters a variety of problems during post-transplant period. Gastroparesis, peptic ulcer disease, and gastritis are most commonly seen stomach related complications in transplant recipients. The delaying in emptying of the stomach (gastroparesis) is most frequently observed in lung, lung-heart, pancreas and kidney transplant recipients (Cashion et al., 2004; Yiannopoulos et al., 2004). The pathogenesis of gastroparesis is multifactorial, which includes damage to vagus nerves, viral infection, and immunosuppressive agents. The un-noticed and severe gastroparesis can lead to electrolyte disturbances in the body, malnutrition, weight loss, esophageal reflux, and poor/inconsistent absorption of the immunosuppressive medication; thereby it can increase the risk of rejections (Yiannopoulos et al., 2004). Gastritis is a condition caused by inflammation and irritation of lining of the stomach, which is another frequently seen stomach related disorder in transplant recipients. Acute Gastritis is more common in transplant patients that present with a sudden mucosal injury or inadequate repair of mucosal injury caused by infections and/or therapeutic drugs (Lauwers et al., 2010).

3.4.1. Etiology and Pathogenesis

The etiologies of gastroparesis and peptic ulcer diseases are already discussed in section 3.3.1. In this part, pathogenesis of gastritis is focused. The microbial infection related damage to the mucous coating, a protective layer of the stomach, is major route cause for gastritis in transplant recipients. In general, transplant patients are most frequently susceptible to *H. Pylori*, Enteric *E. Coli* infections, CMV, HSV and these organisms have been associated with the development of gastritis and peptic ulcer (Helderman and Goral, 2002; Lauwers et al., 2010). The intubation like orogastric tube and naso gastric tubes are placed for several days to weeks in transplant patients for feeding or drain the stomach content. These tubes can cause irritation to stomach and also causes damage to stomach tissue, which resembles peptic ulcer disease. The immunosuppressive medications (MMF) and NSAID (prednisone) could also cause gastritis in transplant recipients.

3.4.2. Diagnosis and Management

Gastritis can be developed without any symptoms. However, in most cases, the symptoms are similar to those seen with ulcers. The commonly seen symptoms are: Patients having burning sensation or pain in the upper abdomen, and it may better after eating. They have a bad taste in the mouth, indigestion and bloating, loss of appetite, and in severe cases loose stools or diarrhea. Vomiting blood or black/tarry stool is an indicator of severe gastritis. The patients with symptoms of gastritis are suggested to perform several clinical laboratory tests for confirmation of gastritis. The blood samples are collected to find the microbial infections. A stool sample is checked for blood, which is a sign of bleeding and the color of stool indicates whether bleeding is from the stomach or other parts of the GI tract. The test may include complete blood count (CBC), which helps to identify if these patients are having anemia. In addition, stools are also checked for any abnormal microbes (especially for bacteria) that could colonize and damaging stomach. The endoscopy or gastroscopy is also performed to detect inflammation, ulcer and tissue damage in the stomach. If it is severe, biopsies from stomach lining tissue are collected for further examination. If symptoms are not severe medications are suggested for 7 to 10 days.

The treatment of gastritis includes a combination of medications and changes in food habit and lifestyle. In general, antacids and drugs that blocks acid production are prescribed to reduce stomach acid, thereby acidity and irritation to the stomach can be decreased. In addition, antibiotics are prescribed if in case gastritis is due to bacterial infections. So the reduction of stomach acid and removal of infectious agents could give time for the healing of stomach tissue. During this treatment, patients should avoid or limit certain foods to increase the healing of stomach and reduce the risk of reversal of gastritis. The nutritional changes such as diet with high fiber are helpful. The foods with high acids (citrus fruits) should be avoided. The foods with high fat contents, spices and carbonated beverages should also be avoided. The chocolates, coffee and caffeine containing products increase the stomach acid production. So these stuffs should be avoided until healing of stomach lesions.

3.5. Colonic Complications

The colon disorders have also been found in a considerable number of SOT recipients. The renal and liver transplant patients are easily susceptible to colonic complications, which occurs in about 10% of these organ recipients. Renal transplant recipients, mainly elder patients, are at high risk for colon disorders. The most predominant complications are inflammatory bowel diseases (various types of colitis and diverticulitis), perforation, and malignancies (Goldberg et al., 2006; Lee et al., 2014).

3.5.1. Inflammatory Bowel Disease (IBD)

Inflammatory bowel disease (IBD) is a T-cell driven chronic inflammatory disease of the intestinal tract, in which ulcerative colitis and Crohn's disease are most commonly found IBD. Ulcerative colitis involves inflammation of the large intestine, whereas Crohn's disease causes inflammation in any part of the digestive tract. In transplant population, IBD usually develops in the later post-transplant period (2-10 years after transplantation) and its prevalence is ten times higher than in the general population. Despite anti-T cell based immunosuppression has been used in transplant patients, the development of denovo IBD as well as recurrent IBD during post-transplant period remains largely unknown (Hampton et al., 2008; Jorgensen et al., 2013). A very high incidence of IBD, especially, ulcerative colitis, has been seen in patients receiving liver transplantation for primary sclerosing cholangitis (PSC), a chronic cholestatic liver disease, characterized by blockage of the bile duct due to inflammation, scarring or fibrosis and subsequent liver failure due to cirrhosis. In these patients, the risk of colorectal cancer is also high (Jorgensen et al., 2013).

The transplant maintenance medications may also play a role in the development of IBD after transplant surgery. The anti-rejection drugs such as TAC and MMF increase the risk of IBD while CsA does not influence the post-transplant IBD development (Jorgensen et al., 2013). In contrast, AZA can prevent post-transplant IBD. Corticosteroids are also having favorable effects on IBD development, but its side effects upon long term usage is an important concern. Hence, some modifications in the ongoing transplant therapeutic regimen are important to control IBD in transplant patients. For example, replacement of TAC and MMF with suitable alternatives (AZA or CsA) and the inclusion of 5-aminosalicylates (mesalamine) could be appropriate to prevent new onset and relapse of IBD in addition to maintenance of transplant (Indriolo and Ravelli, 2014; Jorgensen et al., 2013). Budesonide is a steroid sparing drug, which can also be considered as a first-line of therapy for new onset of denovo IBD during post-transplant period. Anti-TNFα therapy (infliximab) is more effective, but it should be used with careful monitoring (Indriolo and Ravelli, 2014; Jorgensen et al., 2013). A routine endoscopic surveillance and biopsy analysis helps to evaluate the severity and pathological changes. For severe and refractive IBD, particularly in liver transplant for PSC, colectomy is a better strategy to prevent colorectal cancer in these patients (Indriolo and Ravelli, 2014).

Some viral, bacterial and protozoan infection also mimics ulcerative colitis caused by denovo inflammation. Several pathological studies reveal that emergence of colon ulceration (colitis) due to *C. difficile*, CMV or HSV histologically shares many characteristics of IBD, especially, ulcerative colitis (Geboes, 2008). So careful evaluation should be carried out before conclusive therapy. Since colonic mucosa is the predominant site of CMV disease, the colitis caused by CMV begins with watery diarrhea, and progressively causes abdominal pain, fatigue, and rectal bleeding. In patients with these symptoms, a therapy with ganciclovir or valganciclovir may suppress CMV colitis (Garrido et al., 2013). In addition to this, ischemia due to surgical procedures also leads to colitis, which resembles ulcerative colitis (Geboes, 2008).

Among various transplant medications, high usage of MMF causes non-infectious colitis. The MMF colitis is attributed to its active metabolite MPA. In rare cases, non-obstructive colon dilatation and perforation can be seen. MMF is de-esterified to MPA after absorption and conjugated to form glucuronidated MPA, and this inactive metabolite is partially excreted in the bile and then again converted into an active metabolite (MPA) by colonic bacteria. Hence, the increased concentration MMF and its active metabolites in the colon become toxic (Calmet et al., 2015; Lee et al., 2013). It is quite difficult to distinguish MMF-induced colitis from other colon complications because MMF colitis histologically resembles infectious colitis, IBD and ischemic colitis. Recent clinical studies of colon biopsies suggest more than 15 lamina propria eosinophils per HPF, lack of apoptotic microabsecesses and lack of endocrine cell aggregates in lamina propria can be used to separate MMF colitis other types of colitis (Star et al., 2013).

3.5.2. Diverticulitis

Diverticulosis is the formation of bulges/pockets, filled with solid wastes or liquids, in the weakened spots of mucosal walls of the large intestine due to pressure or straining (constipation) during a bowel movement. In general, diverticulosis is asymptomatic, and they are not harming until any infections or damage to diverticula. Colonic diverticular disease is a medical condition, which can be quite commonly seen in the aged population. It is also found in a considerable number of lung, kidney, heart and lung-heart transplant recipients (Oor et al., 2014; Qasabian et al., 2004). Given the fact that transplant patients are highly prone to infections, the inflammation in diverticula (called diverticulitis) caused by infections and/or immunosuppressive agents becomes life threatening in transplant recipients. In most cases, the initial symptoms such as lower abdominal pain and bloating are masked by graft maintenance therapeutics. Over the time, the bulging of diverticula leads to severe diverticulitis, which may depend on the degree the infection or damage to the diverticulum (Oor et al., 2014; Von Rahden and Germer, 2012). The most serious symptoms include severe pain or cramps in the left side of the lower abdomen, diarrhea, mucous stool, painless bleed from the anus.

A severe diverticulitis can cause colon perforation, which is characterized by a puncture or tear in the wall of the colon. This leads to the leak of intestinal materials into abdominal cavity and causes serious infection, and finally results in death due to peritonitis. In the early period after transplantation, the emergence of perforation is associated with CMV infection or heavy doses of immunosuppressive agents, but in a later period (after 6 months) largely attributed to diverticulosis or un-recognized lymphoma (Calmet et al., 2015; Dalla Valle et al., 2005). It is known that long term use of NSAIDs and corticosteroids increases the risk of perforation. So switch to corticosteroid sparing regimens could help to decrease the severity (Calmet et al., 2015; Dalla Valle et al., 2005).

The diagnosis of diverticulitis is usually done by colonoscopy or computed tomography (CT) scan. In the majority of cases, diverticular disorders have been identified when the patients are diagnosed with other problems since diverticulitis symptoms are masked by immunosuppressive regimens (Medina-Fernandez et al., 2015). Both aerobic and anaerobic bacteria are responsible for infections and inflammations of diverticula. Hence, a common approach for the treatment of mild to moderate diverticulitis is oral intake of broad spectrum antibiotics such as metronidazole along with ciproloxacin or trimethoprim-sulfamethoxazole to control infections related diverticulitis. The combination of amoxicillin and clavulanic acid is also effective and it is a better alternative for diverticulitis treatment. The bowel rest is very important during the treatment of diverticulitis. So patients are usually advised to take liquid diet to manage and avoid further worsening of diverticulitis (Medina-Fernandez et al., 2015). The acute and severe diverticulitis does not respond to any therapeutics hence immediate resection of the colon is important to avoid death in these patients.

4. Other GI Associated Complications in Transplant Recipient

4.1. Biliary Tract Disorders

Biliary complications are more common in liver transplantation, especially in pediatric liver transplants. The major complications of biliary tracts are biliary casts, biliary stricture and choledocholithiasis. The leakage of bile contents is frequent within 3 months of the post-transplant period, mainly due to T-Tube removal, a tube used to reconstruct biliary tract during liver transplantation (Feier et al., 2015). Among these, the biliary stricture is an important concern in liver transplant recipients. Both anastomotic and non-anostomotic biliary stricture are seen in transplant recipients. The anostomotic biliary stricture is due to fibrotic healing and non-anostomotic biliary stricture is due to hepatic artery thrombosis and cytotoxic injury of bile salts. The treatment option for this condition is a reconstruction of the biliary tract or stenting of the bile duct by endoscopic retrograde cholangiopancreatography (ERCP) or percutaneous transhepatic cholangiography (PTCD) (Arain et al., 2013; Verdonk et al., 2006).

Cholelithiasis is a formation of gallstone in the biliary tract, which is another common biliary complication developing in transplant patients. This condition is frequently reported in liver, heart and renal transplant recipients. In the case of kidney transplantation, pre-existing conditions play an important role in the formation of gallstones, in particular, renal transplantation for diabetic nephropathy (Sutariya and Tank, 2014). In these patients, laparoscopic cholecystectomy provides a better outcome from post-transplant cholelithiasis (Coelho et al., 2010). The cardiac transplant patients are having a risk for cholelithiasis during post-transplant period so preemptive cholecystectomy has been carried out in the majority of heart recipients (Englesbe et al., 2005). Retrospective studies indicate that prophylactic cholecystectomy during heart transplantation reduced mortality rate and this procedure is also cost effective compared with treatment for acute choleccystitis, biliary colic or biliary pancreatitis after heart transplantation (Englesbe et al., 2005; Gupta et al., 2000). Infections and immunosuppressive medications are also playing a vital role in the development of gallstone disorders. In patients under long term treatment with CsA or TAC, the incidence of cholelithiasis is relatively high (Alberu et al., 2001; Stief et al., 2009).

4.2. GI Malignancies

The post-transplant malignancy in the GI tract is becoming an important cause of late mortality among the transplant population (Buell et al., 2005; Sampaio et al., 2012). The depressed native antiviral activity and suppressed immunosurveillance of neoplastic cells due to immunosuppressive agents are responsible for high risk of cancer development in transplant recipients (Buell et al., 2005). Population based cancer a study from different centers worldwide confirms that transplant recipients are at high risk for oral and colorectal malignancies. A Swedish study found that transplant patients are 6 fold risks for oral cavity cancer (Adami et al., 2003). Another study showed that the transplant patients are 10 to 20 time's higher risk for rectal cancer. This is mainly due to immunosuppression mediated aggravation of human papillomavirus (HPV) (Rice et al., 2009; Sampaio et al., 2012). Several clinical investigations suggest that mTOR inhibitors based therapeutics can reduce the incidence of post-transplant malignancies (Monaco, 2009). However, a careful selection of immunosuppressive medication should be carried out based on the transplanted organ and prehistory of malignancy. For example, TAC reduces the incidence of anogenital cancer, but it increases the risk of oropharyngeal cancer in transplant recipients with HPV infections (Madeleine et al., 2013).

The post-transplant lymphoproliferative disorder (PTLD) is one of the most common malignancies in transplant recipients since GI tract is abundant of lymphoid tissue. The most common GI site of PTLD is a colon, followed by the small intestine and stomach (Green, 2001; Rubin, 2001). The PTLD incidence is higher in pediatric transplant recipients compared to adult patients. More than 80% of post-transplant lymphomas are associated with B-lymphocytes (Green, 2001). The viral infections by EBV and CMV are important risk factors for the development of PTLD (Wasson et al., 2006). The abdominal pain with evidence of intestinal bleeding is a sign for the possibility of GI tract PTLD. The gold standard for diagnosis of GI tract PTLD is radiographic imaging and histological analyses of tissue biopsy. The Contrast material-enhanced CT scan and magnetic resonance imaging (MRI) are helpful to identify staging of disease (Borhani et al., 2009; Shitrit et al., 2005).

The treatment strategy for PTLD is based on the severity of disease, blood viral load and the requirement of immunosuppressive drugs for the survival of transplanted organs (Green, 2001; Ishii, 2002). The standard therapy typically consists of reduction of immunosuppressive agent and administration of antiviral agents (acyclovir, ganciclovir, or foscarnet) to manage viral load. In addition, most of the PLTD patients have CD20 positive lymphocytes hence administration of more specific CD20 monoclonal antibody (rituximab) could help with quick recovery (Oertel et al., 2005). The surgical treatment is a rare condition. The intestinal obstruction, perforation, and GI bleeding are the indication for emergency surgical resection, which can provide better relief. However, it reduces only 50% risk of death (Shitrit et al., 2005). Chemotherapy also used in under certain conditions like patients failed to respond to surgical excision, but there is high risk for severe toxic and septic complications in this regimen.

Conclusion

The disorders of the GI tract system are unavoidable in solid organ transplant patients and it significantly contributes to morbidity and mortality in the transplant community. The etiology of most GI disorder is an infection, immunosuppressive therapeutics, and pre-existing conditions (cancer, autoimmune diseases). In the early post-transplant period, most of the complications are related to upper GI tract. This includes diarrhea, esophagitis, gastritis, gastroparesis, GERD and peptic ulcer. The disorders like IBD, gastrointestinal malignancies, diverticulitis, and GI tract PTLD are seen in the late post-transplant period. Early diagnosis and prompt intervention are necessary to avoid fatal outcomes and early mortality associated with GI complications. The routine microbiological observations by using multiplex-PCR are crucial to avoid infections related GI complications. The endoscopy, laparoscopy, and/or CT scans evaluation are more helpful to characterize the nature of GI disorders. For infection related GI disorders, an appropriate antimicrobial (antibiotics, antiviral or antifungal) agent as well as ulcer prophylaxis, has to be included in the therapeutic regime with cognizance of adverse effects of these approaches. The careful adjustment of dose (dose splitting/reduction of dose) or temporary withdrawal of ongoing immunosuppressive regimen is also required to boost up treatment of GI complications. In addition, the knowledge of interactions between transplant maintenance drugs and therapeutics used for treating GI disorders is essential to avoid graft dysfunction and rejections. The changes in food habit and lifestyles, such as intake of high fiber and liquid diet, having a small volume of food at regular intervals, avoid high-fat diet, alcohol and smoking can help to prevent and manage GI disorders developed during the post-transplant period.

References

Abdulrahman IS, Al-Quorain AA, Prevalence of gastroesophageal reflux disease and its association with Helicobacter pylori infection in chronic renal failure patients and in renal transplant recipients. *Saudi J Gastroenterol*, 2008; 14: 183-6.

Adami J, Gabel H, Lindelof B, Ekstrom K, Rydh B, Glimelius B, Ekbom A, Adami HO, Granath F, Cancer risk following organ transplantation: a nationwide cohort study in Sweden. *Br J Cancer,* 2003; 89: 1221-7.

Aiyangar A, Rajput P, Shah BV, Mycophenolate induced diarrhoea. *J Assoc Physicians India,* 2010; 58: 192-4.

Al-Absi AI, Cooke CR, Wall BM, Sylvestre P, Ismail MK, Mya M, Patterns of injury in mycophenolate mofetil-related colitis. *Transplant Proc,* 2010; 42: 3591-3.

Alberu J, Gatica M, Cachafeiro-Vilar M, Robles-Diaz G, Bezaury P, Paz-Pinedo F, Vargas-Vorackova F, Asymptomatic gallstones and duration of cyclosporine use in kidney transplant recipients. *Rev Invest Clin,* 2001; 53: 396-400.

Albuquerque A, Cardoso H, Ribeiro A, Rios E, Silva R, Magalhaes J, Macedo G, Herpes and cytomegalovirus esophagitis. *Endoscopy,* 2012; 44 Suppl. 2 UCTN: E242-3.

Angarone M, Ison MG, Diarrhea in solid organ transplant recipients. *Curr Opin Infect Dis,* 2015; 28: 308-16.

Arns W, Noninfectious gastrointestinal (GI) complications of mycophenolic acid therapy: a consequence of local GI toxicity? *Transplant Proc,* 2007; 39: 88-93.

Arslan H, Inci EK, Azap OK, Karakayali H, Torgay A, Haberal M, Etiologic agents of diarrhea in solid organ recipients. *Transpl Infect Dis,* 2007; 9: 270-5.

Aulagnon F, Scemla A, Dewolf S, Legendre C, Zuber J, Diarrhea after kidney transplantation: a new look at a frequent symptom. *Transplantation,* 2014; 98: 806-16.

Basseri B, Conklin JL, Pimentel M, Tabrizi R, Phillips EH, Simsir SA, Chaux GE, Falk JA, Ghandehari S, Soukiasian HJ, Esophageal motor dysfunction and gastroesophageal reflux are prevalent in lung transplant candidates. *Ann Thorac Surg,* 2010; 90: 1630-6.

Bhat M, Watt KD, Mammalian target of rapamycin inhibition after solid organ transplantation: can it, and does it, reduce cancer risk? *Clin Transplant,* 2015; 29: 654-63.

Borhani AA, Hosseinzadeh K, Almusa O, Furlan A, Nalesnik M, Imaging of posttransplantation lymphoproliferative disorder after solid organ transplantation. *Radiographics,* 2009; 29: 981-1000; discussion 1000-2.

Bouza E, Loeches B, Munoz P, Fever of unknown origin in solid organ transplant recipients. *Infect Dis Clin North Am,* 2007; 21: 1033-54, ix-x.

Bravo C, Gispert P, Borro JM, De La Torre M, Cifrian Martinez JM, Fernandez Rozas S, Zurbano Goni F, Group MS, Prevalence and management of gastrointestinal complications in lung transplant patients: MITOS study group. *Transplant Proc,* 2007; 39: 2409-12.

Buell JF, Gross TG, Woodle ES, Malignancy after transplantation. *Transplantation,* 2005; 80: S254-64.

Calmet FH, Yarur AJ, Pukazhendhi G, Ahmad J, Bhamidimarri KR, Endoscopic and histological features of mycophenolate mofetil colitis in patients after solid organ transplantation. *Ann Gastroenterol,* 2015; 28: 366-373.

Cashion AK, Holmes SL, Hathaway DK, Gaber AO, Gastroparesis following kidney/pancreas transplant. *Clin Transplant,* 2004; 18: 306-11.

Chung MC, Wu MJ, Chang CH, Muo CH, Yu TM, Ho HC, Shu KH, Chung CJ, Increased risk of post-transplant malignancy and mortality in transplant tourists: a nationwide population-based cohort study in Taiwan. *Medicine* (Baltimore), 2014; 93: e344.

Cianciolo G, Feliciangeli G, Comai G, Stefoni S, [Protonic pump inhibitors in kidney transplant patients: efficacy and safety]. *Minerva Urol Nefrol,* 2007; 59: 207-15.

Coelho JC, Contieri FL, De Freitas AC, Da Silva FC, Kozak VN, Da Silva Junior AS, [Laparoscopic cholecystectomy in transplant patients]. *Rev Col Bras Cir,* 2010; 37: 23-6.

Coste JF, Vuiblet V, Moustapha B, Bouin A, Lavaud S, Toupance O, De Rougemont A, Benejat L, Megraud F, Wolak-Thierry A, Villena I, Chemla C, Le Magrex E, De Champs C, Andreoletti L, Rieu P, Leveque N, Microbiological diagnosis of severe diarrhea in kidney transplant recipients by use of multiplex PCR assays. *J Clin Microbiol,* 2013; 51: 1841-9.

Dalla Valle R, Capocasale E, Mazzoni MP, Busi N, Benozzi L, Sivelli R, Sianesi M, Acute diverticulitis with colon perforation in renal transplantation. *Transplant Proc,* 2005; 37: 2507-10.

Danziger-Isakov L, Gastrointestinal infections after transplantation. *Curr Opin Gastroenterol,* 2014; 30: 40-6.

Davies NM, Grinyo J, Heading R, Maes B, Meier-Kriesche HU, Oellerich M, Gastrointestinal side effects of mycophenolic acid in renal transplant patients: a reappraisal. *Nephrol Dial Transplant,* 2007; 22: 2440-8.

Davis CS, Shankaran V, Kovacs EJ, Gagermeier J, Dilling D, Alex CG, Love RB, Sinacore J, Fisichella PM, Gastroesophageal reflux disease after lung transplantation: pathophysiology and implications for treatment. *Surgery,* 2010; 148: 737-44; discussion 744-5.

Dongari-Bagtzoglou A, Dwivedi P, Ioannidou E, Shaqman M, Hull D, Burleson J, Oral Candida infection and colonization in solid organ transplant recipients. *Oral Microbiol Immunol,* 2009; 24: 249-54.

Echenique IA, Penugonda S, Stosor V, Ison MG, Angarone MP, Diagnostic yields in solid organ transplant recipients admitted with diarrhea. *Clin Infect Dis,* 2015; 60: 729-37.

Enderby C, Keller CA, An overview of immunosuppression in solid organ transplantation. *Am J Manag Care,* 2015; 21: s12-23.

Englesbe MJ, Dubay DA, Wu AH, Pelletier SJ, Punch JD, Franz MG, Gallbladder disease in cardiac transplant patients: a survey study. *Arch Surg,* 2005; 140: 399-403; discussion 404.

Feier FH, Da Fonseca EA, Seda-Neto J, Chapchap P, Biliary complications after pediatric liver transplantation: Risk factors, diagnosis and management. *World J Hepatol,* 2015; 7: 2162-70.

Fortunato GA, Machado MM, Andrade CF, Felicetti JC, Camargo Jde J, Cardoso PF, Prevalence of gastroesophageal reflux in lung transplant candidates with advanced lung disease. *J Bras Pneumol,* 2008; 34: 772-8.

Frye JW, Peura DA, Managing gastroesophageal reflux disease - comparative efficacy and outcomes of dexlansoprazole MR. *Ther Clin Risk Manag,* 2015; 11: 1649-56.

Garces JC, BK Virus-Associated Nephropathy in Kidney Transplant Recipients. *Ochsner J,* 2010; 10: 245-9.

Garrido E, Carrera E, Manzano R, Lopez-Sanroman A, Clinical significance of cytomegalovirus infection in patients with inflammatory bowel disease. *World J Gastroenterol,* 2013; 19: 17-25.

Gautam A, Gastrointestinal complications following transplantation. *Surg Clin North Am,* 2006; 86: 1195-206, vii.

Geboes K, Crohn's disease and solid organ transplantation. *Gastroenterol Hepatol* (NY), 2008; 4: 877-8.

Gil-Vernet S, Amado A, Ortega F, Alarcon A, Bernal G, Capdevila L, Crespo JF, Cruzado JM, De Bonis E, Esforzado N, Fernandez AM, Franco A, Hortal L, Jimenez C, Group MS, Gastrointestinal complications in renal transplant recipients: MITOS study. *Transplant Proc,* 2007; 39: 2190-3.

Ginsburg PM, Thuluvath PJ, Diarrhea in liver transplant recipients: etiology and management. *Liver Transpl,* 2005; 11: 881-90.

Goldberg HJ, Hertz MI, Ricciardi R, Madoff RD, Baxter NN, Bullard KM, Colon and rectal complications after heart and lung transplantation. *J Am Coll Surg,* 2006; 202: 55-61.

Green M, Management of Epstein-Barr virus-induced post-transplant lymphoproliferative disease in recipients of solid organ transplantation. *Am J Transplant,* 2001; 1: 103-8.

Gumbo T, Hobbs RE, Carlyn C, Hall G, Isada CM, Microsporidia infection in transplant patients. *Transplantation,* 1999; 67: 482-4.

Gupta D, Sakorafas GH, Mcgregor CG, Harmsen WS, Farnell MB, Management of biliary tract disease in heart and lung transplant patients. *Surgery,* 2000; 128: 641-9.

Hagerty JA, Ortiz J, Reich D, Manzarbeitia C, Fungal infections in solid organ transplant patients. *Surg Infect* (Larchmt), 2003; 4: 263-71.

Hampton DD, Poleski MH, Onken JE, Inflammatory bowel disease following solid organ transplantation. *Clin Immunol,* 2008; 128: 287-93.

Hanif FM, Luck NH, Abbas Z, Aziz T, Hassan SM, Mubarak M, Prevalence and Characteristics of Duodenal Villous Atrophy in Renal Transplant Patients Presenting With Persistent Diarrhea in a Developing Country. *Exp Clin Transplant,* 2015.

Hasler WL, Gastroparesis--current concepts and considerations. *Medscape J Med,* 2008; 10: 16.

Helderman JH, Goral S, Gastrointestinal complications of transplant immunosuppression. *J Am Soc Nephrol,* 2002; 13: 277-87.

Herrero JI, Benlloch S, Bernardos A, Bilbao I, Castells L, Castroagudin JF, Gonzalez L, Irastorza I, Navasa M, Otero A, Pons JA, Rimola A, Suarez F, Casanovas T, Otero E, Rodriguez M, Serrano T, Otero S, Lopez I, Miras M, Prieto M, Group MS, Gastrointestinal complications in liver transplant recipients: MITOS study. *Transplant Proc,* 2007; 39: 2311-3.

Hocevar SN, Paddock CD, Spak CW, Rosenblatt R, Diaz-Luna H, Castillo I, Luna S, Friedman GC, Antony S, Stoddard RA, Tiller RV, Peterson T, Blau DM, Sriram RR, Da Silva A, De Almeida M, Benedict T, Goldsmith CS, Zaki SR, Visvesvara GS, Kuehnert MJ, Microsporidia Transplant Transmission Investigation T, Microsporidiosis acquired through solid organ transplantation: a public health investigation. *Ann Intern Med,* 2014; 160: 213-20.

Honda H, Dubberke ER, Clostridium difficile infection in solid organ transplant recipients. *Curr Opin Infect Dis,* 2014; 27: 336-41.

Indriolo A, Ravelli P, Clinical management of inflammatory bowel disease in the organ recipient. *World J Gastroenterol,* 2014; 20: 3525-33.

Ishii KK, [Rapid diagnosis of infectious complications after transplantation]. *Rinsho Byori,* 2002; 50: 1055-60.

Joo YB, Jung HS, Baeg MK, Lee WH, Lee HJ, Yang CW, Cytomegalovirus esophagitis presents as chest pain in a renal transplant recipient. *Korean J Intern Med,* 2013; 28: 497-9.

Jorgensen KK, Lindstrom L, Cvancarova M, Karlsen TH, Castedal M, Friman S, Schrumpf E, Foss A, Isoniemi H, Nordin A, Holte K, Rasmussen A, Bergquist A, Vatn MH, Boberg KM, Immunosuppression after liver transplantation for primary sclerosing cholangitis influences activity of inflammatory bowel disease. *Clin Gastroenterol Hepatol,* 2013; 11: 517-23.

Kellar CA, Solid organ transplantation overview and delection criteria. *Am J Manag Care,* 2015; 21: S4-11.

Khan MQ, Nizami IY, Khan BJ, Al-Ashgar HI, Lung transplantation triggered "jackhammer esophagus": a case report and review of literature. *J Neurogastroenterol Motil,* 2013; 19: 390-4.

Kim IS, Lee H, Park JC, Shin SK, Lee SK, Lee YC, Increased incidence of endoscopic erosive esophagitis in solid organ transplant recipients. *Gut Liver,* 2012; 6: 349-54.

Kim JJ, Marks SD, Long-term outcomes of children after solid organ transplantation. *Clinics* (Sao Paulo), 2014; 69 Suppl. 1: 28-38.

Lauwers GY, Fujita H, Nagata K, Shimizu M, Pathology of non-Helicobacter pylori gastritis: extending the histopathologic horizons. *J Gastroenterol,* 2010; 45: 131-45.

Lee JT, Dunn TB, Sirany AM, Melton GB, Madoff RD, Kwaan MR, Colorectal surgery after kidney transplantation: characteristics of early vs. late posttransplant interventions. *J Gastrointest Surg,* 2014; 18: 1299-305.

Lee LY, Ison MG, Diarrhea caused by viruses in transplant recipients. *Transpl Infect Dis,* 2014; 16: 347-58.

Lee S, De Boer WB, Subramaniam K, Kumarasinghe MP, Pointers and pitfalls of mycophenolate-associated colitis. *J Clin Pathol,* 2013; 66: 8-11.

Leroy S, Isapof A, Fargue S, Fakhoury M, Bensman A, Deschenes G, Jacqz-Aigrain E, Ulinski T, Tacrolimus nephrotoxicity: beware of the association of diarrhea, drug interaction and pharmacogenetics. *Pediatr Nephrol,* 2010; 25: 965-9.

Lipson DA, Berlin JA, Palevsky HI, Kotloff RM, Tino G, Bavaria J, Kaiser L, Long WB, Metz DC, Lichtenstein GR, Giant gastric ulcers and risk factors for gastroduodenal mucosal disease in orthotopic lung transplant patients. *Dig Dis Sci,* 1998; 43: 1177-85.

Madeleine MM, Finch JL, Lynch CF, Goodman MT, Engels EA, HPV-related cancers after solid organ transplantation in the United States. *Am J Transplant,* 2013; 13: 3202-9.

Mahmud N, Klipa D, Ahsan N, Antibody immunosuppressive therapy in solid-organ transplant: Part I. *MAbs*, 2010; 2: 148-56.

Maltzman JS, Koretzky GA, Azathioprine: old drug, new actions. *J Clin Invest,* 2003; 111: 1122-4.

Mathis AS, Managed care implications of improving long-term outcomes in organ transplantation. *Am J Manag Care,* 2015; 21: s24-30.

Mayer AD, Dmitrewski J, Squifflet JP, Besse T, Grabensee B, Klein B, Eigler FW, Heemann U, Pichlmayr R, Behrend M, Vanrenterghem Y, Donck J, Van Hooff J, Christiaans M, Morales JM, Andres A, Johnson RW, Short C, Buchholz B, Rehmert N, Land W, Schleibner S, Forsythe JL, Talbot D, Pohanka E et al., Multicenter randomized trial comparing tacrolimus (FK506) and cyclosporine in the prevention of renal allograft rejection: a report of the European Tacrolimus Multicenter Renal Study Group. *Transplantation,* 1997; 64: 436-43.

Medina-Fernandez FJ, Diaz-Jimenez N, Gallardo-Herrera AB, Gomez-Luque I, Garcilazo-Arsimendi DJ, Gomez-Barbadillo J, New trends in the management of diverticulitis and colonic diverticular disease. *Rev Esp Enferm Dig,* 2015; 107: 162-70.

Modi P, Pal B, Modi J, Kumar S, Sood A, Menon M, Robotic assisted kidney transplantation. *Indian J Urol,* 2014; 30: 287-92.

Mohammed A, Neujahr DC, Gastroesophageal reflux disease and graft failure after lung transplantation. *Transplant Rev* (Orlando), 2010; 24: 99-103.

Monaco AP, The role of mTOR inhibitors in the management of posttransplant malignancy. *Transplantation,* 2009; 87: 157-63.

Munoz P, Fernandez NS, Farinas MC, Epidemiology and risk factors of infections after solid organ transplantation. *Enferm Infecc Microbiol Clin,* 2012; 30 Suppl. 2: 10-8.

Oertel SH, Verschuuren E, Reinke P, Zeidler K, Papp-Vary M, Babel N, Trappe RU, Jonas S, Hummel M, Anagnostopoulos I, Dorken B, Riess HB, Effect of anti-CD 20 antibody rituximab in patients with post-transplant lymphoproliferative disorder (PTLD). *Am J Transplant,* 2005; 5: 2901-6.

Oor JE, Atema JJ, Boermeester MA, Vrouenraets BC, Unlu C, A systematic review of complicated diverticulitis in post-transplant patients. *J Gastrointest Surg,* 2014; 18: 2038-46.

Pant C, Deshpande A, Larson A, O'connor J, Rolston DD, Sferra TJ, Diarrhea in solid-organ transplant recipients: a review of the evidence. *Curr Med Res Opin,* 2013; 29: 1315-28.

Parfitt JR, Jayakumar S, Driman DK, Mycophenolate mofetil-related gastrointestinal mucosal injury: variable injury patterns, including graft-versus-host disease-like changes. *Am J Surg Pathol,* 2008; 32: 1367-72.

Ponticelli C, Passerini P, Gastrointestinal complications in renal transplant recipients. *Transpl Int,* 2005; 18: 643-50.

Qasabian RA, Meagher AP, Lee R, Dore GJ, Keogh A, Severe diverticulitis after heart, lung, and heart-lung transplantation. *J Heart Lung Transplant,* 2004; 23: 845-9.

Reimer C, Bytzer P, [Adverse events associated with long-term use of proton pump inhibitors]. *Ugeskr Laeger,* 2012; 174: 2289-93.

Rice JP, Spier BJ, Cornett DD, Walker AJ, Richie K, Pfau PR, Utility of colonoscopy in the evaluation of diarrhea in solid organ transplant recipients. *Transplantation,* 2009; 88: 374-9.

Rosolowski M, Kierzkiewicz M, Etiology, diagnosis and treatment of infectious esophagitis. *Prz Gastroenterol,* 2013; 8: 333-7.

Rubin RH, Gastrointestinal infectious disease complications following transplantation and their differentiation from immunosuppressant-induced gastrointestinal toxicities. *Clin Transplant,* 2001; 15 Suppl. 4: 11-22.

Ryan EA, Paty BW, Senior PA, Shapiro AM, Risks and side effects of islet transplantation. *Curr Diab Rep,* 2004; 4: 304-9.

Saidi RF, Current status of liver transplantation. *Arch Iran Med,* 2012; 15: 772-6.

Sampaio MS, Cho YW, Qazi Y, Bunnapradist S, Hutchinson IV, Shah T, Posttransplant malignancies in solid organ adult recipients: an analysis of the US National Transplant Database. *Transplantation,* 2012; 94: 990-8.

Schaier M, Scholl C, Scharpf D, Hug F, Bonisch-Schmidt S, Dikow R, Schmitt WH, Schwenger V, Zeier M, Sommerer C, Proton pump inhibitors interfere with the immunosuppressive potency of mycophenolate mofetil. *Rheumatology* (Oxford), 2010; 49: 2061-7.

Shitrit D, Shitrit AB, Dickman R, Sahar G, Saute M, Kramer MR, Gastrointestinal involvement of posttransplant lymphoproliferative disorder in lung transplant recipients: report of a case. *Dis Colon Rectum,* 2005; 48: 2144-7.

Snydman DR, Posttransplant microbiological surveillance. *Clin Infect Dis,* 2001; 33 Suppl. 1: S22-5.

Star KV, Ho VT, Wang HH, Odze RD, Histologic features in colon biopsies can discriminate mycophenolate from GVHD-induced colitis. *Am J Surg Pathol,* 2013; 37: 1319-28.

Steger AC, Timoney AS, Griffen S, Salem RR, Williams G, The influence of immunosuppression on peptic ulceration following renal transplantation and the role of endoscopy. *Nephrol Dial Transplant,* 1990; 5: 289-92.

Stief J, Stempfle HU, Gotzberger M, Uberfuhr P, Kopple M, Lehnert P, Kaiser C, Schiemann U, Biliary diseases in heart transplanted patients: a comparison between cyclosporine A versus tacrolimus-based immunosuppression. *Eur J Med Res,* 2009; 14: 206-9.

Sutariya V, Tank A, An audit of laparoscopic cholecystectomy in renal transplant patients. *Ann Med Health Sci Res,* 2014; 4: 48-50.

Torricelli FC, Watanabe A, David-Neto E, Nahas WC, Current management issues of immediate postoperative care in pediatric kidney transplantation. *Clinics* (Sao Paulo), 2014; 69 Suppl. 1: 39-41.

Tzvetanov I, Bejarano-Pineda L, Giulianotti PC, Jeon H, Garcia-Roca R, Bianco F, Oberholzer J, Benedetti E, State of the art of robotic surgery in organ transplantation. *World J Surg,* 2013; 37: 2791-9.

Vaziri S, Pezhman Z, Sayyad B, Mansouri F, Janbakhsh A, Afsharian M, Najafi F, Efficacy of valganciclovir and ganciclovir for cytomegalovirus disease in solid organ transplants: A meta-analysis. *J Res Med Sci,* 2014; 19: 1185-92.

Wasson S, Zafar MN, Best J, Reddy HK, Post-transplantation lymphoproliferative disorder in heart and kidney transplant patients: a single-center experience. *J Cardiovasc Pharmacol Ther,* 2006; 11: 77-83.

Watson CJ, Dark JH, Organ transplantation: historical perspective and current practice. *Br J Anaesth,* 2012; 108 Suppl. 1: i29-42.

Yiannopoulos A, Shafazand S, Ziedalski T, Berry GJ, Robbins RC, Theodore J, Faul JL, Gastric pacing for severe gastroparesis in a heart-lung transplant recipient. *J Heart Lung Transplant,* 2004; 23: 371-4.

Zhang Y, Ruiz P, Solid organ transplant-associated acute graft-versus-host disease. *Arch Pathol Lab Med,* 2010; 134: 1220-4.

In: Disorders of Gastrointestinal Systems … ISBN: 978-1-63485-366-8
Editors: S. Rajagopal, S. Murugan and R. Saravanan

Chapter 13

PHARMACOLOGICAL REVIEW OF PROTON PUMP INHIBITORS

Prakash Srinivasan Timiri Shanmugam[1,*], PhD, Senthilkumar Sankararaman[2], MD, and Uma Anitha[3], MTech

[1]Department of Biochemistry and Molecular Biology,
Louisiana State University Health Sciences Center-Shreveport, Louisiana, US
[2]Department of Pediatrics, Pediatric Gastroenterology division,
Rainbow Babies and Children's Hospital Cleveland, Ohio, US
[3]School of Bio Science and Technology, VIT University, Vellore, Tamil Nadu, India

ABSTRACT

Acid-related diseases include a variety of disorders that can affect the esophagus, stomach and duodenum. It is a broad term used to describe a range of conditions in which acid is involved in the generation of symptoms and/or complications. Proton pump inhibitors (PPIs) were introduced in 1980 and, since then there has been a sharp increase in their usage in the western world. It is the first-choice therapy in the management of a variety of upper gastrointestinal (GI) conditions, particularly gastroesophageal reflux disease (GERD) by inhibiting the gastric H^+/K^+ adenosine triphosphatase via covalent binding to the cysteine residues of the proton pump. This chapter addresses the pharmacological action of PPI in acid-related diseases, indications for PPI use, the adverse effects/risks involved with its use, and some conditions in which their use is controversial.

Keywords: proton pump inhibitor, H^+/K^+ adenosine triphosphatase, histamine-2 receptor

---

* Corresponding author: Dr. Prakash Srinivasan Timiri Shanmugam, PhD. Department of Biochemistry and Molecular Biology, Louisiana State University Health Sciences Center-Shreveport, Shreveport, Louisiana 71130, US. Ph: + (1) 318-675-9105, fax: + (1) 318-675-5180, email: prakashsrini2002@yahoo.com.

INTRODUCTION

Proton pump inhibitors (PPIs) are the most effective drugs to reduce gastric acid secretion and are the most commonly prescribed class of medications worldwide. PPIs are acid-activated prodrugs which reduce the gastric acid secretion by inhibiting the H^+/K^+ adenosine triphosphatase (ATPase). H^+/K^+ ATPase are also known as the proton pump. Because of covalent binding, the inhibitory effects of PPIs last much longer than their plasma half-life. Apart from many short-term applications, maintenance therapy with PPIs is recommended and increasingly used in certain diseases, such as Zollinger-Ellison syndrome and severe gastroesophageal reflux disease (GERD). GERD with erosive esophagi is or Barrett's esophagus benefit from long-term PPI. The combination of PPIs and antibiotics also eradicates *Helicobacter pylori*. In this chapter, we review the pharmacological action, indications and adverse effects of PPI.

PHYSIOLOGY OF GASTRIC ACID SECRETION

Gastric acid is produced in the stomach by the parietal cells. The normal human stomach contains approximately one billion parietal cells which secrete 0.16 M hydrochloric acid (HCl). The number of parietal cells determines the maximum secretory rate and also accounts for the individual variability of acid production (Hersey et al. 1995). The parietal cells are predominantly located in the middle and lower parts of the gastric glands in the fundus and body (termed the oxyntic part) of the stomach. Secretion of acid from a parietal cell into the lumen is an energy demanding process where the parietal cell must spend a large amount of energy to concentrate the hydrogen ions. This energy comes from adenosine triphosphate (ATP) which is produced by the numerous mitochondria located within the cell. When the parietal cell pumps H^+ into the lumen, it is exchanged for K^+ across the mucosal membrane (Glynn et al. 1990). This active transport is catalyzed by the H^+/K^+ ATPase which is also called the gastric proton pump. This proton pump comprises the final process of acid secretion by which hydrochloric acid (HCl) is secreted in to the gastric lumen. HCl aids in the digestive process and also provides a sterile environment in the stomach.

Acid secretion by the parietal cells is a complex process which is regulated by paracrine, endocrine and neural pathways. Neural stimulation occurs via the involvement of the vagal nerve which activates in response to the smell, sight or taste of food. The physiological stimuli for acid secretion include acetylcholine, gastrin and histamine. Acetylcholine (ACh) is released by postganglionic neurons of the vagus and stimulates hydrogen ion secretion via muscarinic M3 receptors on the parietal cells. ACh also stimulates gastrin release which in turn produces acid secretion (Hersey et al. 1995; Sachs 1997; Waldum et al. 1993). ACh activates phospholipase C (PLC), which catalyzes the formation of inositol triphosphate (IP_3). IP_3 causes the release of intracellular Ca^{2+} and activates calmodulin kinases.

Histamine is the chief paracrine transmitter and a potent stimulator of acid secretion. It is ubiquitous in many tissues including the entire gastrointestinal (GI) tract. Histamine is produced by the enterochromaffin-like (ECL) cells in the GI tract. In the stomach, the ECL cells are located close to the parietal cells. Histamine acts on the H2 receptors which are located on the basolateral aspect of the parietal cell membrane. In parietal cells, histamine binds to the H2 receptors, leading to elevation of intracellular cyclic AMP concentrations and activation of protein kinase A (PKA). One effect of PKA activation is the phosphorylation of cytoskeletal proteins involved in the transport of the gastric H^+/K^+ ATPase from cytoplasm to the plasma membrane, i.e., from the vesicular and/or tubular vesicular membrane to the canaliculus. In the canaliculus, the gastric H^+/K^+ ATPase can access potassium chloride (KCl) in the extracellular region and exchange the intracellular protons (H^+) with the extracellular K^+ ions, which represent the gastric acid secretion.

Gastrin stimulates acid secretion by directly stimulating the parietal cells as well as stimulating the release of histamine from the ECL cells. Gastrin is produced by the G cells which are located in the antral part of the stomach. Gastrin has a trophic effect on the ECL cells and also regulates the proliferation of ECL cells. By binding to the gastrin/CCK-2 receptors on the parietal cells, gastrin stimulates the PLC similar to ACh and activates a further cascade of events resulting in increased acid production. Increased gastrin levels (hypergastrinemia) results in an increase in the number of ECL cells (hyperplasia) which in turn leads to an increase in the blood levels of chromogranin-A (CgA) (Hersey et al. 1995; Sachs 1997; Waldum et al. 1993). These three regulatory pathways are well coordinated either to stimulate or inhibit acid production. The release of histamine is the most important positive regulatory mechanism of the gastric acid secretion as histamine enhances acid production directly and, gastrin also stimulates the ECL cells to produces histamine.

When activated by stimuli such as histamine and ACh, the parietal cell undergoes dramatic morphologic changes from the resting status to the stimulated state. In the parietal cells, the gastric H^+, K^+ - ATPase which pumps gastric acid, are present in cytoplasmic tubular membranes in the resting state and in the stimulated state. They are noted in the microvilli of the expanded secretory canaliculus. This morphologic change is thought to result from fusion of cytoplasmic vesicles with rudimentary microvilli to form the elongated microvilli of the expanded secretory canaliculus (Forte et al. 1983; Sawaguchi et al. 2005). The gastric H^+/K^+ ATPase moves from the tubulovesicles to the apical membrane in the canaliculus of the stimulated state and secretes gastric acid by an electroneutral, ATP-dependent hydrogen-potassium (H^+/K^+) exchange (Sachs et al. 1976). This enzyme utilizes the extracellular K^+ and secretes acid by the exchange of cytoplasmic hydrogen ions with these K^+ ions. Thus, they are also considered a proton pump and this activity in the parietal cell represents the final step of acid secretion. The parietal cell H^+/K^+ ATPase is a member of the family of ion-motive transport enzymes which includes F1, V and P ATPases. P ATPases are subdivided into P1 or P2 types based on the number of transmembrane segments. H^+/K^+ ATPase and Na^+/K^+ ATPase belong to P2 subtype.

Gastric Acid Suppressive Therapies

More than a century ago, the initial discoveries of gastrin followed by that of histamine, lead to tremendous progress in understanding their role in the regulation of acid secretion (Malfertheiner et al. 2006). The initial management strategy for acid-related diseases was acid neutralization by compounds such as calcium carbonate, aluminum hydroxide and magnesium hydroxide which are called antacids. Even though antacids provided good symptom relief, their effects were only temporary. A dramatic improvement in the management of acid related disorders was accomplished four decades ago with the invention of histamine type 2 (H2) receptor antagonists (Black et al. 1972; Fellenius et al. 1981).

The first H2 receptor antagonists introduced on the market was cimetidine in 1977 (Okabe et al. 1977), followed by ranitidine, famotidine and nitrazidine. These agents are specific antagonists that inhibit gastric acid secretion by blocking the H2 receptors on the basolateral membrane of the parietal cells. The H2 receptor antagonists are not able to inhibit meal-induced acid secretion, and are only suitable for acid suppression during periods of basal acid secretion (Black et al. 1972). Hence, a dosage at bedtime is generally recommended (Gledhill et al. 1983). Adverse reactions are relatively rare. However, there are some clinically important interactions between H2 receptor antagonists and other drugs such as ketoconazole, metoprolol and theophylline. Another limitation in clinical use is the development of tachyphylaxis (Nwokolo et al. 1990). Due to the partial inhibition of acid production, H2 receptor antagonists showed only limited healing effects in GERD which prompted the researchers to explore the inhibition of the proton pump as the most potent target for acid suppression (Fellenius et al. 1981). PPIs are the preferred first line therapy as they produce more complete and longer lasting acid suppression than H2 receptor antagonist (Sachs 1997). The first PPI introduced in 1989 was omeprazole and the other PPIs available on the market include lanzoprazole, pantoprazole, esomeprazole, and rabeprazole. All PPIs share a common motif and vary in their substitutions. These medications effectively inhibit the final pathway for acid secretion in the parietal cells.

PHARMACOKINETICS OF PPI

PPI are rapidly absorbed in the duodenum after oral administration with peak concentrations occurring two to four hours after administration. Since these drugs are acid-labile, they must be formulated in an enteric coating to avoid rapid degradation the stomach (Stedman et al. 2000). Both symptom control and healing in acid related disorders correlate well to the degree of acid suppression (Burget et al. 1990). PPIs also have a slightly more preferable safety profile with fewer interactions with other drugs when compared with H2 receptor antagonists (Scarpignato et al. 2006). PPIs are effective when the parietal cell is inhibited for post prandial acid production. These drugs should be taken prior to a meal for optimal control of the acid secretion and to avoid therapeutic failure (Hatlebakk et al. 2000; Wolfe et al. 2000). Therefore the administration of PPIs is recommended 0.5-1.0 hour before a meal to enhance the absorption and availability. Since PPIs require an acid environment for activation, simultaneous administration of PPI with other acid suppressing medications such as H2 receptor antagonists, prostaglandins or somatostatin analogous (octreotide) is not recommended.

In most individuals, once daily dosing is sufficient to produce the desired level of acid inhibition. However, occasionally a second dose is necessary and should preferably be administered prior to the evening meal. PPIs are metabolized by the polymorphic cytochrome P450 system (Andersson 1996; Meyer 1996; Tucker 1994; Andersson et al. 1993). Most PPIs are predominantly metabolized by the S-mephenytoin hydroxylase and to varying degrees by nifedipine hydroxylase (Meyer 1996; Tucker 1994; Andersson et al. 1993). However, in contrast to the other PPIs, pantoprazole has a lower affinity to the cytochrome P450 (Huber et al. 1995; Kromer et al. 1990; Simon et al. 1991). In addition to metabolism by the cytochrome P450 system, pantoprazole is also metabolized by a cytosolic sulphotransferase (Meyer 1996; Kromer et al. 1990; Simon et al. 1991; Sharma et al. 1984; Robert et al. 1991; Wallace et al. 1991).

Omeprazole, lansoprazole and pantoprazole are mainly metabolized via the isoenzyme CYP2C19, while esomeprazole mainly involves CYP3A4. Inactive metabolites are excreted via urine and feces. Omeprazole is converted to hydroxyl and 5-O-demethyl metabolites by CYP2C19 and to the sulfone by CYP3A4 (Furuta et al. 2005). Omeprazole is a racemic mixture of two enantiomers, R-omeprazole and S-omeprazole. Each enantiomer showed a different affinity to the CYP enzyme. R-omeprazole was more sensitive to CYP2C19 while S-omeprazole was less sensitive (Abelo et al. 2000; Andersson et al. 2001). Therefore S-omeprazole provided a better plasma level of the drug. Clinicians should be aware of the interaction between PPI and drugs that are metabolized through CYP2C19 and/or CYP3A4 including ketoconazole, atazanavir and clopidogrel. PPIs also affect the absorption of drugs which are dependent on low pH like gefitinib. PPIs do not require dose adjustment in hepatic and renal failures. PPI interacts with many antiviral agents. Concurrent use of PPIs and rilpivirine is not recommended due to reduced plasma levels of rilpivirine and subsequent decreased therapeutic effect of rilpivirne.

Since PPIs are acid-activated prodrugs, it is important to keep the PPI plasma levels high untill the beginning of gastric acid secretion. Maintaining a high plasma level of the drug is significantly affected by the character of the metabolism. According to the metabolic rate of omeprazole, individuals are classified as homozygous extensive metabolizer (homoEM), heterozygous extensive metabolizer (heteroEM) and poor metabolizer (PM). PMs exhibit a three to tenfold higher area under the plasma concentration curve (AUC) than homo EM, while hetero EMs exhibit a two to three fold higher AUC (Klotz et al. 2004; Klotz 2006). Hence, slow metabolizers show a greater acid-suppressive effect of PPI than rapid metabolizers.

PHARMACODYNAMICS OF PPI

All PPIs are substitute benzomidazole derivates, and they function as prodrugs and accumulate in the acid space of the parietal cell where they are converted to active sulphenamides by an acid catalyzed reaction. All PPIs are weak bases (pyridines) and in contact with the acidic environment in the gastric glands, they are protonated and accumulated in the secretory canaliculus which is the highly acidic space in the parietal cell. Within the acidic space, PPIs are transformed and bind covalently and almost irreversibly to the proton pump leading to a specific and sustained inhibition of acid secretion. By covalent binding at cysteines near the ion pathway, the sulphenamides inhibit the proton pump (H^+/K^+ ATPase) irreversibly, resulting in marked inhibition of both basal and stimulated gastric acid secretion (Fellenius et al. 1981). PPIs only bind to active proton pumps, therefore only activated parietal cells will be inhibited, and a resting parietal cell will escape inhibition (Sachs 1997). So with the first dose of PPI, the acid suppression is incomplete and suboptimal. Two-thirds of maximal acid production is inhibited after five continuous days of administration of PPI due to constant recruitment of active proton pumps and their successive inhibition. The ability of the parietal cell to secrete acid is restored when a new proton pump is converted on the canalicular surface. Similarly on discontinuation, maximal acid output is restored in 24-48 hours due to restoration of new proton pumps.

APPROVED INDICATIONS FOR PPI USE

Increased acid secretion is often found in patients with a duodenal ulcer (Sachs G et al. 2000). Inhibiting the acid secretion heals the ulcer, and the more the secretion is inhibited, the quicker the healing process will be (Huang JQ et al. 1996). In the case of gastric ulcer, acid secretion is either normal or reduced (Wolfe MM et al. 1988). Nonetheless, inhibition of acid secretion does help in ulcer healing and reduces relapses (Huang JQ et al. 1996). Reduced acid secretion in gastric ulcers is caused by the accompanying gastritis (Duplessis DJ 1965). Gastric ulcers generally need a longer period of treatment (usually eight weeks) before healing, compared with duodenal ulcers (usually four weeks) (Huang JQ et al. 1996). It is well accepted that the *Helicobacter pylori* infection is an important factor in the development of peptic ulcer diseases, particularly the duodenal ulcer (Bonagura AF et al. 1996). Not all patients with peptic ulcer diseases are *Helicobacter pylori* positive, but those who are positive will benefit from an eradication regimen consisting of a PPI plus antimicrobial agents. A seven-day regimen is recommended by consensus guidelines (Malfertheiner P et al. 2002).

Non-steroidal anti-inflammatory drugs (NSAID) are known to increase the risk of dyspepsia and peptic ulcers, with up to 25% of long-term NSAID users developing ulcer disease (Cheatum 1999). NSAID use results in gastric mucosal damage with even a reduced acid load (Schoen RT et al. 1989). Therefore, adverse events that influence the GI tract are common among NSAID users, where the predominant GI side effects are gastroduodenal ulcers, erosions and dyspeptic symptoms (Butt JH et al. 1988). According to the 2009 American College of Gastroenterology guidelines, patients taking daily NSAID long term should be considered for preventive therapy with PPI (Lanza et al. 2009). PPI have been shown to have a prophylactic effect against ulcers and dyspeptic symptoms in patients on long-term treatment with NSAIDs (Ekstrom P et al. 1996; McCarthy DM 2001). Patients who have experienced a gastric ulcer bleed and use of both a cyclooxygenase-2 inhibitor and a PPI have no recurrent events at all (Chan et al. 2007). In the setting of active ulcer disease, an appropriate course of PPI therapy (four weeks for duodenal ulcers and eight weeks for gastric ulcers) should be used in addition to discontinuing the NSAID.

GERD is among the most common gastrointestinal disorders in people in the western world (Dent J et al. 2005). Erosive esophagitis (EE) is a common complication of GERD, and shows a range from 20% to 40% of cases. It is widely recognized that patients with EE develop complications (e.g., bleeding, strictures, Barrett esophagus). The diagnosis of GERD is usually based on a history of "typical" symptoms such as heartburn and acid regurgitation, with the symptoms ranging from mild to atypical, making diagnosis of this condition difficult at times difficult. According to the Montreal definition, GERD symptoms have to be troublesome or severe enough to cause a clinically significant impairment of the patient's health-related quality of life (Vakil N et al. 2006). PPIs provide healing of erosive esophagitis and relief of symptoms in patients with GERD, with intragastric pH > 4.0 positively correlating with healing of EE (Katz et al. 2007; Armstrong 2004). Studies have shown that

PPIs healed EE in at least 84% of patients with daily use with 12-month maintenance success rates ranging from 78% to 82% with daily use. Use of PPIs in Barrett esophagus can provide symptomatic benefits with regard to heartburn relief, prevention of stricture formation, and more effective and faster healing of esophagitis and esophageal ulcers than an H2 antagonist (Triadafilopoulos 2000). The use of PPIs for the prevention of stress ulcers has been well-defined in critical care patients.

Maintaining an intragastric pH above four has been widely accepted as the benchmark for the efficiency of anti-secretary agents which are used in the treatment of pathological reflux (Lambert R 1997). The degree of mucosal healing is directly related to the proportion of time during the 24 hour period for which intragastric pH is maintained above four. Distinct advantages in terms of healing and symptom relief have been shown for PPIs over H2 receptor antagonists in the control of GERD symptoms as well as in the healing of esophagitis (Jones R et al. 2001). PPI offers, according to 33 randomized controlled trials, a healing rate of approximately 78% in patients with esophagitis (DeVault KR et al. 1999). PPI are also used in the treatment of patients with Zollinger-Ellison syndrome. In some countries, these drugs are also approved for treatment of ulcer-like symptoms, and this indication is probably based on the results from the Bond and Opera studies, showing the benefit of PPI compared with placebo in patients with ulcer-like dyspepsia (Talley NJ et al. 1998). PPIs are also used to treat PPI-responsive eosinophilia, an entity similar to eosinophillic esophagitis.

NON-APPROVED INDICATIONS FOR PPI USE

The use of PPI for functional dyspepsia is common although the usage to manage dyspepsia is controversial. There is little evidence that excess acid secretion is involved in the etiology of this condition (Moayyedi P et al. 2006), and the natural history of functional dyspepsia remains poorly defined (Agreus L et al. 2001; Talley NJ et al. 1992). It has been shown that the placebo response in functional dyspepsia is high and is at least 30% to 40% (Thompson WG 2000). It has also been demonstrated that treatment with PPI has a limited therapeutic effect over placebo (Talley NJ et al. 1998; Wong WM et al. 2002). Patients with uninvestigated dyspepsia may, according to some guidelines, be recommended a single dose therapy of H2 receptor antagonists for two to four weeks to assess the response in patients without alarming symptoms. Endoscopy is recommended only for the elderly and patients with persistent or rapidly recurring symptoms (Talley NJ et al. 1998).

PPI are often prescribed as ulcer prophylaxis together with corticosteroids in a variety of conditions treated with corticosteroids. There has been some controversy about whether the use of corticosteroids is associated with an increased risk for peptic ulcer. Earlier data indicated that the use of corticosteroids was associated with the development of a peptic ulcer, although only in a minority of patients (Messer J et al. 1983). Recent studies have found no association between corticosteroid use and the development of a peptic ulcer. It has been demonstrated that only patients on corticosteroids who are concomitantly treated with NSAID are at increased risk for development of a peptic ulcer compared to patients taking only corticosteroids (Conn HO et al. 1976; Piper JM et al. 1997). The use of PPIs for the prevention of stress ulcers has been well-defined in critical care patients. In recent years, this practice has become increasingly common in hospitalized patients (Nardino RJ et al. 2000).

With little or no evidence to support the PPI use, this usage for prevention of stress ulcer in general medicine patients are currently not recommended (Howden CW 1999; Raynard B et al. 1999). PPIs are not approved for GERD in infants less than one year of age but are frequently used by clinicians.

Adverse-Effects of PPIs

The most frequently reported short-term primary adverse effects of PPI on the order of 1% to 5% are headache, nausea, vomiting, flatulence, diarrhea, constipation, abdominal pain and rash. Secondary adverse effects associated with long-term use include osteoporosis, increased risk of enteric infections, altered metabolism of other medications, and formation of gastric polyps/carcinoid.

Patients treated with a PPI develop secondary hypergastrinemia and subsequently on longer term develop ECL cell hyperplasia. The widespread and chronic use of PPIs has raised concerns over the potential risk of the development of ECL carcinoids when exposed to life-long and potent acid inhibition. During the early development phase of the PPIs, it was shown that female rats developed gastric carcinoids when exposed to life-long PPI therapy. However, in retrospect this was found to be a species-specific effect related to a 10 times higher gastrin production in rats compared to humans. There have been case reports arguing for a plausible association between PPI use and gastric carcinoids in humans (Jianu et al. 2012). However, these case reports can be argued as being coincidental given the low prevalence of gastric carcinoids and the high prevalence of PPI use. More robust data comes from randomized controlled trial study in which 158 GERD patients undergoing laparoscopic anti-reflux surgery were compared to 180 patients treated with esomeprazole for five years. This study found that despite a continued proliferative drive on enterochromaffin-like cells during esomeprazole treatment, no dysplastic or neoplastic lesions were found and no safety concerns were raised (Fiocca et al. 2012). PPIs have now been available for 25 years and post-marketing surveillance and prospective studies do not support a causal relationship between long-term PPI use and an increased risk of GI cancer.

PPI use leads to diminished acid secretion, diminished somatostatin release, and thus increased G-cell release of gastrin and hypergastrinemia. Gastric cells can become hyperplastic and form fundic gland polyps (FGPs) in 7% to 10% of patients taking PPIs for ≥12 months. Such polyps are benign and typically regress with the discontinuation of PPI.

Gastric acid plays a principal role in sterilizing contents entering the digestive tract. Thus, reduction in gastric acid has been associated with an increased risk of both enteric and systemic infections, particularly *Clostridium difficile (C. difficile)* colitis. The risks of prescribing PPIs to individuals at risk for *C. difficile*, including the immunocompromised elderly, hospitalized patients and those taking cyclic antibiotics should be weighed against the benefits. These concerns have led the Food and Drug Administration (FDA) to issue a safety announcement regarding the use of PPIs and the incidence of *C. difficile*, stating that a diagnosis of *C. difficile* should be considered for people taking PPIs who develop diarrhea that does not improve.

In recent years, retrospective observational studies have indicated an association between PPI use and hypomagnesaemia. In patients receiving diuretics or digoxin, before initiation of

PPIs for long-term therapy, serum magnesium levels should be obtained and monitored periodically. PPIs are used for gastric protection in patients using clopidogrel and acetylsalicylic acid. It is debatable whether PPI (especially omeprazole) blunts the cardiovascular protective effects of clopidogrel as has been shown in pharmacodynamic studies. However, high quality observational studies and one randomized controlled trial study have not reported a significant increase in cardiovascular events for PPI users as compared to non-PPI users (Bhatt et al. 2010).

There have also been reports of an association between PPIs and Community-Acquired Pneumonia (CAP). Abnormal gastric colonization and increased microorganisms associated with increased gastric pH leading to aspiration are theoretical risks of PPI use. PPI therapy started within 30 days was associated with an increased risk for CAP, although longer-term use did not show a significant increase (Sarkar et al. 2008). Rebound dyspepsia, after discontinuation of PPIs, has been documented as a known entity. Some studies have linked the use of PPI to an increased risk of community acquired pneumonia, *C. difficile* diarrhea and campylobacter jejuni gastroenteritis. Long-term PPI use affects bone metabolism due to reduced calcium absorption. Many studies have shown the association of long-term PPI use and an increased risk of hip fractures especially in the older population (Yu et al. 2011). Iron and vitamin B12 malabsorption has also been reported with long-term PPI use.

Challenges Associated with the Use of PPIs

a) Refractory symptoms to PPI treatment
b) The vast majority of patients with erosive disease show complete healing of esophagitis (Bardhan 1995) and improved quality of life when treated with PPIs (Havelund et al. 1999). However, a significant proportion of GERD patients have persistent symptoms despite therapy with PPIs. This is more commonly observed in patients with non-erosive reflux disease (NERD) (Fass et al. 2005; Castell et al. 2002). In a survey of 11,000 patients with chronic heartburn only 58% reported being totally satisfied with their anti-reflux treatment (Crawley et al. 2000). Approximately 30% (range 25-40%) of patients with GERD symptoms are either not completely satisfied with PPI therapy or their symptoms persist despite treatment (Fass et al. 2005). Inadequate response to PPI therapy among GERD patients has been reported to be increasingly encountered in both primary and secondary care (Fass et al. 2005; Sgouros et al. 2006). Although patients with persistent problems despite acid suppressive therapy have been presented as a considerable problem, the PPI dose and duration of therapy is controversial before a patient is considered to be refractory to PPIs (Bredenoord et al. 2007). The medical literature does not offer an accepted definition for PPI failure (Fass 2007). The underlying mechanisms for PPI refractory reflux symptoms have not yet been fully identified. One important reason for treatment failure is lack of compliance, and in one study, only 55% patients with GERD took their PPI once daily for four weeks as prescribed. A proposed mechanism for treatment is persistence of weakly acid reflux. Weakly acid reflux is the reflux of gastric content into the esophagus with a pH between four and seven. It has been suggested that weakly acid reflux is associated with classic GERD

symptoms (Vela et al. 2001). Another possible mechanism for treatment failure is visceral hypersensitivity (Fass 2007).

c) Rebound acid hyper secretion

Rebound acid hyper secretion is defined as an increase in gastric acid secretion above pre-treatment levels following discontinuation of acid suppressive therapy. Rebound acid hyper secretion after withdrawal of H2 receptor antagonist treatment is well-established phenomenon and occurs between two to ten days after withdrawal. Whether occurrence of rebound acid hyper secretion also applies after withdrawal of PPI therapy is an issue that has been addressed in a number of studies (Gillen et at 1999; Gillen et al. 2004; Waldum et al. 1996; Prewett et al. 1991; Bell et al. 2001; Lind et al. 1983; Sharma et al. 1987; Sharma et al. 1984). However, these studies present conflicting data. Some studies have found no evidence for rebound acid hyper secretion after discontinuation of PPI therapy (Bell et al. 2001; Lind et al. 1983; Sharma et al. 1987; Sharma et al. 1984). However, more recent studies suggest that there is an increase in acid secretory capacity after PPI therapy discontinuation in *H. pylori* negative subjects.

H. pylori positive subjects are less likely to experience rebound problems and this is probably due to the interaction between *H. pylori* colonization and acid production. *H. pylori* positive subjects have a mucosal inflammation which releases inflammatory mediators such as interleukin-1. Interleukin-1 is a potent suppressor of the production of gastric acid, and it is also suggested that bacteria may have a direct suppressive effect on the parietal cells (Robert et al. 1991; Wallace et al. 1991). Rebound phenomena in *H. pylori* positive patients may be masked at least two weeks after treatment by persisting oxyntic gastritis (Eissele et al. 1997; Kuipers et al. 1995).

The exact mechanism of the acid rebound phenomenon remains unknown. However, there are four proposed mechanisms for the acid rebound hyper secretion. These are: up regulation of H2 receptors, hypergastrinaemia-stimulating histamine release by ECL cells, increase of parietal cell mass, and up regulation of H^+/K^+-ATPase activity (Nwokolo et al. 1990; Fullarton et al. 1991; Fullarton et al. 1989; Jones et al. 1988; Sandvik et al. 1997; Wilder-Smith et al. 1990). The development of ECL hypergastrinemia is probably associated with treatment duration since hyperplasia happens over time. PPIs block the proton pump irreversibly taking a number of days to generate fully. Therefore, the rebound acid hyper secretion might be expected first after a number of days following cessation. The duration of rebound acid hyper secretion remains unknown, although it is suggested that after treatment for 4-12 months, the rebound of hyper secretion measured with gastric acid output studies has lasted for at least eight weeks but less than 26 weeks (Fossmark et al. 2005; Gillen et al. 1999; Lind et al. 1983). Studies have suggested that CgA is useful in the evaluation of ECL-hyperplasia (Waldum et al. 1996), as well as the possibility of gastrin being used to measure the rebound acid hyper secretion (Hunfeld et al. 2007; Raghunath et al. 2005).

After withdrawal of PPI therapy, the rebound acid hyper secretion has been proposed to lead to difficulties for some patients in ceasing treatment with PPIs. This might be due to the resurgence of symptoms induced by acid rebound hyper secretion. The discontinuation of H2 receptor antagonist is accompanied by the onset of dyspeptic symptoms in previously asymptomatic subjects (Smith et al. 1999). According to this hypothesis, rebound acid hyper secretion may lead to a physical "dependency" on acid suppressive therapy. Although many studies have been performed to evaluate the rebound of acid after withdrawal of PPIs, the clinical relevance of rebound hyper secretion after treatment with PPI remains unknown.

REFERENCES

Abelo A, Andersson TB, Antonsson M, Naudot AK, Skanberg I and Weidolf L. Stereoselective metabolism of omeprazole by human cytochrome P450 enzymes. *Drug Metab Dispos*., 2000; 28: 966-972.

Agreus L, Svardsudd K, Talley NJ, Jones MP and Tibblin G. Natural history of gastroesophageal reflux disease and functional abdominal disorders: a population-based study. *Am J Gastroenterol*., 2001; 96: 2905-14.

Andersson T, Hassan-Alin M, Hasselgren G, Rohss K and Weidolf L. Pharmacokinetic studies with esomeprazole, the (S)-isomer of omeprazole. *Clin Pharmacokinet*., 2001; 40: 411-426.

Andersson T, Miners JO, Veronese ME, Tassaneeyakul W, Meyer UA, Birkett DJ. Identification of human liver cytochrome P450 isoforms mediating omeprazole metabolism. *Br J Clin Pharmacol* 1993; 36:521-30.

Andersson T. Pharmacokinetics, metabolism and interactions of acid pump inhibitors. Focus on omeprazole, lansoprazole and pantoprazole. *Clin Pharmacokinet* 1996; 31:9-28.

Armstrong D. Gastric pHVthe most relevant predictor of benefit in reflux disease. *Aliment Pharmacol Ther*., 2004;20:19Y26.

ASHP Therapeutic Guidelines on Stress Ulcer Prophylaxis. ASHP Commission on Therapeutics and approved by the ASHP Board of Directors on November 14, 1998. *Am J Health Syst Pharm*., 1999; 56:347-79.

Bardhan KD. The role of proton pump inhibitors in the treatment of gastrooesophageal reflux disease. *Aliment Pharmacol Ther*., 1995; 9 Suppl. 1:15-25.

Bell N, Karol MD, Sachs G, Greski-Rose P, Jennings DE, Hunt RH. Duration of effect of lansoprazole on gastric pH and acid secretion in normal male volunteers. *Aliment Pharmacol Ther*., 2001; 15:105-13.

Bhatt DL, Cryer BL, Contant CF, Cohen M, Lanas A, Schnitzer TJ et al. Clopidogrel with or without omeprazole in coronary artery disease. *N Engl J Med*., 2010; 363(20):1909-17.

Black JW, Duncan WA, Durant CJ, Ganellin CR and Parsons EM. Definition and antagonism of histamine H 2-receptors. *Nature* 1972; 236:385-90.

Bonagura AF and Dabezies MA. Helicobacter pylori infection. The importance of eradication in patients with gastric disease. *Postgrad Med*., 1996; 100:115-6.

Bredenoord AJ, Dent J. Proton pump inhibitor-therapy refractory gastro-oesophageal reflux disease patients, who are they? *Gut*., 2007; 56:593-4.

Burget DW, Chiverton SG and Hunt RH. Is there an optimal degree of acid suppression for healing of duodenal ulcers? A model of the relationship between ulcer healing and acid suppression. *Gastroenterology*. 1990; 99:345-51.

Butt JH, Barthel JS and Moore RA. Clinical spectrum of the upper gastrointestinal effects of nonsteroidal anti-inflammatory drugs. Natural history, symptomatology, and significance. *Am J Med*., 1988; 84:5-14.

Castell DO, Kahrilas PJ, Richter JE, Vakil NB, Johnson DA, Zuckerman S et al. Esomeprazole (40 mg) compared with lansoprazole (30 mg) in the treatment of erosive esophagitis. *Am J Gastroenterol.*, 2002; 97:575-83.

Chan FK, Wong VW and Suen BY et al. Combination of a cyclo-oxygenase-2 inhibitor and a proton-pump inhibitor for prevention of recurrent ulcer bleeding in patients at very high risk: a double-blind, randomised trial. *Lancet.*, 2007; 369:1621Y1626.

Cheatum D, Arvanitakis C and Gumpel M et al. An endoscopic study of gastroduodenal lesions induced by nonsteroidal anti-inflammatory drugs. *Clin Ther.*, 1999;21:992Y1003.

Conn HO and Blitzer BL. Nonassociation of adrenocorticosteroid therapy and peptic ulcer. *N Engl J Med.*, 1976; 294:473-9.

Crawley JA, Schmitt CM. How satisfied are chronic heartburn suffers with their prescription medications? Results of the patient's unment study. *JCOM.*, 2000;7:29-34.

Dent J, El-Serag HB, Wallander MA and Johansson S. Epidemiology of gastrooesophageal reflux disease: a systematic review. *Gut.* 2005; 54:710-7.

DeVault KR and Castell DO. Updated guidelines for the diagnosis and treatment of gastroesophageal reflux disease. The Practice Parameters Committee of the American College of Gastroenterology. *Am J Gastroenterol.*, 1999; 94:1434-42.

Duplessis DJ. Pathogenesis of Gastric Ulceration. *Lancet.* 1965; 1:974-8.

Eissele R, Brunner G, Simon B, Solcia E and Arnold R. Gastric mucosa during treatment with lansoprazole: Helicobacter pylori are a risk factor for argyrophil cell hyperplasia. *Gastroenterology.*, 1997; 112:707-17.

Ekstrom P, Carling L, Wetterhus S, Wingren PE, Anker-Hansen O and Lundegardh G et al. Prevention of peptic ulcer and dyspeptic symptoms with omeprazole in patients receiving continuous non-steroidal anti-inflammatory drug therapy. A Nordic multicentre study., *Scand J Gastroenterol.* 1996; 31:753-8.

Fass R, Shapiro M, Dekel R, Sewell J. Systematic review: proton-pump inhibitor failure in gastro-oesophageal reflux disease--where next? Aliment *Pharmacol Ther.*, 2005; 22:79-94.

Fass R. Proton-pump inhibitor therapy in patients with gastro-oesophageal reflux disease: putative mechanisms of failure. *Drugs.*, 2007; 67:1521-30.

Fellenius E, Berglindh T, Sachs G, Olbe L, Elander B and Sjostrand SE et al. Substituted benzimidazoles inhibit gastric acid secretion by blocking (H+ + K+)ATPase. *Nature* 1981; 290:159-61.

Fiocca R, Mastracci L, Attwood SE, Ell C, Galmiche JP and Hatlebakk J et al. Gastric exocrine and endocrine cell morphology under prolonged acid inhibition therapy: results of a 5-year follow-up in the LOTUS trial. *Aliment Pharmacol Ther.*, 2012; 36(10):959-71.

Forte JG, Forte TM and Black JA et al. Correlation of parietal cell structure and function. *J Clin Gastroenterol* 1983;5(Suppl. 1):17-27 [PubMed: 6228573].

Fossmark R, Johnsen G, Johanessen E and Waldum HL. Rebound acid hypersecretion after long-term inhibition of gastric acid secretion. *Aliment Pharmacol Ther.*, 2005; 21:149-54.

Fullarton GM, Macdonald AM and McColl KE. Rebound hypersecretion after H2-antagonist withdrawal--a comparative study with nizatidine, ranitidine and famotidine. *Aliment Pharmacol Ther.*, 1991; 5:391-8.

Fullarton GM, McLauchlan G, Macdonald A, Crean GP and McColl KE. Rebound nocturnal hypersecretion after four weeks treatment with an H2 receptor antagonist. *Gut.*, 1989; 30: 449-54.

Furuta T, Shirai N, Sugimoto M, Nakamura A., Hishida A and Ishizaki T. Influence of CYP2C19 pharmacogenetic polymorphism on proton pump inhibitor-based therapies. *Drug Metab Pharmacokinet.*, 2005; 20: 153-167.

Gillen D, Wirz AA and McColl KE. Helicobacter pylori eradication releases prolonged increased acid secretion following omeprazole treatment. *Gastroenterology.*, 2004; 126: 980-8.

Gillen D, Wirz AA, Ardill JE and McColl KE. Rebound hypersecretion after omeprazole and its relation to on-treatment acid suppression and Helicobacter pylori status. *Gastroenterology.*, 1999; 116:239-47.

Gledhill T, Howard OM, Buck M, Paul A and Hunt RH. Single nocturnal dose of an H2 receptor antagonist for the treatment of duodenal ulcer. *Gut.* 1983; 24:904-8.

Glynn IM and Karlish SJ. Occluded cations in active transport. *Annu Rev Biochem* 1990; 59: 171-205.

Hatlebakk JG, Katz PO, Camacho-Lobato L, Castell DO. Proton pump inhibitors: better acid suppression when taken before a meal than without a meal. *Aliment Pharmacol Ther.* 2000; 14:1267-72.

Havelund T, Lind T, Wiklund I, Glise H, Hernqvist H, Lauritsen K et al. Quality of life in patients with heartburn but without esophagitis: effects of treatment with omeprazole. *Am J Gastroenterol.*, 1999; 94:1782-9.

Hersey SJ and Sachs G. Gastric acid secretion. *Physiol Rev* 1995 Jan; 75(1):155-89.

Howden CW. Use of proton-pump inhibitors in complicated ulcer disease and upper gastrointestinal tract bleeding. *Am J Health Syst Pharm.*, 1999;56 (23 Suppl. 4):S5-11.

Huang JQ and Hunt RH. pH, healing rate and symptom relief in acid-related diseases. *Yale J Biol Med.*, 1996; 69:159-74.

Huber R, Kohl B, Sachs G, Senn-Bilfinger J, Simon WA and Sturm E. Review article: the continuing development of proton pump inhibitors with particular reference to pantoprazole. *Aliment Pharmacol Ther* 1995; 9:363-78.

Hunfeld NG, Geus WP and Kuipers EJ. Systematic review: Rebound acid hypersecretion after therapy with proton pump inhibitors. *Aliment Pharmacol Ther.*, 2007; 25:39-46.

Jianu CS, Fossmark R, Viset T, Qvigstad G, Sordal O and Marvik R et al. Gastric carcinoids after long-term use of a proton pump inhibitor. *Aliment Pharmacol Ther.*, 2012;36(7): 644-9.

Jones DB, Howden CW, Burget DW, Silletti C and Hunt RH. Alteration of H2 receptor sensitivity in duodenal ulcer patients after maintenance treatment with an H2 receptor antagonist. *Gut.*, 1988; 29:890-3.

Jones R and Bytzer P. Review article: acid suppression in the management of gastrooesophageal reflux disease--an appraisal of treatment options in primary care. *Aliment Pharmacol Ther.*, 2001; 15:765-72.

Katz PO, Ginsberg GG and Hoyle PE et al. Relationship between intragastric acid control and healing status in the treatment of moderate to severe erosive esophagitis. *Aliment Pharmacol Ther.*, 2007;25:617Y628.

Klotz U, Schwab M and Treiber G. CYP2C19 polymorphism and proton pump inhibitors. *Basic Clin Pharmacol Toxicol.*, 2004; 95: 2-8.

Klotz U. Clinical impact of CYP2C19 polymorphism on the action of proton pump inhibitors: a review of a special problem. *Int J Clin Pharmacol Ther.*, 2006; 44: 297-302.

Kromer W, Postius S, Riedel R, Simon WA and Hanauer G, Brand U et al. BY 1023/SK&F 96022 INN pantoprazole, a novel gastric proton pump inhibitor, potently inhibits acid secretion but lacks relevant cytochrome P450 interactions. *J Pharmacol Exp Ther* 1990; 254:129-35.

Kuipers EJ, Uyterlinde AM, Pena AS, Hazenberg HJ, Bloemena E and Lindeman J et al. Increase of Helicobacter pylori-associated corpus gastritis during acid suppressive therapy: implications for long-term safety. *Am J Gastroenterol.*, 1995; 90:1401-6.

Lambert R. Review article: current practice and future perspectives in the management of gastro-esophageal reflux disease. *Aliment Pharmacol Ther.*, 1997; 11:651-62.

Lanza FL and Chan FK, Quigley EM. Practice parameters committee of the American College of Gastroenterology. Guidelines for prevention of NSAID-related ulcer complications. *Am J Gastroenterol.*, 2009;104: 728Y738.

Lind T, Cederberg C, Ekenved G, Haglund U, Olbe L. Effect of omeprazole--a gastric proton pump inhibitor--on pentagastrin stimulated acid secretion in man. *Gut.*, 1983; 24:270-6.

Malfertheiner P, Fass R, Quigley EM, Modlin IM, Malagelada JR and Moss SF et al. Review article: from gastrin to gastro-oesophageal reflux disease--a century of acid suppression. *Aliment Pharmacol Ther* 2006; 23:683-90.

Malfertheiner P, Megraud F, O'Morain C, Hungin AP, Jones R and Axon A et al. Current concepts in the management of Helicobacter pylori infection--the Maastricht 2-2000 Consensus Report. *Aliment Pharmacol Ther.*, 2002; 16:167-80.

McCarthy DM. Prevention and treatment of gastrointestinal symptoms and complications due to NSAIDs. *Best Pract Res Clin Gastroenterol.*, 2001; 15:755-73.

Messer J, Reitman D, Sacks HS, Smith H, Jr. and Chalmers TC. Association of adrenocorticosteroid therapy and peptic-ulcer disease. *N Engl J Med.*, 1983; 309:21-4.

Meyer UA. Interaction of proton pump inhibitors with cytochromes P450: consequences for drug interactions. *Yale J Biol Med* 1996; 69:203-9.

Moayyedi P, Soo S, Deeks J, Delaney B, Innes M and Forman D. Pharmacological interventions for non-ulcer dyspepsia. *Cochrane Database Syst Rev.*, 2006(4):CD001960.

Nardino RJ, Vender RJ and Herbert PN. Overuse of acid-suppressive therapy in hospitalized patients. *Am J Gastroenterol.*, 2000; 95:3118-22.

Nwokolo CU, Smith JT, Gavey C, Sawyerr A and Pounder RE. Tolerance during 29 days of conventional dosing with cimetidine, nizatidine, famotidine or ranitidine. *Aliment Pharmacol Ther.*, 1990; 4 Suppl. 1:29-45.

Okabe S, Takeuchi K, Urushidani T and Takagi K. Effects of cimetidine, a histamine H2-receptor antagonist, on various experimental gastric and duodenal ulcers. *Am J Dig Dis* 1977; 22:677-684.

Piper JM, Ray WA, Daugherty JR and Griffin MR. Corticosteroid use and peptic ulcer disease: role of nonsteroidal anti-inflammatory drugs. *Ann Intern Med.*, 1991; 114:735-40.

Prewett EJ, Hudson M, Nwokolo CU, Sawyerr AM, Pounder RE. Nocturnal intragastric acidity during and after a period of dosing with either ranitidine or omeprazole. *Gastroenterology.*, 1991; 100:873-7.

Raghunath AS, O'Morain C and McLoughlin RC. Review article: the long-term use of proton-pump inhibitors. *Aliment Pharmacol Ther.*, 2005; 22 Suppl. 1:55-63.

Raynard B and Nitenberg G. [Is prevention of upper digestive system hemorrhage in intensive care necessary?]. *Schweiz Med Wochenschr.*, 1999; 129:1605-12.

Robert A, Olafsson AS, Lancaster C and Zhang WR. Interleukin-1 is cytoprotective, antisecretory, stimulates PGE2 synthesis by the stomach, and retards gastric emptying. *Life Sci.*, 1991; 48:123-34.

Sachs G, Chang HH and Rabon E et al. A nonelectrogenic H+ pump in plasma membranes of hog stomach. *J Biol Chem* 1976;251:7690-7698 [PubMed: 12175].

Sachs G, Shin JM, Munson K, Vagin O, Lambrecht N and Scott DR et al. Review article: the control of gastric acid and Helicobacter pylori eradication. *Aliment Pharmacol Ther.*, 2000; 14:1383-401.

Sachs G. Proton pump inhibitors and acid-related diseases. *Pharmacotherapy* 1997; 17:22-37.

Sandvik AK, Brenna E and Waldum HL. Review article: the pharmacological inhibition of gastric acid secretion--tolerance and rebound. *Aliment Pharmacol Ther.*, 1997; 11:1013-8.

Sarkar M, Hennessy S and Yang YX. Proton-pump inhibitor use and the risk for community-acquired pneumonia. *Ann Intern Med.*, 2008; 149:391Y398.

Sawaguchi A, Aoyama F and Ide S et al. The cryofixation of isolated rat gastric mucosa provides new insights into the functional transformation of gastric parietal cells: an in vitro experimental model study. *Arch Histol Cytol* 2005; 68:151-160 [PubMed: 1627602 1].

Scarpignato C, Pelosini I and Di Mario F. Acid suppression therapy: where do we go from here? *Dig Dis* 2006; 24:11-46.

Schoen RT and Vender RJ. Mechanisms of nonsteroidal anti-inflammatory drug-induced gastric damage. *Am J Med.*, 1989; 86:449-58.

Sgouros SN, Mantides A. Refractory heartburn to proton pump inhibitors: epidemiology, etiology and management. *Digestion.*, 2006; 73:218-27.

Sharma B, Axelson M, Pounder RP, Lundborg P, Ohman M, Santana A et al. Acid secretory capacity and plasma gastrin concentration after administration of omeprazole to normal subjects. *Aliment Pharmacol Ther.*, 1987; 1:67-76.

Sharma BK, Walt RP, Pounder RE, Gomes MD, Wood EC, Logan LH. Optimal dose of oral omeprazole for maximal 24 hour decrease of intragastric acidity. *Gut.*, 1984; 25:957-64.

Simon WA, Budingen C, Fahr S, Kinder B and Koske M. The H+, K(+)-ATPase inhibitor (BY1023/SK&F96022) interacts less with cytochrome P450 than omeprazole and lansoprazole. *Biochem Pharmacol* 1991; 42:347-55.

Smith AD, Gillen D, Cochran KM, El-Omar E and McColl KE. Dyspepsia on withdrawal of ranitidine in previously asymptomatic volunteers. *Am J Gastroenterol.*, 1999; 94:1209-13.

Stedman CA and Barclay ML. Review article: comparison of the pharmacokinetics, acid suppression and efficacy of proton pump inhibitors. *Aliment Pharmacol Ther* 2000; 14: 963-78.

Talley NJ, Meineche-Schmidt V, Pare P, Duckworth M, Raisanen P and Pap A et al. Efficacy of omeprazole in functional dyspepsia: double-blind, randomized, placebocontrolled trials (the Bond and Opera studies). *Aliment Pharmacol Ther.*, 1998; 12:1055-65.

Talley NJ, Silverstein MD, Agreus L, Nyren O, Sonnenberg A and Holtmann G. AGA technical review: evaluation of dyspepsia. American Gastroenterological Association. *Gastroenterology.*, 1998; 114:582-95.

Talley NJ, Weaver AL, Zinsmeister AR and Melton LJ, 3rd. Onset and disappearance of gastrointestinal symptoms and functional gastrointestinal disorders. *Am J Epidemiol.*, 1992; 136: 165-77.

Thompson WG. Placebos: a review of the placebo response. *Am J Gastroenterol.*, 2000; 95: 1637-43.

Triadafilopoulos G. Proton pump inhibitors for Barrett's oesophagus. *Gut.*, 2000;46:144Y14 6.

Tucker GT. The interaction of proton pump inhibitors with cytochromes P450. *Aliment Pharmacol Ther* 1994; 8 Suppl. 1:33-8.

Vakil N, van Zanten SV, Kahrilas P, Dent J and Jones R. The Montreal definition and classification of gastroesophageal reflux disease: a global evidence-based consensus. *Am J Gastroenterol.*, 2006;101:1900-20.

Vela MF, Camacho-Lobato L, Srinivasan R, Tutuian R, Katz PO, Castell DO. Simultaneous intraesophageal impedance and pH measurement of acid and nonacid gastroesophageal reflux: effect of omeprazole. *Gastroenterology.*, 2001; 120:1599-606.

Waldum HL, Arnestad JS, Brenna E, Eide I, Syversen U and Sandvik AK. Marked increase in gastric acid secretory capacity after omeprazole treatment. *Gut.*, 1996; 39:649-53.

Waldum HL, Brenna E, Kleveland PM, Sandvik AK and Syversen U. Review article: the use of gastric acid-inhibitory drugs--physiological and pathophysiological considerations. *Aliment Pharmacol Ther.* 1993; 7:589-96.

Wallace JL, Cucala M, Mugridge K, Parente L. Secretagogue-specific effects of interleukin-1 on gastric acid secretion. *Am J Physiol.*, 1991; 261:G559-64.

Wilder-Smith CH, Ernst T, Gennoni M, Zeyen B, Halter F and Merki HS. Tolerance to oral H2-receptor antagonists. *Dig Dis Sci.*, 1990; 35:976-83.

Wolfe MM and Sachs G. Acid suppression: optimizing therapy for gastroduodenal ulcer, gastroesophageal reflux disease, and stress-related erosive syndrome. *Gastroenterology* 2000; 118(2 Suppl. 1):S9-31.

Wolfe MM and Soll AH. The physiology of gastric acid secretion. *N Engl J Med.*, 1988; 319:1707-15.

Wong WM, Wong BC, Hung WK, Yee YK, Yip AW and Szeto ML et al. Double blind, randomised, placebo controlled study of four weeks of lansoprazole for the treatment of functional dyspepsia in Chinese patients. *Gut.*, 2002; 51:502-6.

Yu EW, Bauer SR, Bain PA, Bauer DC. Proton pump inhibitors and risk of fractures: a meta-analysis of 11 international studies. *Am J Med.*, 2011 Jun; 124(6):519-26.

In: Disorders of Gastrointestinal Systems … ISBN: 978-1-63485-366-8
Editors: S. Rajagopal, S. Murugan and R. Saravanan

Chapter 14

IMPACT OF GUT MICROFLORA ON HUMAN HEALTH AND DISEASES

Sabina Fatima[1,*], MSc, and Senthilkumar Rajagopal[2], PhD
[1]Department of Microbiology, Dr. NTR University of Health Sciences, Vijayawada, AP, India
[2]Department of Biotechnology, Rayalaseema University, Kurnool, AP, India

ABSTRACT

A virtually sterile human body gets colonized by myriad of microbes soon after birth that makes up the human microbiome. The gut of infant is first colonized by maternal and environmental bacteria during the passage of birth canal and continues to be populated through feeding and other contacts thereafter. The gastrointestinal tract mucosal layer act as an interface between the gut lumen of the host and microflora. Intestinal and colonic microbiota has been regarded as solitary, planktonic and non-interacting. However, sessile bacteria forming quorum sensing mediated biofilms in the mucus layer of the gut are likely to play a pivotal role in health and disease. The dominant intra luminal species implicated in the formation of quorum are non sporing anaerobes, gram positive cocci, gram negative bacilli and other diverse flora. The bacterial species constitute a microbial ecosystem in the magnitude of 10^{14} cells/mm, which account for the vast majority of total cells associated with the human digestive system. Detection of quorum sensing mediated biofilm production is a marker of pathogenic potential of colonizers and commensals hence should not be discarded as mere intestinal or colonic flora of the gastrointestinal system. Other areas of interest in this regard are surgical site and device associated infections.

Keywords: microbiota, microbiome, planktonic, sessile, biofilms, quorum sensing

* Corresponding author: Sabina Fatima, PhD. Department of Microbiology, Dr. NTR University of Health Sciences, Vijayawada. A.P. E-mail: ssaabina@gmail.com.

1. Introduction

The key role of gut flora in health and disease has been invoked in the context of disorders of the gastrointestinal system. The true diversity and function of the human gut microbiota as well as the extent and nature of microbial interactions with the mammalian host or with other microorganisms is taken into account to diagnose the gastrointestinal disorders. The term gut microflora describes the vast collection or the ecological community of commensal symbiotic and pathogenic microorganisms inhabiting the niches of the human gastrointestinal system in close association. This has established the importance of the gut microbiome in the disease pathogenesis for numerous systemic disorders of gastrointestinal system.

1.1. Gut Microbiota in Beneficial Role

Gastrointestinal system microflora forms an important component of the microbial ecosystem. Gut bacteria play a vital role in human health, such as supplying essential nutrients, synthesizing vitamin K, aiding in the digestion of cellulose, promoting angiogenesis, secretion of hormones, enzymes and enteric nerve function. Gut flora form a protective layer in the form of biofilm communities on the mucosa to protect the gastrointestinal lining from the adverse effects of pathogens, food or toxins. Through these mechanisms, the gut microbiota can be seen to play a critical role in protecting the digestive system of the host from colonization by pathogenic species. Moreover some intestinal bacteria produce a variety of substances, ranging from relatively non specific fatty acids and peroxides to highly specific bacteriocins, which can inhibit or kill other potentially pathogenic bacteria of the same or other species, while certain strains produce proteases capable of denaturing bacterial toxins. However, the gut flora can also be potentially harmful due to the change of their composition when the gut ecosystem undergoes alterations leading to disorders of gastrointestinal system. In humans, the composition of the gut flora is influenced not only by age but also by diet and socioeconomic conditions of the individuals.

1.2. Gut Microbiota in Gastrointestinal Disorders

The extent of the consequences of qualitative and quantitative disturbances in the gut flora or the interaction between the flora and the host has been relatively obvious. When the normal flora are eliminated or suppressed by a course of long term broad spectrum antibiotics, the commensal flora of the digestive tract become opportunistic to cause diseases of the gastrointestinal system. The classic example of this is antibiotic associated diarrhea and its clinical manifestations of anaerobic bacterium *Clostridium difficile* colitis. Similar perturbations in the gut flora is involved in a devastating form of intestinal inflammation that may occur in newborns and especially premature infants, which is known as necrotizing enterocolitis. In other situations, bacteria may simply alter the habitat and become pathogenic in the due course of time, leading to disorders ranging from autoimmunity, obesity, stress related psychiatric disorders to carcinomas. If motility of the bowel is impaired or gastric acid secretion is drastically reduced, an environment conducive to the proliferation of commensal organisms in the small intestine that are normally confined to the colon results. The consequence is the syndrome of small bowel bacterial overgrowth. In other situations, the immunologic interaction between the flora and the host cells is disturbed, and the host may recognize the constituents of the normal flora as pathogenic and may mount an inappropriate inflammatory response which also ultimately leads to conditions such as inflammatory bowel disease. The frustrated phagocytes release enormous amount of proinflammatory cytokines leading damage to the intestinal epithelium which renders the gut wall leaky and permits bacteria from the vicinity of the gut to gain access to the sub mucosal compartments or even to the systemic circulation, with the associated potential to cause gut sepsis [1].

In order to treat gastrointestinal disorders, the invention of antibiotics has been a milestone in the history of medicine. It was assumed, with the advent of antibiotics, a new era of therapeutics has dawned which promised to be a potential tool for abolition of gut related infections, but the emergence of myriad multidrug resistant super bugs in the digestive tract at swifter rate, witnessed the fall of antibiotics. Bacteria embedded in a hydrated biomass acquire resistant traits to high concentration of broad spectrum standard antibiotics as a part of the survival instinct. In a revolutionized manner, gut microbial population can survive antibiotic concentrations up to several magnitudes higher than needed to eradicate planktonic bacteria of same species in the gastrointestinal system. The association between biofilm production and drug resistance in the digestive tract has been documented for primary infections, gut sepsis as well as surgical site nosocomial infections.

Higher living creatures came into existence from a single cell through the fundamentals of evolution according to the Darwinian Theory. The interactions between cells in the digestive tract resulted in multi-cellularity from uni-cellularity. The same laws of evolution have been exploited by bacteria in the gut through quorum sensing, which is a bacterial cell to cell communication that involves production, detection and response to extracellular signaling molecules called auto inducers. Auto inducers accumulate in the gut environment as the bacterial population density in the digestive tract increases. Bacteria monitor this information to track, changes in their cell numbers to collectively alter gene expression within the gastrointestinal tract. Quorum sensing activities are beneficial when performed by groups of bacteria acting in synchrony when residing in the mucosa of the digestive tract. Processes controlled by quorum sensing include sporulation, competence for nutrition, antibiotic production, and biofilm formation and virulence factor expressions. The evolution of sophisticated communication systems in bacteria could therefore have been one of the early steps in the development of social activities resulting in multicellular nature of the unicellular microbes in the gut. The process of dynamic quorum sensing mechanism bestows bacteria in the digestive tract the qualities of eukaryotic behaviour. Research elucidated that communication occurs within and between bacterial species that elicit specific responses from the digestive system inherent immunity of the host. The nature of chemical signals, the relay mechanisms, target genes modulated by bacterial quorum sensing is unique in its own right but similarities bound to exist as the ability to communicate is fundamental for a synchronized behavior in the gut lumen. Quorum sensing mechanism renders bacteria to infect the gastrointestinal system of the host as a whole community at a high cell density. Pathogenic bacteria proliferate within the mammalian host digestive tract in a quiescent mode asymptomatically, until a threshold population is achieved, enough to overwhelm the host immune defenses or antimicrobials. At high cell density, activation of ample arsenal of virulence determinants takes place in the gut enabling the bacteria to make a concerted attack in coordination. A network of three dimensional community architecture of a coherent multilayered biofilm develops, which function as a eukaryotic manner, when the sensory information from auto inducers transduce within the gut lumen.

On one hand pathogenic biofilm dwellers exhibit an altruistic and symbiotic behavior through kin selection for the progeny to flourish in harmony, on the other hand bacteria engaged in quorum sensing adopt competitive social conflicts between co-operator species of the gut flora that produce and detect quorum signals to respond accordingly and social cheaters that no longer participate in quorum sensing. The phenomenon enables pathogens to persist as reservoirs of infections, resulting in recrude scence even after the device is explanted from the body [2].

1.3. Rationale

A new era in medical science has emerged with the realization of the critical role of the gut micro-biota, in health and disease. Central to the interaction between the microbiota and host is the manner in which bacteria and most likely other microorganisms contained within the gut communicate with the host cells and participate in a variety of metabolic processes of mutual benefit to the host and the microbe. Although the approach is still in its infancy, some important insights have already been gained about how the microbiota might influence a number of disease processes both within and distant from the gut. The discovery lay the groundwork for the development of therapeutic strategies [3].

2. Foreign Body Related Infections of the Gastrointestinal Tract

The introduction of mucous membrane traversing urethral catheters facilitated an easy access to the urinary tract, from the disease management point of view. Catheters composed of biopolymers are frequent and indispensable for the assessment of non invasive kidney function monitoring through urine samples and therapeutic purposes. Extensive use of Foley catheters form an integral part of medical interventions required for the patient care. The catheters may have to be implanted *in situ* for long periods in the urethral orifice for various nonpyogenic conditions, but colonization may subsequently revoke local or systemic pyogenic infections. Hence the very purpose has been hampered due to catheter induced sepsis ultimately ending up in life threatening complications like septic shock rather than disease management. It is hypothesized that the primary colonists of a biofilm comprise of gut mucous membrane flora initially, later pathogens or environmental microbes join the matrix thus leading to a polymicrobial consortium. It has been implicated that gut commensal bacterial species transform into pathogens and diverse phenotypes by expression of virulence determinants on abiotic materials as soon as the device is implanted. The associated infections are recalcitrant and refractory due to the secretion of protective exopolymeric matrix by the bacteria embedded in an adherent biofilm. Conditioning of inert surfaces and interfaces of catheter biopolymers serve as substrates to which unicellular planktonic bacteria attach irreversibly and transform into interacting sessile, glycocalyx secreting forms executing multicellular behaviours. The minimal infecting dose of inoculum for abiotic material is multifold lower than biotic surfaces, owing to the fact that an inert biomaterial mounts a poor and delayed immune response from the host. The rate of colonization by gut, metal, perennial or faucal commensal flora and primary invading pathogens ultimately results in the development of catheter associated urinary tract infection.

The extent of pathogenicity is directly proportional to the duration of catheter *in situ* apart from other risk factors like implementation of aseptic procedures, catheter manipulations or maintenance, surrounding environment, etc. The shedding of daughter cells and shearing of micro colonies from the mature gut biofilm by dispersion seed other sections of the catheter or gut mucosa in contact. Peripheral biofilm cells translocate to other niches of the digestive tract to disseminate and establish infection in the gastrointestinal system. This necessitates the prolonged and high-dose wide spectrum antibiotic therapy as well as the elimination of infected foreign material which were the only cornerstones of the therapy so far. Gastrointestinal delivery systems have been charged to comply with zero tolerance for preventable hospital acquired infections. Enormous efforts have been devoted to analyze the microbiology and genetics of quorum sensing mediated gut biofilms but their evolution remained virtually unexplored. An insight is mandatory into understanding interactions in biofilms to pave way towards better quality of medical care of devices implanted in gut by using non bactericidal approaches that attenuate virulence by anti-infective strategies [4, 5].

3. Problem Survey

Epidemiological studies revealed that almost all long term gut implanted devices get infected due to glycocalyx enclosed biofilms. Thus it sets a significant negative drawback to the healthcare system, necessitating prolonged hospital stay which can adversely affect the quality of life, thereby causing substantial economic burden. As a result, a vicious cycle initiates, contributing to the increased morbidity and mortality.

4. Scope of Research

Rapidly evolving advances in analytic techniques in microbiology, genetics and molecular biology, the true diversity of microorganisms that inhabit the gastrointestinal tract of humans commonly referred to as the human gut microbiota is being revealed and its contributions to homeostasis in health and to the pathogenesis of gastrointestinal disorders is appreciated recently. Gut-commensal microbiota interactions play a fundamental role in promoting homeostatic functions in the digestive tract such as immunomodulation, up regulation of cyto protective genes, prevention and regulation of apoptosis, and maintenance of barrier function. As a consequence, the study of gut ecology now has emerged as one of the most active and exciting fields in biology and medicine. It is in this context diet and broad spectrum antibiotic therapy alters or modifies the microbiota. A high prevalence of multidrug resistant traits among gastrointestinal pathogenic or commensal bacteria within biofilm mode of existence necessitates impetus to explore therapeutic alternatives which are secured with respect to long term effect. WHO has warned the commencement of post antibiotic era due to widespread pan drug resistance among clinical pathogens?

Conventional antibiotics are bactericidal or bacteriostatic, less penetrative through slime and develop multi drug resistant traits in microbes of gastrointestinal system. Alternative perspectives for the development of novel pharmaceutical and prophylactic strategies such as anti-biofilms and anti-quorum sensing are promising. The anti-pathogenic agents work on the principle of anti-infective or anti-virulence strategies where the bacteria on the whole are not targeted but the biofilms and quorum sensing cascade mechanisms were interfered. It has been discovered that a wide spectrum of organisms in the digestive system utilize quorum sensing to control virulence factors expression, thus by blocking signaling mechanisms, pathogenic organisms could be rendered avirulent. Biofilm production is a marker of pathogenic potential of colonizers and commensals, hence should not be considered as mere gut flora [6, 7].

Presently numerous investigations were taken up to explore the burden of quorum sensing mediated biofilms on gut mucous membranes and gastrointestinal access devices. Quorum sensing has been touted as an ideal target for antivirulence therapy lowering the potential for unwanted off target effect in the gastric cells of the host. Appreciating quorum sensing systems as a mean to alleviate or prevent infection has been met with optimism in the wake of antibiotic resistance that impedes treatment of the gastrointestinal disorders.

5. Future Perspective

In view of the inevitability of losing combat against bacteria, it has been envisaged that it is time to make peace. The bacteria are not targeted on the whole directly but infectious cascades in the gut would be interrupted at various stages, which consequently inhibit pathogenicity by agents with anti-quorum sensing or anti-biofilm activities. It is achieved by virtue of not exerting selective pressures or suppress gut commensal flora unlike antibiotics. Alternative therapy by anti-pathogenic agents attenuates the virulence which is considered as an anti-infective strategy which does not alter the balance of beneficial and harmful bacteria in the gastrointestinal tract. Language molecules of bacteria are diffusible and their accumulation correlates with cell density and contain information about the metabolic potential of the gut environment and the presence of other constituent species of bacteria. The use of the diverse assortment of communication chemical molecules as sources of information exemplifies the acuity with which bacteria sense, integrate and modulate behavior in response to ever fluctuating environments in the digestive tract. These microbial tactics have spurred growing interest to design and implement anti-pathogenic strategies suggesting that continued research aimed at deciphering these chemical languages which could have enormous clinical applications in the management of the disorders of gastrointestinal system. By extrapolation it is supposed that still vast numbers of signaling organic molecules await discovery. The research has just begun to eavesdrop on a microbial agora, a bustling polyglot of microbial dialogues in the vicinity of the digestive tract, each with its own biological story to tell. Progress has already been made, but the future of gastrointestinal system quorum sensing mediated biofilm research and management of disorders relies upon collaborative multidisciplinary efforts to explore the core in order to unravel and tackle the complexities of the microbial world on human health and disease [8, 9].

6. Historical Backgrounds of Biofilms

Traditionally bacteria were considered as freely suspended cells, but it is realized that most exist in micro ecosystems with other organisms. The concept of biofilm dates back to Anton Van Leeuwenhoek (1632-1723), the Father of Microscopy, who scraped slime from dental plaque and observed "animalcules" through primitive microscope. This was possible perhaps, because biofilm structure can be sufficiently thick to be visible to the naked eye. Biofilm is defined as a functional consortium of cells, embedded in a self produced extracellular polymeric matrix adherent to living or synthetic surfaces [10].

7. Gastrointestinal System Biofilms

The term biofilm and slime are often used interchangeably. There is a general consensus that planktonic bacteria exists only transiently in the gastrointestinal tract and the majority of the population form biofilms as it confers a survival advantage to microorganisms in the digestive tract. Biofilm formation is a developmental process by which bacteria undergo a regulated lifestyle, switch from nomadic unicellular to a sedentary multicellular state subsequently resulting in structured communities and cellular differentiation of growth. Biofilms of gastrointestinal tract were found to be composed of gram positive, gram negative bacteria and diverse flora. It may initially consist of single species, but longer exposure inevitably lead to multispecies biofilms. Biofilm formation is a ubiquitous phenomenon which initiates soon after birth and all biofilms regardless of their location, share several common features. Biofilm formations occurs in sequential steps, such as gastrointestinal surface conditioning, bacterial adhesion (reversible then irreversible), biofilm maturation and dispersion. The adherence factors like 'microbial surface components recognizing adhesive matrix molecules (MSCRAMM), Biofilm associated proteins (BAP), Accumulation associated proteins (AAP) mediate a crucial role. A multitude of biofilm associated genes like *ica* (intracellular adhesion) gene cluster, etc., and bacterial components such as clumping factor (clf), teichoic acid facilitate adhesion and immobilization in the gut lumen. Further attachment is reinforced by bacterial cellular appendages such as LPS, pili and fimbriae. Gastrointestinal environmental cues such as nutrition, optimum temperature, pH, osmolarity, and iron and oxygen availability are the contributing parameters. A biofilm matures by active cell division, microbial aggregation, extracellular matrix production, host protein accumulation and colonization by secondary invaders and diverse flora forming apolymicrobial miniature ecosystem in the gastrointestinal tract. Synergistic mechanisms come into play due to consumption of oxygen by aerobes which locally increase the redox potential allowing anaerobes to flourish thereby forming a mixed species gut biofilm. Confocal laser scanning microscopy established a spatially heterogeneous mosaic model of towers or mushroom shaped architecture. The structures interspersed with cell clusters, voids for oxygen, and fluid-filled channels for the transport of nutrients, hydration and cellular metabolic byproducts.

The organization of colloidal stability, polar interactions and distribution of ionic charges is maintained in a heterogenous environment in coalescing mass as explained by extended X-DLVO theory in a highly structured biofilm. Up regulation of specific genes of virulence determinants takes place at this stage, such as production of toxins, antibiotics, and drug resistance, etc. Exopolysaccharide (EPS) or extracellular polymeric matrix is an integral feature of biofilm. It is present in the form of viscous gel due to hydrated organic polymers which impart a slimy sticky consistency to a gut biofilm. It acts as a physical and chemical barrier to phagocytosis, opsonisation, stress, temperature, pH., osmotic fluctuations, oxidation, desiccation, diffusion of antimicrobials and shield against other detrimental conditions in the digestive tract. The matrix is anionically charged thus inhibit cationic based antibiotics like aminoglycosides. Some examples of a polymeric biofilm matrix components produced by bacteria in the gut include the mucopolysaccharide, alginate that predominates the matrix of mucoid strains of *Pseudomon asaeruginosa*. Colanic acid is the primary EPS component of *Escherichia coli* which consists of hexasaccharide subunits with fucose and glucuronic acid. Colony migration factor (Cmf), an extracellular slime material, from wild type *Proteus mirabilis* is an acidic compound composed of tetrasaccharide repeating units. In addition the matrix provides a structural scaffold to physically hold the biofilm together and facilitates diffusion of quorum sensing signals within the gut lumen. Dispersion is the critical stage of the biofilm life cycle that contributes to persistence, translocation, bacterial survival, reattachment, disease transmission and to promote genetic diversity. Mechanism of dispersion is divided into two categories namely Active and Passive.

Active dispersal refers to mechanisms that are initiated by the bacteria themselves and is mediated by bacterial enzymes, hyaluronidase, rhamnolipids, DNAse, etc., whereas passive dispersal is the detachment of biofilm cells by external forces such as fluid shears and abrasion. The distinct modes of erosion are continuous release of cells or cell clusters, seeding dispersal also known as central hollowing is the rapid release of fragments forming cavities in biofilm structure. Sloughing off is the sudden detachment of a segment of a microcolony [11, 12].

8. Quorum Sensing among Gut Microbes

Quorum sensing is defined as the cell to cell communication system mediated by self produced signal molecules, enabling bacteria to sense critical threshold density to coordinate gene expression for synchronized activities within communities in the gut. The phenomenon of quorum sensing was described first in marine luminous bacteria *Vibrio fischeri* and *Vibrio harveyi* to regulate bioluminescence. However, it has been recognized that quorum sensing controlled gene expression is widely distributed among vast genera of gram positive and gram negative taxonomic groups occupying various niches of the gastrointestinal system. The output is the coordination of genes responsible for critical physiological and pathological activities including the formation of biofilms, sepsis and drug resistance, etc. Traditionally, bacteria was regarded as free floating, solitary, non-interacting reclusive forms in the gut environment. Bacterial patho-physiology and antimicrobial therapies were focussed towards homogenous cultures comprising of single species. The conventional view of microbiology of planktonic bacteria has altered due to the emergence of social behaviour among microbes in the gastrointestinal system. The sub discipline termed as sociomicrobiology was introduced in the context of polymicrobial communities within the gut or elsewhere in the body where bacteria are sessile, interacting either interspecies or intraspecies, displaying a multicellular cooperative lifestyle *en massse.*

The evolutionary theory of microbes considered the dynamic transition and social networking as an evolutionary step of bacteria towards eukaryotic nature. Almost all known quorum sensing systems depend on three basic principles. First, the gut residing bacteria engaged in quorum sensing constitutively produce, secrete and detect low molecular weight diffusible chemical signaling molecules termed as pheromones or quoromones or autoinducers as they induce their own synthesis. Autoinducers are synthesized intracellular and released outside the cells of the gastrointestinal system. Signaling molecules get specifically detected by receptors of other bacteria of the digestive system only at aquorate. As the number of cells in a population increase, the extracellular concentration of auto inducer in the vicinity increases. Second, the cumulative production of auto inducers above the critical threshold concentration enables detection and response by other bacteria of the gut flora. The inducer gets internalized and binds to cognate receptors inside the gastrointestinal cells either in the cytoplasm or cell membrane. Third the autoinducer-receptor complex activate the transcription of specific target genes and trigger signal transduction cascades that result in population wide changes and thereby modifies the bacterial phenotypes of the gut flora. There is a low likelihood of a bacterium detecting its own secreted inducer. For gene transcription activation, the cell must encounter signaling molecules secreted by other cells in the environment. When similar strains are in the vicinity, diffusion reduces the concentration of the inducer in the surrounding medium to negligible, hence the bacteria produce meagre amount of inducer at a low cell density (LCD).

However, as the population of the gut flora or pathogen grows, the concentration attains a threshold, causing more inducer to be synthesized. This forms an auto inducing positive feedback loop, the receptor becomes fully activated and the cell switches to high cell density (HCD) mode. The feed foreword auto induction loop promotes synchrony in the population to induce upregulation of specific genes, causing all bacteriae to begin transcription at approximately the same time. As a result of the coordinated behavior the protein expression is paramount and the system conserves substantial energy and results in a robust patho-physiological gut metabolism. Thus, quorum sensing enables cells in a population to function in unison and enforce synchrony in collective behaviors such as biofilm formation toxins, antibiotic production, drug resistance, sporulation and competence for DNA uptake which are critical for microbial survival in the digestive tract. The fundamental steps involved in detecting and responding to fluctuations in cell number are analogous in all known quorum sensing systems [13, 14].

8.1. Interaction of Microbes in the Gastrointestinal System

Auto Inducer - II is an interspecies mediator of cell to cell communication, widespread among phylogenetic range of gastrointestinal gram positive and gram negative genera. Thus AI-2 is a universal signal molecule. Production of autoinducer is endogenous but AI-2 respond to autoinducers produced by many other bacteria in the vicinity. It is evident that AI-2 is involved in the control of transcription of genes encoding pathogenicity islands of critical activities such as virulence factor expression, antibiotics resistance, biofilm formation, expression of recombinant proteins in various gastrointestinal disorders [15].

8.2. Multilingual Dialogues among the Gut Bacteria

The Gammaproteobacteria classes, which include genus, widely prevalent in the digestive tract such as, *Escherichia*, *Klebsiella, Salmonella*, *Shigella, and Enterobacter species* encode an orphan quorum sensing communication homolog named as SDI A (suppressor of cell division inhibitor). SDI A has a role role in biofilm formation, quorum sensing, antibiotic resistance due to activation of efflux pumps, Indolesignalling, etc. Extracellular death factor (EDF) is a unique suicide inducing peptide based signaling linking programmed cell death with quorum sensing which have been described in *E. coli* and several prokaryotes due to few unknown stable toxins [16].

8.3. Autoinducer-3-Interkingdom Communication in the Gut

AI-3 is the communication of the bacteria with host cells. Prokaryotes and eukaryotes coexist in commensal and pathogenic relationships in the gastrointestinal tract than any other system of the human body, consequently coevolving to sense and respond to each other's signaling molecules. Autoinducer (AI-3) is an aromatic signaling molecule produced by human intestinal microflora as well as certain enteric pathogens. The mammalian host stress hormone epinephrine and norepinephrine signal the system and activate virulence gene transcription, facilitating eukaryotic and prokaryotic communication in the gut. Epinephrine or norepinephrine signaling pathway is involved in host-bacteria cross talk and rely on the host's adrenergic network. Enterohaemorrhagic *Escherichia coli* like pathogenic organisms sense autoinducer-3 produced by gastro intestinal mucous flora and epinephrine or norepinephrine hormones produced by the host through Histidine Kinases (HK). HK constitute the predominant family of signaling proteins acting in concert with a Response Regulator (RR) protein for flagellar motility, toxin expression, intestinal lesions, bloody diarrhea, etc. AI-3 regulate the transcription of genes encoding the Leucocyte Enterocyte Effacement (LEE) in a type III secretion system (TTSS) in Enterohaemorrhagic *Escherichia coli* [17].

9. Multidrug Resistance in Gastrointestinal Biofilms

A trend of antibiotic resistance has been most steadily emerging in clinical pathogens and commensals of the gut. Bacteria in biofilms acquire inherent resistance to antimicrobial agents as compared to their planktonic counterparts in the vicinity of the digestive tract. The hypothesis prevailing the mechanism of intrinsic multidrug resistance conferred by the biofilm environment in the gut include exopolysaccharide barrier, selection pressure, restricted penetration, retarded diffusion, over expression of stress responsive genes, mutations, structural heterogeneity, persisters, reduced metabolic activity, efflux pumps, etc. Reduced susceptibility to antimicrobial agents can be due to nutrient limitation and oxygen gradient within the biomass leading to slow growth, reduced metabolic rate (Growth advantage in stationary phase-GASP), enzymatic degradation, modified targets, starved state of bacteria and lateral exchange of genes, transposons and plasmids due to ideal niches provided in a close proximity of the digestive tract leading to the spread of resistance markers and therapeutic failure. Negatively charged molecules within the biomass bind to antimicrobial agents resulting in lesser permeability and emergence of phenotypic ally and genetically heterogeneous subpopulation of the organisms in the gastrointestinal system. Furthermore result in differentiation of subpopulation of biofilm cells into resistant dormant cells in the gut.

Established biofilms dwellers in the gut can tolerate antibiotics at concentration of thousand times, needed to inactivate genetically equivalent planktonic bacteria of the gut. Bacteria enjoy multiple benefits due to community mode of growth such as cooperative, unselfish or altruistic behaviors. Even after the death phase of older population of cells, the next generation takeover as resistant mutants, known as "evolutionary cheaters" [18, 19].

10. Biofilms on Biomaterials Implanted in the Gastrointestinal System

Invasion and colonization is the default mode of existence for microbes, more so on abiotic material rather than living tissues due to the inertness of biomaterials to mount an immune response and unexposure to the antibodies in the blood. Biofilms on implanted medical devices in the gastrointestinal tract act as a foci for persistent infections ensuing adhesion and co-aggregation. The most commonly used urethral catheters are indispensable in modern day medical practice to provide bladder access. Foleyurinary catheters implanted in post-operative patients to reduce mobility and cases with urinary bladder dysfunction to avoid urinary retention or to manage a neurogenic bladder. The physical size of the catheter and therefore the size of the defect in the intrinsic host defences are likely to be correlated with increased risk. Catheter composition and gauge size may also influence the risk of infection. It is hypothesized that the physicochemical properties of the surface ensue bacterial adhesion rapidly to hydrophobic, non polar surfaces of catheter biomaterials such as Teflon, silicone, latex and plastic than to hydrophilic materials such as elastomer, glass or metals. Silicon catheters facilitate frequent microbial adherence than polyurethane or polyvinyl chloride. Urinary catheters made of tubular latex or hydrogel coated biosurface readily acquire conditioning and colonization by microbes. Biofilms are shown to be universally present associated with either the exterior of the catheter or inner lumen. The bacterial growth and activity enhance substantially with contact to a surface leading to narrowing or bottle effect of the area.

Endogenous microflora of the host originates from the perineum or anus at the insertion site; migrate along the external surface of the device and from the hub, into the urine through inner lumen. Exogenous source of infection include environmental air borne pathogens or shedding of microbes due to manipulations of the device implanted in the gastrointestinal system by health care personnel. Almost all bacteria exist in a biofilm in the natural ecosystem and synthetic surfaces of the gut. Virtually all indwelling catheters in the urethra get colonised by microorganisms embedded in a matrix which account for larger proportion of health care infections of the intestinal tract. In this context the revised definition of the biofilm is an 'assemblage of microbially derived sessile community characterized by viable microbes, irreversibly attached to a substratum or interface or to each other and embedded in a self produced glycocalyx of extracellular polymeric substances exhibiting an altered phenotype with respect to growth rate and gene transcription. As a result of adherence and multiplication acute exacerbations occur that metastasize to other niches of the digestive tract in an ascending fashion [20].

Uropathogensif firmly attach to the Foley catheter surface migrate to uroepithelium and change phenotypically. The entrapped bacteria replicate to form microcolonies that eventually mature into biofilms. Gut bacteria use flagellum mediated motility and twitching *via* type IV pili to facilitate the dissemination of infection from the initial colonization site of the catheter surface to the urinary tract aiding in biofilm formation. Magnesium and calcium ions lead to encrustationin established biofilms on bio-polymeric surfaces. Antibacterial host defences in the urine are found to be present like Tamm-Horsfall proteins, high pH due to organic acids, polymorphonuclear neutrophils, and secretory immunoglobulin A (SIgA) in the gut to ward off biofilm. In general organisms contained within a slimy biomass get protection from the mechanical flushing of urine, intestinal peristalsis and migrating motor complex host defences and antibiotics. Additionally, as a foreign body, the catheter mechanically damage urinary epithelium. Catheter drainage is imperfect and latent bacteria may remain in the bladder as stable residents which proliferate from time to time. These species comprise up to 15% of recalcitrant nosocomial infections of the gastrointestinal system [21].

11. Laboratory Diagnosis of Disorders of Gastrointestinal System

Culture dependent and genomic strategies largely diagnose the potential for the biological activity or the disease state of commensal or pathogenic bacteria respectively. Real time analysis of the intestinal microbiome is essential in future for the development and monitoring of interventional personalized therapeutic strategies. Conventional routine non invasive clinical microbiology lab diagnosis can be facilitated by samples of faecal cultures, urine cultures and extracted devices or catheters.

11.1. Processing of Relevant Specimens of Gastrointestinal Tract

Laboratory Processing of Catheterized Urine or Clean Catch Mid Stream Urine Specimen

Macroscopic examination: Turbidity, haematuria, sediment, crystals or flakes should be looked to arrive at a presumptive diagnosis of gastrointestinal etiology.

Microscopic observation: Wet mount of uncentrifuged urine was observed under 40X magnification of light microscope.

11.2. Standard Loop Technique

A fixed volume calibrated loop of 4 mm diameter which delivers a standardized 0.01 ml of uncentrifuged urine should be used. Surface treading onto all quadrants of 5% sheep blood agar and MacConkeys agar plates to isolate discrete colonies. The Agar plates should be incubated aerobically and in CO_2 at 37°C, examined at 24, 48 and 72 hours in an incubator.

Interpretation of Standard Loop Technique

After incubation the colony forming units per ml should be enumerated, the total bacterial count per ml obtained after multiplication by 100 provides the semi-quantities estimation. If no growth is detected, plates were reincubated for another 24 hours, before reported as negative for culture.

A colony count of 10^5 colony forming units/ml or greater give a presumptive estimate, which was the cut off criterion for urinary tract infection.

11.3. Urinalysis for Pyuria Estimation

Pyuria is the hallmark of inflammation. The presence of polymorphonuclear neutrophils (PMNs) should be detected and enumerated in uncentrifuged urine specimen [22].

This method of screening urine correlates fairly well with infection in the gastrointestinal system and is the best indicator of the host's state.

Microscopic Interpretation

>1 pus cell/7 HPF, corresponded to a significant pyuria of 10^4 WBC/ml.

WBC Grading:

Few = 1-10 pus cells/High power field
Moderate = 11-40 pus cells/High power field
Plenty = >40 pus cells/High power field

Fecal cultures should be performed by inoculating 1 gm of faeces in enrichment broth such as selenite F broth in order to suppress the normal flora of the gut and to isolate the pathogens of the gastrointestinal system.

12. Identification of Isolated Bacteria

Presumptive preliminary identification of bacteria can be inferred by conventional laboratory techniques. Morphology of the discrete colonies on the routine plating media followed by Grams stain, motility, biochemical reactions and carbohydrate fermentation of the bacteria isolated from the specimens of the gastrointestinal system [23].

13. Antibiotic Susceptibility Testing

Antibiotic sensitivity testing evaluated the *in vitro* interactions between antibiotic and microorganism, in controlled conditions that would be appropriate for use *in vivo* to predict or monitor the therapy of the disorders of gastrointestinal tract. Existence within a gut biofilm represents a basic survival mechanism by rendering bacteria inherently resistant to standard antibiotics. The antibiogram of each isolated bacteria should be determined using therapeutically relevant antibiotics. The representative antibiotics among different classes should be used such as carbapenem-imipenem (30 μg), β lactam or β lactamase inhibitor combination-pipercillin (100 μg), tazobactam (10 μg), Aminoglycoside-amikacin (30 μg) or tobramycin (30 μg), fluoroquinolones-ciprofloxacin (5 μg) or norfloxacin (10 μg), cephalosporinsie. 1st generation-cephalexin (30 μg), 2nd generation-cefuroxime (30 μg), 3rd generation-cefotaxime (30 μg), 4th generation-cefepime (30 μg). Nitrofurantoin (300 μg) for uropathogens and glycopeptide-vancomycin (30 μg) for gram positive cocci isolated from gastrointestinal system specimens should be tested. Apart from these other antibiotics administered empirically should also be included for susceptibility testing. Kirby Bauer disc diffusion method is a feasible test to be performed on Mueller Hinton agar by commercially available antibiotic discs according to the norms of clinical laboratory standards institute guidelines [24].

14. Laboratory Diagnosis of Quorum Sensing Mediated Disorders of Gastrointestinal System

14.1. Quorum Sensing Detection of Gut Bacteria by Phenotypic Bioassays

Chromobacterium violaceum strains are used as a control for bioassay detection of the quorum sensing chemical, acyl homoserine lactone mediated activity by plate streaking protocol. The purple pigment violacein is produced under the regulation of acyl homoserine lactone dependent quorum sensing mechanism among gut commensal and pathogenic bacteria. Another approach is by using a bioreporter strain of *Agrobacterium tumefaciencs* as biosensor organism where quorum sensing can be detected by the use of a reporter gene [25].

14.2. Quorum Sensing Detection of Gut Bacteria by Genotypic Assays

Cutting edge scientific and technological research has given rise to a gamut of analytical tools that were previously unimaginable. With advancements in genetic research, techniques of molecular biology have been used to manipulate and investigate biological elements. Among them is Polymerase Chain Reaction (PCR) to amplify and mutate DNA, gel electrophoresis to purify and analyze DNA. PCR, the gene amplification technique has revolutionized molecular biology by unique attributes of sensitivity and specificity with degrees of flexibility. PCR assay specifically amplify a fragment of target DNA sequence using thermos table polymerase and a pair of oligonucleotide primers. PCR is both a thermodynamic and an enzymatic process for a high yield of specific product under optimal conditions as each reaction component and concentration can affect the results.

To complement the bioflm ecology of the gastrointestinal system, isolated organisms should be studied in order to identify the genes required for quorum sensing. A molecular approach to the identification of Autoinduer-2 in various bacteria isolated from the gut is to be carried out by polymerase chain reaction assay. The amplified product held the diagnostic information of interest [26, 27, 28].

15. Future Outlooks

A microbiologist not only needs to address system biology from a cellular perspective but also synthetic ecology in the wake of detrimental effects of biofilms on biomaterials in clinical situations. Measurement of the metabolic effects by gene expression studies to determine the role of environmental cues for cellular differentiation of the microbes developing like multicellular with a quick adaptation to the constantly changing conditions is the need of the hour. Quorum sensing connects bacterial behaviors to an interacting and structured microbial community including both cooperativity and competition among several pathogenic bacteria. As the exploration of biology goes deeper and wider qualitative experiments and descriptive methods will not be enough to understand the complexity of living systems. *In vivo* experiments and integrated systematic analyses are becoming more and more indispensable to obtain a comprehensive understanding of biological systems to reveal the underlying principles like biofilm kinetics studies and time dependent assays. There is a belief that quorum sensing is an appropriate therapeutic target to reduce the issues of off target effects traditionally associated with antibiotic treatment. Unfortunately, the biological efficiency is not fully appreciated as to whether human beings can overcome or subvert the agents, but will steer future studies. Considering the widespread availability of quorum sensing in gut bacteria, manipulations of the involved processes could result in generation of engineered catheter or device surface modifications to be used for the above purposes with more specificity [29, 30].

Conclusion

A gastroenterologist always seeks to introduce emerging opportunities for synthetic biology and therapeutic developments pertaining to disorders of gastrointestinal system. To detect the universal characteristic nature of quorum sensing in clinically isolated bacteria from the various samples of gastrointestinal system is the need of the day. Emphasis should be placed on developing rigorous analyses of how bacteria communicate within and between species and on how a host talks back in the vicinity of the gastrointestinal tract. The key now for understanding these complex and fascinating bacterial languages is to decipher the impact of the words. The answers will undoubtedly provide new insights and surprises by unifying the concepts clinically regarding the mammalian gut. Finally, this forum has covered few issues and opportunities in the area of human health and disease of gastrointestinal system.

REFERENCES

[1] Eamonn M. M. Quigley, Gut Bacteria in Health and Disease, *Gastroenterology and hepatology*, 2013, 9: 560-569.

[2] Davey M E, O'Toole GA. Microbial biofilms from ecology to molecular genetics. *Microbial molecular biology Review*. 2000, 64:847-867.

[3] Backhed F, Ley R.E, Sonnenburg J L, Peterson, D.A, Gordon J.I. "Host-Bacterial Mutualism in the Human Intestine." *Science*, 2005, 307: 1915-1920.

[4] Costerton J.W, P.S. Stewart and E.P. Greenberg. Bacterial biofilms: a common cause of persistent infections. *Science*. 1999, 284:1318-1322.

[5] ThienFah C. Mah and George A. O'Toole. Mechanism of biofilm resistance to antimicrobial agents. *Trends in Microbiology*. 2001, 9:34-39.

[6] Habash M, Ried G. Microbial biofilms: their development and significance for medical device related infections. *Journal of clinical Pharmacology*. 1999, 39:887-98.

[7] Waters C M, Bassler B L. Quorum sensing: cell to cell communication in bacteria. *Annual Review cell Development Biology*. 2005, 21:319-46.

[8] Miller M B, Bassler B L. Quorum sensing in bacteria. *Annual Review Microbiology*. 2001, 55:165-99.

[9] Diggle SP, Griffin AS, Campbell GS, West SA. Cooperation and conflict in quorum sensing bacterial populations. *Nature*. 2007, 450:411-414.

[10] Danese P. N, Pratt L. A. and Kolter R. Biofilm formation as a developmental process. *Methods in Enzymology*. 2001, 2:19-26.

[11] Flemming, H.C. and Wingender J. The biofilm matrix. *Nature Reviews Microbiology*. 2010, 8:623-633.

[12] Sutherland I W. Biofilm exopolysaccharides: A strong and sticky framework. Microbiology. 2001,147:3-9.

[13] Costerton J W, K. J. Cheng, G. G. Geesey, T. I. Ladd, J. C. Nickel, M. Dasgupta, T. J. Marrie. Bacterial biofilms in nature and disease. *Annual Review Microbiology*. 1987, 41: 435-464.

[14] Federle, M.J, Bassler B.L. Interspecies communication in bacteria. *Journal of Clinical Investigation*. 2003, 112:1291-1299.

[15] Bassler, B. L and R. Losick. Bacterially Speaking. *Cell*. 2006, 125: 237-246.

[16] Vipin Chandra Kalia and Hemant J Purohit. Quenching the quorum sensing system: potential antibacterial drug targets. *Critical Reviews in Microbiology*. 2011, 37: 121-140.

[17] Nicola C. Reading and Vanessa Sperandio. Quorum sensing: the many languages of bacteria. *FEMS Microbiology Letters*. 2006, 254:1-11.

[18] Hogan D, Kolter R. Why are bacteria refractory to antimicrobials? *Current Opinion Microbiology*. 2002, 5:472-477.

[19] Matthew R. Parsek and E.P. Greenberg. Sociomicrobiology: the connections between quorum sensing and biofilms. *Trends in Microbiology*. 2005, 13:27-33.

[20] Antunes L C, Ferreira R.B, Buckner M M, Finlay, B.B. Quorum sensing in bacterial virulence. *Microbiology*. 2010, 156:2271-2282.

[21] Taga M.E, Bassler B.L. Chemical communication among bacteria. *Proceedings of National academy of Sciences*. 2003, 100:14549-14554.

[22] W. E. Stammand and T. M. Hooton. "Management of urinary tract infections in adults." *New England Journal of Medicine*. 1993, 329:1328-1334.

[23] Thomas M Hooton. Nosocomial urinary tract infection. Mandell, Douglas and Bennett's, *Principles and practice of infectious diseases*. 8th edition. Elsevier. ISBN: 978-1-4557-4801-3, 304:3333-3346.

[24] Performance standards for Antimicrobial susceptibility testing; Twenty third information supplement. *Clinical and laboratory standards institute*. 2013, 33:M100-S23.

[25] Dr. Kendra Rumbaugh. Bioassays of Quorum Sensing compounds using *Agrobacterium tumefaciens* and *Chromobacterium Violaceum*, *Quorum Sensing: Methods and Protocols*, 2011, 692:3-19.

[26] Mullis K B. The unusual origin of the polymerase chain reaction. *Scientific American*. 1990, 262:56-65.

[27] Mullis K B, Faloona F A. Specific synthesis of DNA *in vitro via* a Polymerase catalyzed reaction. *Methods in Enzymology*. 1987,155:335-350.

[28] Donald Voet and Judith G. Voet. *Biochemistry*. John Wiley and Sons. ISBN 978-0471586517. 1995, 2:877-878.

[29] Andrew B. Shreiner, John Y. Kao and Vincent B. Young, The gut microbiome in health and in disease. *Current opinion gastroenterology*. 2015; 31: 69-75.

[30] Elliot TSJ. Plastic devices: New fields for old microbes. *Lancet*. 1988, 331:30-31.

In: Disorders of Gastrointestinal Systems ... ISBN: 978-1-63485-366-8
Editors: S. Rajagopal, S. Murugan and R. Saravanan

Chapter 15

ROLE OF ENZYMES ON GASTROINTESTINAL TRACT

Saranya Natarajan* and Geethalakshmi Sundararaman
Division of Bioscience, Nehru Arts and Science College, Coimbatore, Tamilnadu, India

ABSTRACT

Enzymes are a vital component of the digestive process. Enzymes are meticulous for each and every activity of life. They are complex protein molecules that provoke and expedite the speed of chemical reactions in other compounds. They are found throughout the human body, and are essential for digesting food, regulating biochemical reactions, generating energy, and repairing tissues, organs, and cells. Enzymes can be categorized into two groups: digestive and metabolic. Digestive enzymes are secreted along the entire gastrointestinal tract, and break down polymeric macromolecules in to their smaller building blocks that can be absorbed and assimilated by the body. Metabolic enzymes are responsible for the structuring, repairing, and remodeling of all cells. The three main groups of enzymes involved in digestion are amylase, protease and lipase enzymes. The lack of enzyme production results in a range of chronic disorders.

Keywords: digestive enzymes, gastrointestinal tract, amylase, lipase, protease

1. INTRODUCTION

The gastrointestinal tract (GI) is an elongated pipe extending from the mouth to the anus with a number of specialized regions. Most of the nutrients in food have to be digested before they can be assimilated. Digestion involves the hydrolysis of polysaccharides, oligosaccharides, proteins and lipids in enzyme-catalyzed reactions. The yield of hydrolysis, such as monosaccharides, amino acids, free fatty acids and monoacylglycerols, can then be absorbed. Some nutrients, vitamins and minerals for instance, are absorbed without the need

* Corresponding author: Mrs. Saranya Natarajan, PhD., Assistant professor, Division of Bioscience, Nehru Arts and Science College, Coimbatore, Tamilnadu, INDIA. Email:saranbiorythm@gmail.com; Mo: 9047592349.

for digestion. Digestion is the hydrolytic breakdown of nutrient macromolecules and compound lipids to smaller products that can be absorbed. The digestion of food and amalgamation of the liberated nutrients are the major functions of the GIT together with its accessory organs, the pancreas, liver and gall bladder (Henning, 1987).

The hydrolytic reactions are catalyzed by a variety of enzymes: proteases that digest proteins; carbohydrases that digest carbohydrates; lipases that catalyze the hydrolysis of lipids and nucleases that degrade DNA and RNA.

Digestion occurs in the mouth, to a small extent, stomach and small intestine, and most absorption of nutrients occurs in the small intestine and that of water in the large intestine. The peritoneum lines the abdominal cavity and covers the major organs. Folds of the peritoneum, called the mesentery, and mesocolon hold the intestines in place. The GIT has significant roles in the homeostasis of nutrients and in protecting the body against pathogens ingested with the food.

Digestion and absorption, can, of course, only take place after ingestion of food, unlike the homeostatic and protective functions that operate continuously. The GI tract synthesizes and releases various enzymes that perform several important functions, such as breaking down of the food, digestion and assimilation (Fallingborg, 1999).

The food is subjected to enzymatic action; wherein, the solid food is converted in to proteins, fats and carbohydrates, absorbed by the body, and the waste excreted out. The digestive enzymes are divided in to 4 categories. They are: lipolytic enzymes which break down fats in to glycerol and fatty acids, proteolytic enzymes which break down proteins in to amino acids, amylolytic enzymes, break down carbohydrates in to simple sugars and nucleolytic enzyme which break down nucleic acids in to nucleotides.

1.1. Salivary Enzymes

Digestion begins when food first enters the mouth. The first mechanical process occurs with the act of chewing. The body's first enzymes are added to the food with saliva. Saliva is a complex fluid, which persuades oral health through specific and nonspecific physical and chemical properties. The magnitude of saliva in our day by day activities and the medicinal properties it possesses are often taken for decided. When disruptions in the quality or quantity of saliva do occur in an individual, it is likely that he or she will experience detrimental effects on oral and systemic health. Often head and neck radiotherapy has serious and detrimental side effects on the oral cavity including the loss of salivary gland function and a persistent complaint of a dry mouth (xerostomia). Saliva has a myriad of beneficial functions that are essential to our well-being (Twari et al., 2011).

The enzymes present in the mouth are Ptyalin and Amylase, which breaks down carbohydrates in to simple single molecule sugar. Amylase is a member of a class of enzymes that catalyze the hydrolysis of starch into smaller carbohydrate molecules. There are two assortments of amylases, such as alpha and beta, differ in the way they attack the bonds of the starch molecules. Alpha-amylase is widespread among living organisms. In the digestive systems of humans, an alpha-amylase is called ptyalin and is produced by the salivary glands, whereas pancreatic amylase is secreted by the pancreas into the small intestine (Ganong and Barrett, 1995).

Organ	Function
Mouth	**Digestion** starts here! The teeth cut and grind the food, which is mixed with **saliva.** This contains **amylase** to break **starch** down into maltose (sugar).
Oesophagus	Boluses (balls) of food pass through by **peristalsis**, from mouth to stomach.
Stomach	Muscular walls squeeze on food to make it semi-liquid. Gastric juice contains: • **Pepsin (a protease)** to break big proteins down into small protein (polypeptides) • Hydrochloric acid (**HCl**) to maintain an optimum pH (1-2,5). The acid also kills bacteria.
Gall bladder	Stores **bile** used to help in the digestion of **fats.**
Pancreas	Secretes **pancreatic juice** into the duodenum, also makes the hormones **insulin** and **glucagon**.
Liver	Makes **bile**, which is stored on the gall bladder. Bile contains **salts** that emulsify **fats**, forming droplets with a large surface area to make digestion by lipase more efficient. Digested foods are **assimilated** here. For example, glucose is stored as glycogen, surplus amino acids are deaminated.
Small intestine	**Duodenum + Ilium**
Duodenum	The first part of the small intestine. It receives pancreatic juice containing **protease, lipase** and **amylase**. Proteins, fats, starches and complex sugars are broken down into small soluble molecules. The juice also contains sodium hydrogen carbonate, which neutralises acid from the stomach, producing a **pH of 7-8**.
Ileum	The second part of the small intestine. Enzymes in the epithelial lining break down **lactose** and **peptides**. Its surface area is increased by the presence of villi which allow the efficient **absorption** of fully digested food molecules into the bloodstream.
Large intestine	**Colon + Rectum** Only undigested food reaches here. Water absorbed.

Figure 1. Different organs in GI tract and their function.

Alpha-amylase (EC 3.2.1.1) is the most abundant enzyme in the saliva of man and of several vertebrates. In humans, salivary amylase is mainly formed in the parotid gland; its activity is of high inter-individual and intra-individual variability. The physiological functions of α-amylase have not yet been explored completely. It is well known that the enzyme cleaves the α-(1,4)-glycosidic bonds of polysaccharides. Furthermore it plays an important role in initial bioadhesion in man, facilitating carbohydrate metabolism and bacterial adherence at the tooth surface and therewith caries initiation. It is still a matter of interest why humans have such high amounts of salivary amylase (Boehlke et al., 2015).

Ptyalin is mixed with food in the mouth, where it acts upon starches. Although the food remains in the mouth for only a short time, the action of ptyalin continues for up to several hours in the stomach until the food is mixed with the stomach secretions, the high acidity of which inactivates ptyalin. Ptyalin's digestive action depends upon how much acid is in the stomach, how rapidly the stomach contents empty, and how thoroughly the food has mixed with the acid. Under optimal conditions as much as 30 to 40 percent of ingested starches can be broken down to maltose by ptyalin during digestion in the stomach.

When food passes to the small intestine, the remainder of the starch molecules is catalyzed mainly to maltose by pancreatic amylase. This step in starch digestion occurs in the first section of the small intestine (the duodenum), the region into which the pancreatic juices empty. The by-products of amylase hydrolysis are ultimately broken down by other enzymes into molecules of glucose, which are rapidly absorbed through the intestinal wall. Beta-amylases are present in yeasts, molds, bacteria, and plants, particularly in the seeds. They are the principal components of a mixture called diastase that is used in the removal of starchy sizing agents from textiles and in the conversion of cereal grains to fermentable sugars (Mayer et al., 1937).

Human saliva is a complex liquid mixture of about 99% water, the remainder being mainly enzymes, glycoproteins, electrolytes and small organic molecules. It has multiple roles in gastrointestinal tract including bolus formation, enzymatic digestion, and antioxidant action and buffering.

In healthy individuals, the rate of saliva secretion is about 0.3- 0.4 ml/min in resting conditions, but during a meal the salivary glands are stimulated and saliva secretion increases to 1- 2 ml/min. The considerable quantities of saliva are mixed with the food that reaches the stomach.

Among its various physiological functions, human saliva acts as an antioxidant system due to the presence of its antioxidants including uric acid, peroxidase and superoxide dismutase. There are various classes of antioxidants in saliva including non-enzymatic antioxidants, and enzymes such as peroxidase (POD), catalase and superoxide dismutase (SOD). Peroxidase in saliva is secreted by the salivary glands and myeloperoxidases by polymorphonuclear neutrophils. Salivary SOD is a key antioxidant enzyme that efficiently and specifically scavenges O_2 by catalyzing its dismutation to H_2O_2 and O_2. Lactate dehydrogenase (LDH) is an enzyme detectable in cytoplasm of almost every cell and becomes extracellular upon cell death. In an anaerobic condition, pyruvate, the normal product of glycolysis, is reduced to lactate by catalytic action of LDH in the presence of nicotinamide adenine dinucleotide (NAD) as a coenzyme (Langley, 1882).

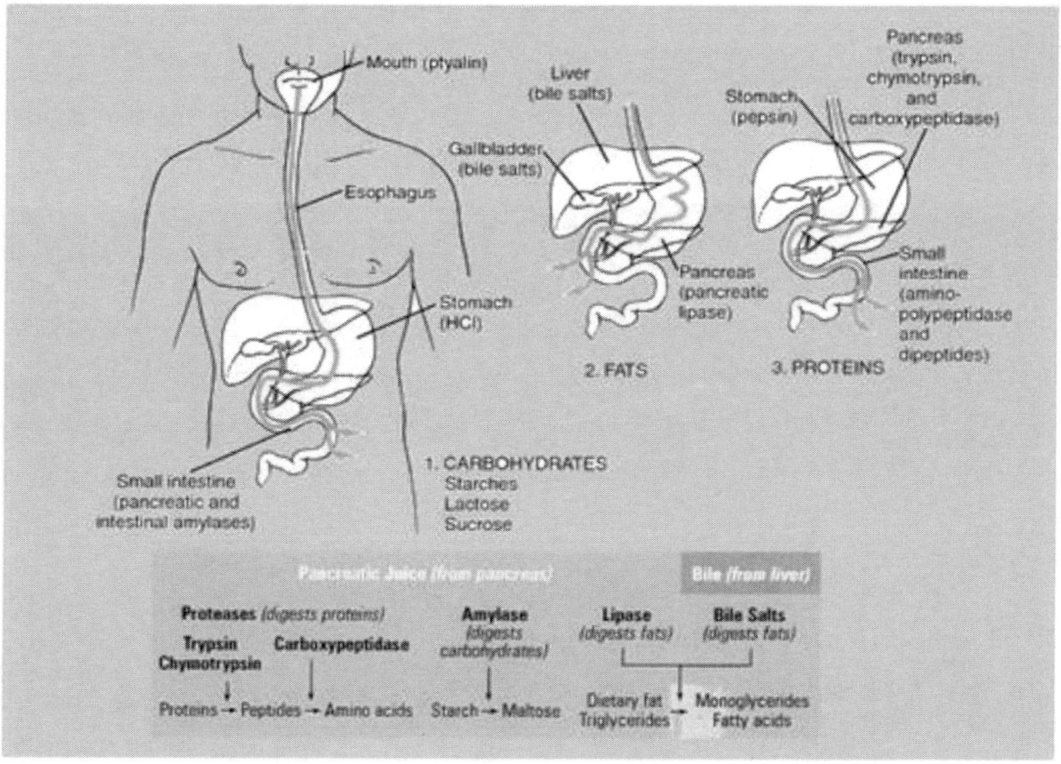

Figure 2. Secretion of various enzymes on gastrointestinal tract.

2. Stomach Enzymes

Pepsin was first documented in 1836 by the German physiologist Theodor Schwann. In 1929, its crystallization and protein character were testimonies by American biochemist John Howard Northrop of the Rockefeller Institute for Medical Research. Glands in the mucous-membrane lining of the stomach formulate and accumulate an inactive protein called pepsinogen. Inclination from the vagus nerve and the hormonal secretions of gastrin and secretin motivate the release of pepsinogen into the stomach, where it is assorted with hydrochloric acid and rapidly rehabilitated to the active enzyme pepsin. The digestive power of pepsin is greatest at the acidity of normal gastric juice (pH 1.5–2.5). In the intestine the gastric acids are neutralized (pH 7), and pepsin is no longer effective (Dunn, 2001).

Pepsin is produced initially as its inactive precursor pepsinogen. This molecule is produced by the chief cells in the body of the stomach, although some is also produced in mucus cells of the stomach glands. At meal time, a variety of stimuli lead to increased release of pepsinogen from these cells, which brings the precursor into contact with hydrochloric acid in the stomach. In the digestive tract pepsin effects only partial degradation of proteins into smaller units called peptides, which then either are absorbed from the intestine into the bloodstream or are broken down further by pancreatic enzymes (Bunell, 1999).

Small amounts of pepsin pass from the stomach into the bloodstream, where it breaks down some of the larger, or still partially undigested, fragments of protein that may have been absorbed by the small intestine. Chronic backflow of pepsin, acid, and other substances from the stomach into the esophagus forms the basis for reflux conditions, particularly gastroesophageal reflux disease and laryngopharyngeal reflux (or extraesophageal reflux). In the latter, pepsin and acid travel all the way up to the larynx, where they can cause damage to the laryngeal mucosa and produce symptoms ranging from hoarseness and chronic cough to laryngospasm (involuntary contraction of the vocal cords) and laryngeal cancer.

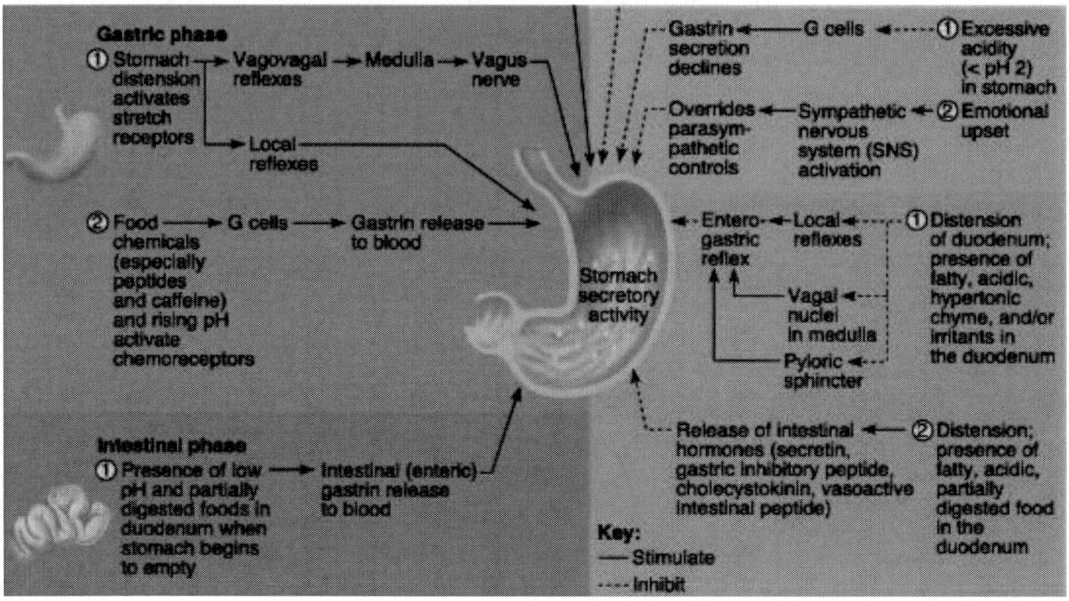

Figure 3. Gastric and Intestinal phase in stomach.

Pepsin is prepared commercially from swine stomachs. Crude pepsin is used in the leather industry to remove hair and residual tissue from animal hides prior to their being tanned. It is also used in the recovery of silver from discarded photographic films by digesting the gelatin layer that holds the silver compound. Food is composed of varying amounts of protein, fats or carbohydrates, and the pepsin enzyme targets the protein portion of a meal. It has a proteolytic function, which means that it slices up large proteins into smaller polypeptides in preparation for absorption in the intestines.

Proteins are made up of long strings of amino acids held together by peptide bonds, and pepsin cuts proteins at certain amino acids, such as glutamic acid, leucine or aspartic acid. Later during digestion, these polypeptide fragments will be further broken down by additional enzymes, such as endopeptidases and exopeptidases, so they can easily cross the intestinal wall into the body. Pepsin's preference for certain amino acids, though, means that some proteins entering the stomach escape cleavage by pepsin. The persistence of these unbroken proteins can lead to disease in certain people. This is exemplified by celiac disease, in which whole gluten proteins of wheat enter the intestines and trigger inflammation (Studdy et al., 1983). Pepsinogen production and release are regulated in part by the nervous system and also by endocrine hormones and the amount of acid in the stomach. People with medical conditions that reduce stomach acid secretion, such as the autoimmune condition achlorhydria, have a reduced pepsin level and are less able to digest proteins efficiently. Significant reduction in stomach acid can also occur with Helicobacter pylori infection of the stomach, following certain gastric surgeries or as a result of medications like proton pump inhibitors.

2.1. Deficient Digestion

A large amount stomach acid is certainly a problem, but so is too diminutive. Stomach acid is indispensable to wind down proteins, so pepsin can work on breaking them apart. Without sufficient stomach acid, proteins are only moderately digested, which means that many inadequately broken down proteins enter the bloodstream causing allergic and autoimmune problems. Enzymes present for predigest can facilitate moderate some of the problem by breaking down some of the proteins without the need for normal levels of stomach acid. But that said, the problem of incomplete protein digestion is only compounded when you use acid reflux medication since you end up with insufficient stomach acid or virtually none in many cases. The less protein that is broken down in the stomach as a result of insufficient stomach acid, the more pancreatic enzymes your pancreas must produce to make up the difference. If the diet is also enzyme deficient, this doubles the stress on the pancreas.

2.2. Malnutrition

Deficient digestion means a universal condition in the elderly, again, aggravated by the use of acid reflux medications. Both iron and vitamin C, for example, require stomach acid for proper absorption. As a result, deficiencies of both nutrients have been noted as side effects from the use of acid reflux medication.

3. Pancreatic Enzymes

Pancreatic enzymes help break down the food components like fats, proteins and carbohydrates. A normal pancreas secretes 8 cups of pancreatic juice into the duodenum per day. This fluid contains pancreatic enzymes to digest and bicarbonate to neutralize stomach acid as it enters the small intestine.

3.1. Types of Pancreatic Enzymes and Their Effects

Pancreas is mutually an endocrine and an exocrine gland, to facilitate it to produce endocrinic hormones circulated into the circulatory system (such as insulin, and glucagon), to control glucose metabolism, and also to secrete digestive/exocrinic pancreatic juice, which is secreted eventually via the pancreatic duct into duodenum. Digestive or exocrine function of pancreas is as significant to the maintenance of health as its endocrine function. Two of the population of cells in the pancreatic parenchyma make up its digestive enzymes (Mallory and Travis, 1973). Ductal cells which is mainly responsible for production of bicarbonate (HCO_3), which acts to neutralize the acidity of the stomach chyme entering duodenum through the pylorus.

Ductal cells of the pancreas are stimulated by the hormone secretin to produce their bicarbonate-rich secretions, in what is in essence a bio-feedback mechanism; highly acidic stomach chyme entering the duodenum stimulates duodenal cells called "S cells" to produce the hormone secretin and release to the bloodstream. Secretin having entered the blood eventually comes into contact with the pancreatic ductal cells, stimulating them to produce their bicarbonate-rich juice. It is interesting to note that secretin also inhibits production of gastrin by "G cells," and also stimulates acinar cells of the pancreas to produce their pancreatic enzyme (Quiroz et al., 2016).

Acinar cells is mainly responsible for production of the inactive pancreatic enzymes (zymogens) that, once present in the small bowel, become activated and perform their major digestive functions by breaking down proteins, fat, and DNA/RNA. Pancreatic juice, composed of the secretions of both ductal and acinar cells, is made up of the following digestive enzymes.

Trypsinogen, which is an inactive (zymogenic) protease that, once activated in the duodenum into trypsin, breaks down proteins at the basic amino acids. Trypsinogen is activated via the duodenal enzyme enterokinase into its active form trypsin. Chymotrypsinogen, which is an inactive (zymogenic) protease that, once activated by duodenal enterokinase, breaks down proteins at their aromatic amino acids. Chymotrypsinogen can also be activated by trypsin.

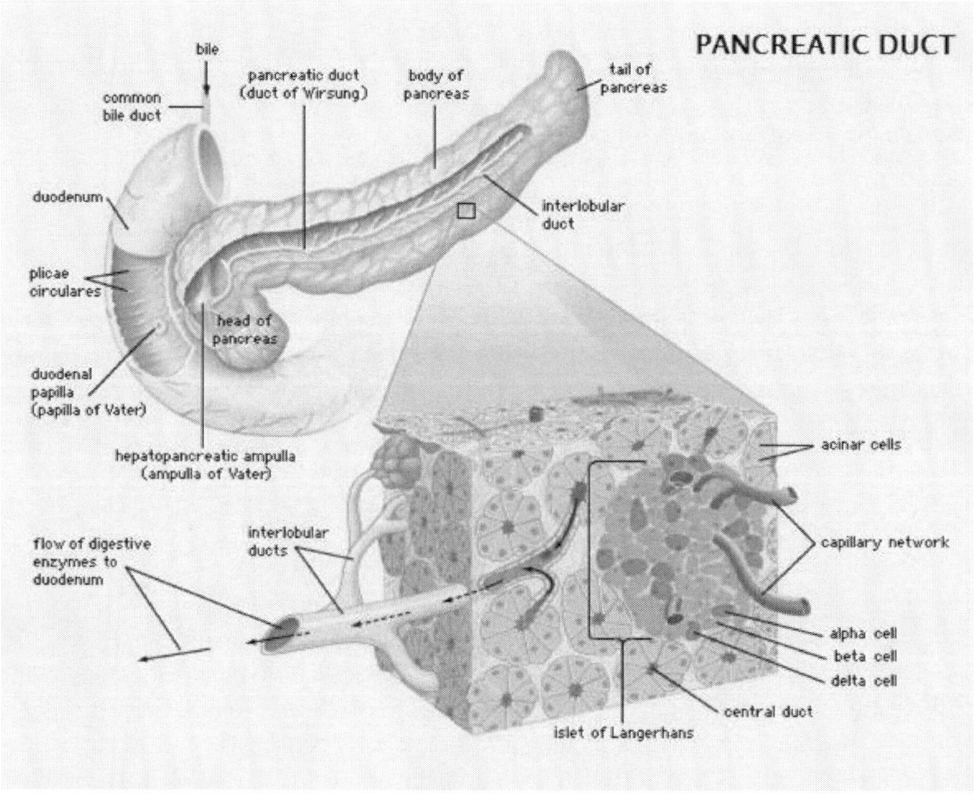

Figure 4. Pancreatic Duct.

Carboxypeptidase, which is a protease that takes off the terminal amino acid group from a protein. Elastases that degrade the protein elastin and some other proteins. Pancreatic lipase that degrades triglycerides into fatty acids and glycerol, Sterol esterase, Phospholipase and Several nucleases that degrade nucleic acids, like DNAase and RNAase Pancreatic amylase that breaks down starch and glycogen which are alpha-linked glucose polymers. Humans lack the cellulases to digest the carbohydrate cellulose which is a beta-linked glucose polymers. Pancreas's exocrine function owes part of its immaculate function to Somatostatin is a hormone produced by the mucosal cells of the duodenum and also the "delta cells" of the pancreas. Somatostatin has a major inhibitory effect, including on pancreatic production.

ENZYME	activity	Deficiency
Lipase	Lipase works with bile from the liver to break down fat molecules so they can be absorbed and used by the body.	Lack of needed fats and fat-soluble vitamins. Diarrhea and/or fatty stools.
Protease	Proteases break down proteins. They help keep the intestine free of parasites such as bacteria, yeast and protozoa.	Allergies or the formation of toxic substances due to incomplete digestion of proteins. Increased risk for intestinal infections.
Amylase	Amylase breaks down carbohydrates (starch) into sugars which are more easily absorbed by the body. This enzyme is also found in saliva.	Diarrhea due to the effects of undigested starch in the colon.

3.2. Reasons to Take Pancreatic Enzymes

The inability of the pancreas to secrete the enzymes needed for digestion is called pancreatic deficiency. This is an important symptom of pancreatic cancer. In the case of pancreatic deficiency, external pancreatic enzyme products are needed to help improve digestion and absorption of food.

Some reasons for pancreatic insufficiency are surgery (pancreatectomy), blockage or narrowing of the pancreatic or biliary duct, pancreatic or duodenal tumors, cystic fibrosis or pancreatitis.

The symptoms include:

- Indigestion
- Large amounts of gas
- Differently colored stools
- Frequent stools
- Cramping after food
- Foul smelling gas or stools
- Greasy/fatty stools
- Loose stools
- Weight loss

Almost 25% of patients who have undergone surgery have mal absorption and have to take supplemental enzymes for their normal life. Patients undergoing radiation therapy along with the Whipple procedure will suffer from mal absorption. In those patients who take supplementary enzymes, fat absorption will not be normal. These patients will be treated for diarrhea to restore adequate nutrition and decrease weight loss.

For those who suffer from weight loss, MCT (Medium Chain Triglyceride) oil may help control mal absorption. MCT oil is a calorie-rich type of fat that restrict usual fat. It is found in coconut oil, palm kernel oil and butter. Oral supplement of MCT promote weight gain, help increase strength and physical activity.

For those patients who suffer from non-operable cancer in the head of the pancreas, bile duct or pancreatic duct blocks are commonly found. For these patients, pancreatic enzyme replacement therapy along with nutritional therapy is followed. Drainage of the bile duct can be given for such patients to avoid weight loss (Gass et al., 2007).

3.3. Sources of Supplemental Pancreatic Enzymes

Pancreatic enzyme supplements can be got through prescription as well as non-prescription forms. Prescribed pancreatic enzyme products are synchronized by the United States Food and Drug Administration (FDA) to ensure their effectiveness, safety and manufacturing consistency. The non-prescribed supplements are classified as dietary supplements and not as drugs and FDA do not organize their production. The manufacturers of such supplements are required to ensure the safety of their products and there is no regulation on manufacturing reliability. Therefore, these products are not recommended for use in patients with pancreatic cancer.

The enzymatic supplements must be recommended based on the type of person. Initially, 10,000 – 20,000 lipase units with snacks and 20,000 – 40,000 lipase units with meals are recommended for all the patients. Assuming 4 meals per day, above 2,500 lipase units per kilogram of body weight per meal should not be exceeded. The dosage can be decided with the recommendation from the physician.

3.4. Taking Pancreatic Enzymes

Since the enzyme supplements are from porcine origin, people who have allergies to porcine meat should consult their physician before taking them. Along with the supplement, acid-reducing medication can be taken to improve the effectiveness. Acid reducing medications include esomeprazole (proton pump inhibitors) and famotidine (H2 blockers). But such prescription is not necessary for all types of supplements (Do et al., 2016).

For better results from pancreatic supplements, some points need to be followed:

- With every meal or snack, additional food that contains fat like meat, dairy, bread and desserts has to be included.
- Smallest dose should be the initial point and adjusted according to the severity.

- The supplement should be taken at the beginning of the meal or snack. This is very important for proper enzyme functioning. When multiple enzymes are taken, some must be taken at the beginning of the meal and the rest at various points throughout the meal.
- Intact tablets and capsules should be taken with liquid along with meal. The tablets should not be crushed or chewed.
- The capsules should not be held in the mouth for a longer time as they may damage the mucous membranes and cause irritation.
- Capsules should not be mixed with milk, custard, ice cream or other dairy products before swallowing as they will destroy enzyme activity.
- They should not be taken with calcium- or magnesium-containing antacids as their activity will be reduced.
- They should be used before expiration date.

3.5. Side Effects of Pancreatic Enzymes

The most common side effect of pancreatic enzymes is constipation. They also cause nausea, abdominal cramps or diarrhea. In case of any allergy, the use of enzymes must be stopped. Pancreatic enzymes may decrease the absorption of iron salts. Pancreatic enzymes help to prevent weight loss and reduce the pancreatic enzyme insufficiency if taken properly (El Kaoutari et al., 2007).

4. Intestinal Enzymes

The jejunum is the middle section of the small intestine. It has a lining which is designed to absorb carbohydrates and proteins. The inner surface of the jejunum, its mucous membrane, is covered in projections called villi, which increase the surface area of tissue available to absorb nutrients from the gut contents. The epithelial cells which line these villi possess even larger numbers of microvilli. The transport of nutrients across epithelial cells through the jejunum includes the passive transport of some carbohydrates and the active transport of amino acids, small peptides, vitamins, and most glucose. The villi in the jejunum are much longer than in the duodenum or ileum.

The three major classes of nutrients that undergo digestion are proteins, lipids (fats), and carbohydrates.

4.1. Proteins

Proteins are degraded into small peptides and amino acids before absorption. Chemical breakdown begins in the stomach and continues through the large intestine. Proteolytic enzymes, including trypsin and chymotrypsin, secreted by the pancreas, cleave proteins into smaller peptides. Carboxypeptidase, a pancreatic brush border enzyme, splits one amino acid at a time. Aminopeptidase and dipeptidase free the end amino acid products.

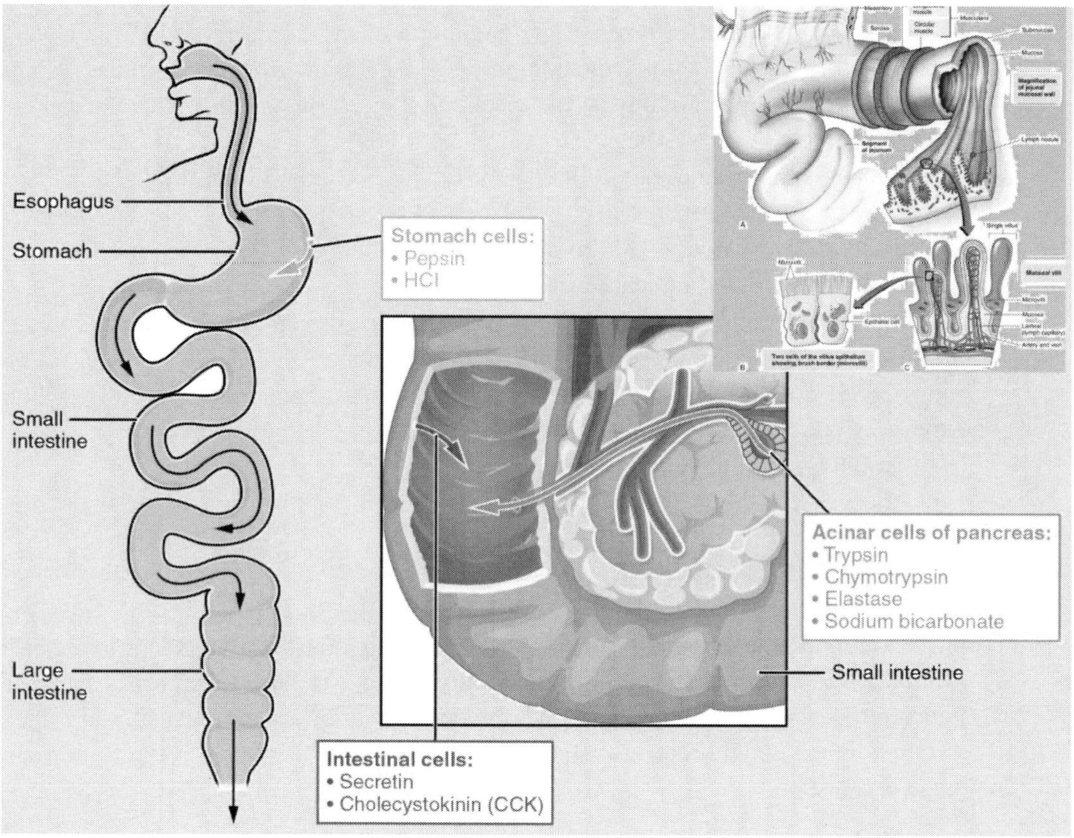

Figure 5. Locations of different enzymes in digestive system.

4.2. Lipids

Lipids (fats) are degraded into fatty acids and glycerol. Pancreatic lipase breaks down triglycerides into free fatty acids and monoglycerides. Pancreatic lipase works with the help of the salts from bile secreted by the liver and the gall bladder. Bile salts attach to triglycerides, helping emulsify them, which aids access by pancreatic lipase; the lipase is water-soluble, but the fatty triglycerides are hydrophobic, tending to orient toward each other and away from the watery intestinal surroundings. The bile salts act as the "main man" that holds the triglycerides in the watery surroundings until the lipase can break them into the smaller components that are able to enter the villi for absorption.

4.3. Carbohydrates

Some carbohydrates are degraded into simple sugars, or monosaccharides (e.g., glucose, galactose) and absorbed by the small intestine. Pancreatic amylase breaks down some carbohydrates (notably starch) into oligosaccharides. Other carbohydrates pass undigested into the large intestine, where they are digested by intestinal bacteria. Brush border enzymes take over from there. The most important brush border enzymes are dextrinase and glucoamylase, which further break down oligosaccharides. Other brush border enzymes are maltase, sucrase, and lactase. Lactase is absent in most adult humans and for them lactose, like most poly-saccharides, is not digested in the small intestine. Some carbohydrates, such as cellulose, are not digested at all, despite being made of multiple glucose units. This is because the cellulose is made out of beta-glucose, making the inter-monosaccharidal bindings different from the ones present in starch, which consists of alpha-glucose. Humans lack the enzyme for splitting the beta-glucose-bonds—reserved for herbivores and bacteria in the large intestine.

The final step in digestion of dietary carbohydrates and proteins occurs right on the face of small intestinal enterocytes, in the immediate vicinity of the transporters which will ferry the resulting sugars and amino acids into the epithelial cells. The enzymes responsible for this terminal stage of digestion are not free in the intestinal lumen, but rather, tethered as integral membrane proteins in the plasma membrane of the enterocyte (Estudante et al., 2013). The apical plasma membrane housing these enzymes is composed of numerous microvilli which extend from the cell and constitute the "brush border." Hence, the enzymes embedded in those microvilli are referred to as brush border enzymes. Various enzymes are secreted which has an important, though not a major role in digestion which include Glucoamylase (Maltase), Sucrase-Isomaltase, Lactase and Peptidases. The following enzymes are produced in the duodenum:

- *Secretin*: This is an endocrine hormone produced by the duodenal "S cells" in response to the acidity of the gastric chyme.
- *Cholecystokinin (CCK):* This is not by definition a hormone; there is new evidence suggesting that CCK works by a very complex neuronal bi-directional pathway. Regardless of its pathway, its eventual role is to increase secretion of acinar cells and increased production of pancreatic juice. CCK also increases gallbladder contraction, causing release of pre-stored bile into the cystic duct, and eventually into the common bile duct and via the ampulla of Vater into the second anatomic position of the duodenum. CCK also decreases the tone of the sphincter of Oddi, which is the sphincter that regulates flow through the ampulla of Vater. CCK also decreases gastric activity and decreases gastric emptying, thereby giving more time to the pancreatic juices to neutralize the acidity of the gastric chyme.
- *Gastric inhibitory peptide (GIP):* This peptide decreases gastric motility and is produced by duodenal mucosal cells.
- *Motilin:* This substance increases gastro-intestinal motility via specialized receptors called "motilin receptors."
- *Somatostatin:* This hormone is formed by duodenal mucosa and also by the delta cells of the pancreas. Its main function is to inhibit a variety of secretory mechanisms. Throughout the lining of the small intestine there are numerous brush border enzymes whose function is to further break down the chyme released from the stomach into absorbable particles. Some of these enzymes include:
- *Erepsin:* It converts peptones and polypeptides into amino acids.
- *Maltase:* It converts maltose into glucose.
- *Lactase:* This is a significant brush border enzyme in that a majority of Middle-Eastern and Asian population lack this enzyme and also this enzyme decreases with

age, and as such lactose intolerance is often a common abdominal complaint in the Middle-Eastern, Asian, and older population, manifesting with bloating, abdominal pain, and osmotic diarrhea. It converts lactose into glucose and galactose.

- *Sucrase:* It converts sucrose into glucose and fructose.

Conclusion

The breakdown of food by various enzymes is the key step in the metabolic process. The knowledge about the activity of various enzymes and their role in digestion will help us to find a remedy for all the digestive problems. Starting from the reaction with saliva, at various stages, the digestion process is executed at various intensities by different concentration of the enzymes. Some may act alone and some can function only when they combine with their counter parts. An in-depth knowledge about the structure and its correlation with the function will provide a greater insight into the structure activity relationship of enzyme soup of the digestive system.

References

Akeson, W. R. and Stahmann, M. A. (1964). A pepsin pancreatin digest index of protein quality evaluation. *Journal of Nutrition*, *83*, 257-261.

Bunnell, T. (1999). The effect of "healing with intent" on pepsin enzyme activity. *Journal of Scientific Exploration*, *13*(2), 139-148.

Do, D. H. T., Kong, F., Penet, C., Winetzky, D. and Gregory, K. (2016). Using a dynamic stomach model to study efficacy of supplemental enzymes during simulated digestion. *LWT-Food Science and Technology*, *65*, 580-588.

Dunn, B. M. (2001). Overview of Pepsin-like Aspartic Peptidases. *Current Protocols in Protein Science*, 21-3.

El Kaoutari, A., Armougom, F., Gordon, J. I., Raoult, D. and Henrissat, B. (2013). The abundance and variety of carbohydrate-active enzymes in the human gut microbiota. *Nature Reviews Microbiology*, *11*(7), 497-504.

Estudante, M., Morais, J. G., Soveral, G. and Benet, L. Z. (2013). Intestinal drug transporters: an overview. *Advanced drug delivery reviews*, *65*(10), 1340-1356.

Fallingborg, J. (1999). Intraluminal pH of the human gastrointestinal tract. *Danish medical bulletin*, *46*(3), 183-196.

Ganong, W. F. and Barrett, K. E. (1995). *Review of medical physiology* (pp. 474-478). Norwalk, CT: Appleton and Lange.

Gass, J., Bethune, M. T., Siegel, M., Spencer, A. and Khosla, C. (2007). Combination enzyme therapy for gastric digestion of dietary gluten in patients with celiac sprue. *Gastroenterology*, *133*(2), 472-480.

Henning, S. J. (1987). Functional development of the gastrointestinal tract. *Physiology of the gastrointestinal tract*, *1*, 285-300.

Langley, J. N. (1882). On the destruction of ferments in the alimentary canal. *The Journal of physiology*, *3*(3-4), 246.

Mallory, P. A. and Travis, J. (1973). Human pancreatic enzymes. Characterization of anionic human trypsin. *Biochemistry*, *12*(15), 2847-2851.

McCarthy, D. M. (2010). Adverse effects of proton pump inhibitor drugs: clues and conclusions. *Current opinion in gastroenterology*, *26*(6), 624-631.

Meyer, J., Golden, J. S., Steiner, N. and Necheles, H. (1937). The ptyalin content of human saliva in old age. *American Journal of Physiology*, *119*, 600-602.

MORRIS, B. J. (1978). Activation of Human Inactive ("Pro-") Renin by Cathepsin D and Pepsin*. *The Journal of Clinical Endocrinology and Metabolism*, *46*(1), 153-157.

Quiroz, A., Ruiz-Cordero, R., Garcia-Buitrago, M. T. and Casillas, J. (2016). Physiology of the Pancreas. In *Multidisciplinary Teaching Atlas of the Pancreas* (pp. 79-89). Springer Berlin Heidelberg.

Schlamowitz, M., Varandani, P. T. and Wissler, F. C. (1963). Pepsinogen and Pepsin: Conformational Relations, Studied by Iodination, Immunochemical Precipitation, and the Influence of Pepsin Inhibitor*. *Biochemistry*, *2*(2), 238-246.

Studdy, P. R., Lapworth, R. U. T. H. and Bird, R. O. G. E. R. (1983). Angiotensin-converting enzyme and its clinical significance--a review. *Journal of clinical pathology*, *36*(8), 938-947.

Tiwari, M. (2011). Science behind human saliva. *Journal of Natural Science, Biology, and Medicine*, *2*(1), 53–58.

In: Disorders of Gastrointestinal Systems ... ISBN: 978-1-63485-366-8
Editors: S. Rajagopal, S. Murugan and R. Saravanan

Chapter 16

CHITOSAN AND ITS DERIVATIVES FOR GASTROINTESTINAL DISORDERS

Subhapradha Namasivayam**, PhD
Faculty of Allied Health Sciences, Chettinad Academy of Research and Education, Kelambakkam, Tamil Nadu, India

ABSTRACT

Marine organisms are rich source of structurally diverse bioactive compounds with various biological activities. Marine polysaccharides present a real potential for natural product discovery and for the delivery of new marine derived products for therapeutic applications. Marine polysaccharide based nonmaterial's is an emerging field with wide range of applications such as targeted drug delivery, cancer therapy, gene therapy, wound dressing, etc., Over the last several years, chitinous polymers, especially chitosan, a co-polymer of (1→4)-2-acetamido-2-deoxy-β-D-glucan and (1→4)-2-amino-2-deoxy-β-D-glucan has received increased attention as one of the promising renewable polymeric materials for their extensive applications in the pharmaceutical, biomedical and food industries. Chitosan possess excellent biological properties such as biodegradation, antibacterial, antioxidant, antitumor and hypocholesterolemic activities. Gastrointestinal disorders have a high prevalence in human societies, in which functional digestive disorders are the most important ones. The gastrointestinal tract is one of the vital organs in the human body, and it is vulnerable to a great diversity of diseases such as parasitic and infectious disorders, diarrhea, reflux, gastroenteritis, constipation, and bloating. This chapter reveals the therapeutic role of chitosan and its derivatives in gastric carcinoma caused by *Helicobacter pylori* infection.

Keywords: chitosan, drug delivery, food industry, gastro intestinal disorders, Nanomaterials

* Corresponding author: Dr. Namasivayam Subhapradha, PhD. Post Doctoral Fellow, Faculty of Allied Health Sciences, Chettinad Academy of Research and Education, Kelambakkam, Tamil Nadu – 603103, India. Email: subhapradha87@gmail.com, mobile: +91 9787483349.

1. INTRODUCTION

The gastro intestinal tract of human is classified into four distinct region starting from mouth, stomach, small intestine and colon. The digestion starts in the mouth where food bolus formed reaching the stomach through esophagus. Stomach secretes Hydrochloric acid that reduces the food pH and the proteins and lipids are digested in stomach with the aid of gastric enzymes. The presence of mucus protects the surface of the mucous membrane from acid attack. Then, the acid chime is secreted in small intestine. Duodenum, the first part of the small intestine receives digestive juices from the pancreas and liver, the chime is neutralized by reacting with sodium bicarbonate ($NaHCO_3$) resulting in a suitable pH for enzyme activities. Two important activities - breakdown of macromolecules and absorption of water and nutrients takes place in the small intestine. The remaining particles not absorbed through digestion reach large intestine, colon absorbs the water and electrolytes as well as the fermentation of polysaccharides and protein by colonic microbial population, re-absorption of bile salts, storage and elimination of feces (Guerra et al., 2012; Pedersen et al., 2013). Small intestine is an important site where the heavy load of microbial population plays a vital role in human health and diseases. The microbial population resides either in the lumen or in the mucus of the intestine but there is no contact with the epithelium. The mucus forms a barrier to prevent colonization in the epithelium by the action of microorganisms and the gastric acid diffusion to the surface of epithelium. The viscosity of mucus is influenced by pH, and increase in pH facilitates the infiltration of microorganisms that can lead to an inflammation in the gastro intestinal tract (Engstrand and Lindberg, 2013).

1.1. Stomach

Some pathogenic microbes can survive in the harsh condition of the gastro intestinal tract especially in stomach. Excellent example of pathogenic organism is *Helicobacter pylori* causing infection in stomach. Nearly 4-7 located flagella at one end and colonize the surface of the epithelium which is located bellow the mucus layer (Izzotti et al., 2009; Lin et al., 2012, 2013; Palacios-Espinosa et al., 2014). The virulence of *H. pylori* is influenced by adherence and colonization of the surface on the gastric epithelial cells, evasion and attenuation of the host defense, and invasion and damaging of the gastric mucosa (He et al., 2014). An increase of stomach normal pH from 1-3 to 4.5-7, makes the environment favorable to its own colonization as well as for the growth and prevalence of other pathogenic bacteria (Chang et al., 2011). Several symptoms and diseases associated with *H. pylori* pathogenicity includes chronic gastritis, duodenal ulcers, gastric cancer, gastro-esophageal reflux, cardiovascular, ocular, neurodegenerative diseases and dermatological disorders (Engstrand and Lindberg, 2013; Izzotti et al., 2009).

1.2. Intestine

Following the stomach, the intestine provides the suitable environment for the colonization of pathogens. *Bacillus cereus*, *Campylobacter* spp., *Staphylococcus aureus*,

Shigella spp., and from Enterobacteriaceae family, *Escherichia coli*, *Listeria monocytogenes*, *Salmonella* spp. and *Yersinia enterocolitica* are some of the important pathogens in intestine. The consumption of the contaminated products leads to two types of food-borne gastro intestinal tract illnesses, the emetic generated by a single peptide toxin and the diarrheal syndrome provoked by enterotoxins produced in small intestine (Ceuppens et al., 2010; Vaz et al., 2012).

1.3. Common Gastrointestinal Disorders

Gastrointestinal disorders are more prevalence in human societies. Gastroenterology care center determines that 50% of the patients are suffered from functional digestive disorders. Gastrointestinal tract is more susceptible to parasitic and infectious disorders such as diarrhea, reflux, gastroenteritis, constipation, and bloating (Kasper et al., 2005).

Diarrhea is defined as "an increase in stool weight of greater than 200 g per day followed by an increase in stool liquidity, stool frequency, perianal problems, and defecation urgency." Diarrhea is a major worldwide health problem, especially among children. Duodenogastric reflux is defined as the upward flow of biliary fluid from the duodenum into the stomach that causes gastritis. The main cause of gastric mucosal injury is due to the presence of bile acids in the duodenum which produce mucosal atrophy and intestinal metaplasia; and in mucosa of esophageous it can develop into intestinal metaplasia and malignancy (Rezaei et al., 2009). Barrett's esophagus is characterized by a chronic inflammation of the esophagus caused by either refluxed stomach acid or internal pressure buildup (Kalish et al., 1984). Gastroenteritis is responsible for 5 million deaths per year worldwide. Gastrointestinal ulcers formed in the stomach is due to increase in acid secretion by various reasons including consumption of non-steroidal anti-inflammatory drugs, alcohol abuse, long starvation, bad eating habits, and severe and persistent stress (Ziaei et al., 2009).

Gas accumulation is one of the most common disorders of the digestive system which refers to a feeling of abdominal distention and elongation accompanied with excessive gas. The prevalence of bloating in Asian countries is about 15-23% whereas in American population is about 15-30% (Vere et al., 2005). Constipation is defined as a delay or severity in passing stools that continues for two weeks or more. The diagnosis of constipation depends on stool consistency, bowel movement times, and severity in passing stools. Constipation is a most common problem of the gastrointestinal tract, which found in about 2-28% of adults and is 3 to 5 times more common in women than men (Chen et al., 2005).

Inflammatory bowel disease is a "chronic condition of the digestive tract and with two subclasses - ulcerative colitis and Crohn's disease" which is characterized by a persistent and instinctive relapsing inflammation that results from the interaction between different substances in the mucosal immune system and microenvironment. Colorectal cancer is extremely common and symptoms include blood in the stool and change in bowel habits.

Gastric cancer is the 2nd important cause of death among the malignant disease worldwide with high death rate in Asia, Europe and South America (Ferlay et al., 2010). Approximately 989,000 new cases of gastric cancer were identified with death rate of 738,000 throughout the world in 2008. In 2015, American Cancer Society predicted 24,590 new cases of gastric cancer with the death rate of 10,720.

1.3.1. Prognosis and Survival Rate

The prognosis of gastric cancer in patients involves the involvement of nodes and extension of tumor beyond the gastric membrane (Siewert et al., 1998). Nearly more than 50% of patients can be alleviated in the case of localized distal gastric cancer. In United States, early stage gastric cancer accounts for only 10 to 20%, whereas the remaining percentage of patients having disease either in the regional site or in the distant sites. At 5 year generally survival rate of gastric cancer ranges from 0% with distributed disease to 50% survival rate with distal gastric cancer. The 5-year survival rate of patients with gastric cancer is only 10 to 15% with apparent localized disease (Adachi et al., 2000).

In India, generally the 5 year survival percent of peoples diagnosed with digestive system cancer is relatively low when compared with more advanced countries. The survival percentage is minimum of 19% in India with the maximum of 58% in South Korea; whereas its average is 25-30% in most countries.

1.3.2. Epidemiology

Gastric cancer is one of the important cancers worldwide, which was the main cause of death due to cancer in the world till 1980 but it was overcome by lung cancer. In recent years, the incidence of gastric cancer is in rapid decline phase because of the recognition of causative agents including pathogens, dietary and other environmental risk factors (Siegel et al., 2014).

According to the report of World Health Organization in 2012, approximately one million peoples having stomach cancer were predicted (952, 000 cases) fetching it the 5th most common cancer in the world next to lung, breast, colorectal and prostate cancer. Table 1 describes the estimated incidence, mortality and prevalence of stomach cancer throughout the world in 2012 (WHO report, 2012). Stomach cancer is the 3rd primary cause of death in both sexes' worldwide (723,000 deaths).

1.3.3. Clinical Presentation and Diagnostic Evaluation

Approximately 90% of gastric cancers are adenocarcinoma, which develops on the glands of the superficial layer or mucosa of the stomach. However, other types of cancer arising from the stomach, including lymphoid tissue lymphomas associated with mucus, which originate from the lymphoid of stomach, and leiomyosarcomas, which arise from the muscles surrounding the mucosa.

The stomach is divided into several anatomic subsites, including the cardia (roughly the top inch of the stomach), fundus, body, pylorus, and the antrum. These areas are distinguished by anatomic demarcations and/or histologic differences. The distinction between adenocarcinomas arising from the cardia (cardia gastric cancer) and other parts of the stomach (noncardia gastric cancer) have different epidemiologic patterns and causes.

Gastrointestinal stromal tumors can form anywhere in the gastro intestinal tract, but most probably found in the stomach or small intestine. The '*American Joint Committee on Cancer (AJCC) Cancer Staging Manual*' describes the dissemination of gastrointestinal tumors in gastro intestinal tract were 60% in stomach, 30% in small intestine, 3% in rectum, 1-2% in colon, <1% in esophagus and rare in omentum/mesentery (Edge et al., 2010).

Table 1. Describes the estimated incidence, mortality and prevalence of gastric carcinoma worldwide in 2012 (WHO report)

Estimated numbers (thousands)	Men			Women			Both sexes		
	Cases	Deaths	5-year prev.	Cases	Deaths	5-year prev.	Cases	Deaths	5-year prev.
World	631	469	1031	320	254	507	952	723	1538
More developed regions	175	107	372	99	68	193	275	175	565
Less developed regions	456	362	659	221	186	315	677	548	974
WHO Africa region (AFRO)	10	10	14	9	8	12	19	18	26
WHO Americas region (PAHO)	52	39	84	34	26	54	85	65	138
WHO East Mediterranean region (EMRO)	15	13	19	9	8	11	23	21	31
WHO Europe region (EURO)	98	75	136	64	51	86	162	126	222
WHO South-East Asia region (SEARO)	60	56	54	30	28	29	91	83	82
WHO Western Pacific region (WPRO)	396	276	724	175	134	315	571	410	1039
IARC membership (24 countries)	232	148	449	124	86	226	355	234	675
US	13	7	20	8	5	12	21	12	32
China	283	221	419	122	104	175	405	325	594
India	43	41	31	20	18	14	63	59	45
European Union (EU-28)	51	35	74	31	23	45	82	58	119

Very rarely gastrointestinal tumors may be formed in the gallbladder, appendix, pancreas, retro peritoneum, and paravaginal tissues. About 40-50% of small intestinal gastrointestinal tumors and 20-25% of gastric tumors are clinically destructive. It has been predicted that 10-25% of patients having metastatic cancer (Joensuu, 2006).

1.3.4. Pathology and Molecular Genetics

When diagnosed clinically, the size of the gastro intestinal tumor from <1 cm to >40 cm, which arise from the muscle wall of the gastro intestinal tract. Small tumor tends to form either subserosal, intramural, or rarely forms polypoid intra-luminal masses whereas large tumor forms external masses attached to the superficial part of the gut involving the muscular layers (Corless and Heinrich, 2008). The morphology of the gastric tumor quite varies and composed of 70% of spindle cells, 20% of epithelioid cells and 10% of mixed spindle and epithelioid cells. The histologic patterns of gastric tumor showed leiomyomas (very low mitotic activity) to leiomyosarcomas (very aggressive-appearing patterns), which may be initiated either from Cajal interstitial cells or the stem cell-precursors.

1.3.5. Risk Factor

Risk factor for the gastric cancer include *Helicobacter pylori* infection, advanced age, male gender, less intake of fruits and vegetables, increased intake of highly salted or preserved foods, chronic atrophic gastritis, pernicious anemia, intestinal metaplasia, gastric adenomatous polyps, cigarette smoking, menetrier disease (giant hypertrophic gastritis), and familial adenomatous polyposis (Edge et al., 2010).

Among these risk factors, *Helicobacter pylori* is one of the most important causative agent responsible for gastric carcinoma, this chapter discussed about the gastric carcinoma *H. pylori* and its inhibition by utilizing the marine polysaccharide chitosan and its derivatives.

2. HELICOBACTER PYLORI

Helicobacter pylori are a spiral-shaped, microaerophilic, gram-negative bacteria inhabitant of gastric mucosa. *H. pylorus is* responsible for various upper gastrointestinal diseases, such as 'chronic gastritis, duodenal and gastric ulcer, gastric adenocarcinoma and mucosa-associated lymphoid tissue lymphoma' and has been categorized as a class 1 carcinogen by "International Agency for Cancer Research (IACR)" in 1994 (Graham and Graham, 2002). *H. pylori* play a major role in terms of public health causing gastro duodenal diseases. It is localized in gastric mucus-secreting cells found in or under a layer of mucus and targets the gastric epithelial cells (Wallis-Crespo and Crespo, 2004). *H. pylori* are present in the stomach of humans in throughout the world. About 70-90% of human carries *H. pylori* in developing countries while the peoples obtain *H. pylori* infection before 10 years of age; whereas the occurrence of infection is low (25-50%) in developed countries (Dunn et al., 1997).

H. pylori were isolated from the patient suffered with peptic ulcer by Warren and Marshall in 1982. Several pathogenic determinants of the organism *H. pylori* were found as 'adhesions, cytotoxins, and different enzymes such as urease, catalase, lipase, protease,' etc. Very potent urease activity is the important enzymatic characteristics of *H. pylori* (Borlace et al., 2008). The urease secreted by *H. pylori* hydrolyses the urea in the gastric juices to form ammonia and bicarbonate which efficiently neutralize the acidic environment and the stomach pH is increased between 4.5 and 7.0 (Bardonnet et al., 2006). *H. pylori* reside mainly in mucosa or at the interface of the mucus layer synthesizing the cytotoxin which alters the reliability of the tight junctions in the epithelium and diminish the stability of the cytoskeleton (Borlace et al., 2008).

The etiology between *H. pylori* infection and its chronic diseases such as gastritis, peptic ulcer and gastric carcinoma has been determined when the organism was first identified. Antibacterial drugs amoxicillin and tetracycline are effective against *H. pylori* at low concentration but single drug treatment is not sufficient to eradicate the infection caused by *H. pylori in vivo*. Because a very minimal dose of drug reaches *H. pylori* resides under the mucosa, the instability of the antibiotic at the low pH of the gastric juice and the stay of drug in stomach is low (Kusters et al., 2006).

While eradicating *H. pylori*, the ultimate concentration of drug not only resides in the gastric juice but also to reach the organism effectively. The Madin–Darby canine kidney MDCK-adapted *H. pylori* superiorly binds with the tight junctions of the epithelial cells and engaged the tight junction scaffolding protein (ZO-1) at the binding site and alters the protein distribution near junctions (Amieva et al., 2003).

To eradicate *H. pylori in vivo*, triple antibiotic therapy for the duration of two weeks is needed. Single drug is not efficient to destroy *H. pylori* when treating *in vivo*, may be due to low residency of the antibiotic at low gastric pH, low penetration of the drug to the mucosa, followed by lumen re-secretion, where adequate amount of drug disseminate to the organism. Two or more antibiotic treatment along with proton pump inhibitor to eradicate *H. pylori* infection showed increased number of therapeutic failures, which highly represent the need of new therapeutic drugs of non-antibiotic materials.

3. Chitosan for Eradicating *H. Pylori* Infection

In order to confine drug at the site of bacterial infection on the gastric epithelium to improve the efficiency of antibacterial compounds, an ideal cationic nanoparticles delivery system consist of polysaccharides (chitosan and heparin) have been utilized (Lin et al., 2009).

Polysaccharides are natural polymers which play a tremendous role in sustaining life. Polysaccharides have the potential to carry the biological information, maintain molecular recognition process on the cell surface due to its structural variability. Polysaccharides are perfect adjuvant for *H. pylori* related diseases. Firstly, polysaccharides are difficult to be absorbed in the alimentary tract and thus avoid possible side effects caused by absorption. Secondly, polysaccharides can increase the viscosity of stomach contents, prolong the time of gastric emptying and reinforce the effect of time dependent antibiotics (Song et al., 2014).

Among the various kind of polysaccharides, cellulose and chitin are the most important biological macromolecules; of which cellulose is produced in many plants, whereas chitin is synthesized especially in lower animals. Cellulose and chitin are the most plentiful organic materials present on Earth and calculated to be synthesized at levels approaching 10^{11} tons per annum.

Chitin is one of the most wide-spread linear biopolymer in nature. It is composed by 2-acetamido-2-deoxy - D-glucopyranose units linked by $\beta(1\rightarrow4)$ glycosidic bonds, functional groups such as hydroxyl, amine and carbonyl present in the polymer chain reacts with hydrogen bonds resulting in the synthesis of micro fibrils (Lehane, 1997). It is a structural polysaccharide present in the exoskeleton of crustaceans, internal bone of cephalopods, arthropods, yeast, fungi in which it provides the mechanical strength to the organisms. It is a super-specialty polymer with unique biological properties which includes antitumor, antimicrobial, antioxidant, biodegradability and biocompatibility and it is utilized for various purposes not only by its plentiful availability but also by novelty of functional material.

The applications of chitosan are mostly based on the polyelectrolytic nature and chelating capacity of the amine groups of the polymer. Amine group present in the chitosan are protonated to NH_3^+ in acidic solution, thus the chelating ability and polyelectrolyte nature is mainly due to the acidity of the NH_3^+ (Park et al., 1983). Chitosan has many useful applications in different fields, mainly because of the amino groups present at C2 position, primary hydroxyl groups at C3 and secondary hydroxyl groups at C6 positions (Furusaki et al., 1996).

Even though chitosan has low transfection efficiency, it is widely used because of its low toxicity when compared with synthetic polymers such as polyethylene imines and lipid based polymer lipofectamine (Lai and Lin, 2009). Another advantage of using chitosan in gene therapy and vaccine design is due to increased Tran- and para-cellular transport across the mucosal epithelium, this property makes it an excellent material for protective mucosal immune response (Janes et al., 2001). These remarkable characteristics, cheap production cost and FDA approval increases the application of chitosan in recent decade (Lin et al., 2007).

Nanoparticles formed from modified chitosan containing thioglycolic acid conjugate and unmodified chitosan for determining the potency of cellular uptake of pDNA were compared and determined that of the transfection efficiency of thiolated chitosan/pDNA nanoparticles was five times higher that the unmodified chitosan/pDNA nanoparticles (Martien et al., 2006). The enzymatic stability of chitosan nanoparticles for delivering pDNA was investigated by adding covalently-bound aurintricarboxylic acid (a nuclease inhibitor present in the gastrointestinal tract); the transfection rate using the Caco-2 cell line was 2.6 times higher than the unmodified chitosan nanoparticles (Martien et al., 2007). Modified aurintricarboxylic acid chitosan showed higher stability with brine solution, enzymes including lysozyme, deoxyribonuclease and freshly collected porcine intestinal fluid. The attachment of aurintricarboxylic acid with chitosan improves the overall stability and transfection of pDNA which could serve as a potential agent for the oral delivery.

Chitosan nanospheres modified with poly (D, L-lactide-co-glycolide) with a nuclear factor kappa B (NF-kB) decoy oligonucleotide were administered to an experimental model having ulcerative colitis. Oligodeoxynucleotides binding sequence of a specific transcription factor served as tools for altering gene expression in living cells and can be used as therapeutic agents. Such constructs targeted to binding NFkB have been used to lower inflammation in an IBD animal model by suppressing various cytokines gene expression (Xiang et al., 2009).

Chitosan nanoparticles for potential application towards the oral administration of a FVIII gene to a FVIII exon 16 knockout mouse models was studied by Bowman et al. (2008) by preparing two types of chitosan with different levels of deacetylation and loaded with three different doses of DNA: 50, 250, and 600 μg were evaluated. Higher concentration of DNA (600 μg) yielded an average transfection efficiency of four times higher than the low concentration of 50 μg. Improvised chitosan nanoparticles could show much greater expression levels of FVIII protein. Alginate–chitosan polyionic complexes serve as another viable option (Yan et al., 2001).

Chitosan microspheres have been used as a binding substance for *Helicobacter pylori* to treat gastric infection (Fernandes et al., 2013). *H. pylori* were removed from infected patients by orally administrating chitosan microspheres, which may be due to the muco-bacterial binding property of chitosan.

Chitosan has been used as a safe drug carrier molecule due to biocompatibility and muco-adhesive property. Positively charged chitosan interact with the negative charge of sialic acid deposits of mucin present in the stomach, which is helpful for releasing drug in low pH, which may be due to the swelling property of chitosan microspheres (He et al., 1999).

The pros and cons of chitosan in eradicating the *H. pyroli* is broad-spectrum antimicrobial effect and higher solubility at acidic pH, respectively. It has been overcome by alternative way of using a crosslinking agent (glutaraldehyde or genipin) (Goncalves et al.,

2013). Lin et al. (2013) utilized two natural cross-linking compounds genipin and glutaraldehyde which inhibits *H. pylori* colonization.

Chitosan microspheres loaded with amoxicillin and metronidazole were delivered at the infectious site of *H. pylori*; the loaded antibiotics were not continuously released at the acid pH of gastric juice. It may be due to the high porous nature of polymeric microspheres leads to the discharge of antibiotics in two hours (Shah et al., 1999). This work clearly demonstrates the sustained release of antibiotics and the interaction between the chitosan microspheres and the mucosa. Portero et al. (2002) utilized the reacetylated chitosan microspheres encapsulated with amoxicillin and metronidazole to evaluate the reduction rate of polymer solubility, delivery of antibiotics and the antimicrobial activity and explained that with short reacetylation period sustained delivery of antibiotic with increased antibacterial activity was obtained.

In another study, chitosan microspheres were encapsulated with amoxicillin and the parameters including stirring speed and polymer and drug ratio were analyzed. While increasing the stirring speed, mucoadhesion and polymer is to drug ratio were decreased. This study determined that amoxicillin was delivered more properly in acidic environment than in basic solutions. High amount of *H. pylori* were destroyed while treating with antibiotic encapsulated in chitosan microspheres than treated with plain antibiotic, it was proven in *in vivo* study by Patel and Patel (2007).

Chitosan microspheres encapsulated with tetracycline have been more stable in acidic medium than amoxicillin. At the pH range between 1.2 and 2.0, chitosan microspheres were dissolve completely and rapidly deliver the antibiotc, but in the pH range of 3.0-5.0 releasing 70% of the drug after 3 h (Hejazi and Amiji, 2002).

Chitosan microspheres loaded with tetracycline utilizing tritiated [^{3}H]-tetracycline and radio-iodinated chitosan microspheres [^{125}I] were analyzed for evaluating the residence time of drug in the gastric juice and the retention profile between the tritiated tetracycline and plain tetracycline (Hejazi and Amiji, 2003). Hejazi and Amiji (2004) studied the effect of cross linking in microsphere production on the gastric residence and found that microspheres formed by chemical cross linking showed more gastric residence time than the microspheres formed by ionic precipitation. *In vivo* studies found that either the plain tertracyline or chitosan microspheres loaded with tetracycline did not showed better reduction against *H. pylori* and also the levels of serum gastrin when compared with the triple antibiotic therapy of using amoxicillin, lansoprazole and clarithromycin (Amiji, 2006). Chitosan have been utilized for the variety of purposes because of its antibacterial and muco-adhesive property enable the polymer to bind, kill and eradicate the bacterium from the stomach. Luo et al. (2009) studied the antibacterial effect of chitosan nanoparticles through both *in vitro* and *in vivo* approaches confirmed that nanoparticles possess high antibacterial effect in eradicating *H. pylori* than the plain chitosan powders. The potential of chitosan microspheres mimicked by ultrathin chitosan film and its effect on the gastric juice was analyzed by Nogueira et al. (2013). Chitosan was considered to an excellent biomaterial in the pH range of 2.6-6 for the gastrointestinal purpose in the absence of urea. When at the higher pH level, the binding of bacteria with the chitosan film was reduced and it was further lowered by the action of pepsin. The death rate of bacteria was high (93%) at low acidic pH 2; whereas more than 75% of organism were eradicated at pH 6 independent of the presence of pepsin and urea.

Chitosan microspheres stabilized with genipicin were much stable in the acidic pH with retaining the binding capacity of microspheres with the mucins of mucosa and found that it was stable for 7 days and its potency remained for 2 hours in the stomach (Fernandes et al., 2013).

The efficacy of chitosan microsphere to diminish the binding efficiency between bacteria and gastric cells were studied and demonstrated that attachment added after and before bacterial gastric cell pre-incubation was 50–76% and in 47-56%, respectively. According to the ISO international standard chitosan microspheres are not found to be cytotoxic even though it reduces 20% of metabolic activity of cells (Goncalves et al., 2013).

Recent studies have pointed out that some native acidic polysaccharides can inhibit the adhesion of *H. pylori* on cells including gastric cells or macrophages (Lutay et al., 2011). In an another study about the adhesion mechanism explained that the adhesion of *H. pylori* to hosts is mediated by bacterial outer membrane proteins (OMPs) and particular oligosaccharide epitopes on gastric mucins (Kenny et al., 2012). Thus the acidic polysaccharides rich in sialylated or sulfated galactoses may possess a strong affinity to *H. pylori*, which compete with host cells or mucins by which it prevents the adhesion of *H. pylori* to hosts.

H. pylori strains stimulate the synthesis of actin filaments in the gastric epithelial cells (human gastric adenocarcinoma cell line). Positive charge of amino groups in the chitosan binds with the negative charge present on the cell surface and tight junction of neighboring epithelial cells stimulate the rearrangement of actin filaments and ZO-1 protein (Hennig et al., 2005).

CONCLUSION

In this chapter, the research work on gastric cancer, its prevalence, *Helicobacter pylori* induced gastric carcinoma and eradication of bacteria using different forms of chitosan and its derivatives both at micro and nano -level. The treatment against *H. pylori* has evolved according to the discovery of morphology and pathogenicity of the bacteria. However, the current therapy still shows various restrictions. This review describes the role of chitosan along with various compounds to inhibit and kill the *H. pylori* in gastric juice. This article provides new insight into the utilization of super-specialty biopolymer chitosan for eliminating gastric cancer.

Table 2. Narrates the different approach of chitosan used for eradicating *H. pylori* infection

S. No	Particle	Nature of drug	References
1.	Chitosan (90% deacetylated)	Probiotic	Ko et al., 2011
2.	Chitosan along with heparin	Phytomedicine	Zhu et al., 2012
3	Chitosan with sodium deoxycholate	Vaccines	Figueiredo et al., 2012
4	Chitosan with alginate and sodium tripolyphosphate	Vaccines	Figueiredo et al., 2012
5	Chitosan nanoparticles with genipin	Carrier molecule	Lin et al., 2013
6	Chitosan/TPP conjugated with ureido	Carrier molecule	Jing et al., 2016

REFERENCES

Adachi, Y, Yasuda, K, Inomata, M, 2000. Pathology and prognosis of gastric carcinoma: well versus poorly differentiated type. *Cancer* 89(7): 1418-24.

Amieva, M.R., Vogelmann, R., Covacci, A., Tompkins, L.S, Nelson, W.J, Falkow, S, 2003. Disruption of the epithelial apical–junctional complex by *Helicobacter pylori* CagA. *Science* 300, 1430-1434.

Amiji, M.M, 2006. Tetracycline-containing chitosan microspheres for local treatment of *Helicobacter pylori* infection, *Cellulose* 14, 3-14.

Bardonnet, P.L, Faivre, V, Pugh, W.J, Piffaretti, J.C, Falson, F, 2006. Gastroretentive dosage forms: overview and special case of *Helicobacter pylori. J. Control Rel.* 111, 1-18.

Borlace, G.N, Butler, R.N, Brooks, D.A, 2008. Monocyte and macrophage killing of *Helicobacter pylori*: relationship to bacterial virulence factors. *Helicobacter*, 13, 380-387.

Bowman, K, Sarkar, R, Raut, S, Leong, K.W, 2008. Gene transfer to hemophilia a mice via oral delivery of FVIII-chitosan nanoparticles. *J. Control. Rel.* 132, 252-259.

Ceuppens, S, Van de Wiele, T, Rajkovic, A, Ferrer-Cabaceran, T, Heyndrickx, M, Boon, N, 2010. Impact of intestinal microbiota and gastrointestinal conditions on the *in vitro* survival and growth of *Bacillus cereus. Int. J Food Microbiol.* 155(3), 241-246.

Chang, C.H, Huang, W.Y, Lai, C.H, Hsu, Y.M, Yao, Y.H, Chen, T.Y, 2011. Development of novel nanoparticles shelled with heparin for berberine delivery to treat *Helicobacter pylori. Acta Biomater.* 7(2), 593-603.

Chen, S.L, Mo, J.Z, Cao, Z.J, Chen, X.Y, Xiao, S.D, 2005. Effects of bile reflux on gastric mucosal lesions in patients with dyspepsia or chronic gastritis. *World J. Gastroentrol.* 11, 2834-2837.

Corless, C.L, Heinrich, M.C, 2008. Molecular pathobiology of gastrointestinal stromal sarcomas. *Annu. Rev. Pathol.* 3, 557-586.

Dunn, B.E, Cohen, H, Blaser, M.J, 1997. *Helicobacter pylori. Clin. Microbiol. Rev.* 10, 720-741.

Edge, S.B., Byrd, D.R., Compton, C.C. 2010. Gastrointestinal stromal tumor. *AJCC Cancer Staging Manual.* 7th ed., Springer, New York, pp. 175-80.

Engstrand, L, Lindberg, M, 2013. *Helicobacter pylori* and the gastric microbiota. *Best Prac. Res. Clin. Gastroenterol.* 27(1), 39-45.

Ferlay, J, Shin, H.R, Bray, F, Forman, D, Mathers, C, Parkin, D.M, 2010. Estimates of worldwide burden of cancer in 2008: GLOBOCAN 2008. *Int. J. Cancer* 127, 2893-2917.

Fernandes, M, Goncalves, I.C, Nardecchia, S, Amaral, I.F, Barbosa, M.A, Martins, M.C, Modulation of stability and mucoadhesive properties of chitosan microspheres for therapeutic gastric application. *Int. J. Pharm.* 454, 116-124.

Figueiredo, L, Calado, C.C.R, Almeida, A.J, Gonçalves, L.M.D, 2012. Protein and DNA nanoparticulate multiantigenic vaccines against *H. pylori*: *in vivo* evaluation, 2nd Portuguese Meeting in Bioengineering (ENBENG), Coimbra, 2012.

Furusaki, E, Ueno, Y, Sakairi, N, Nishi, N, Tokura, S, 1996. Facile preparation and inclusion ability of chitosan derivative bearing carboxymethyl-β-cyclodextrin. *Carbohydr. Polym.* 9, 29-34.

Goncalves, I.C, Magalhaes, A, Fernandes, M, Rodrigues, I.V, Reis, C.A, Martins, M.C, 2013. Bacterial-binding chitosan microspheres for gastric infection treatment and prevention, *Acta Biomater*. 9, 9370-9378.

Graham, S.K, Graham, D.Y., 2002. Contemporary diagnosis and management of *H. pylori* associated gastrointestinal diseases, second edition, *Handbooks in Health Care Co*, US, pp. 40-125.

Guerra, A, Etienne-Mesmin, L, Livrelli, V, Denis, S, Blanquet-Diot, S, Alric, M, 2012. Relevance and challenges in modeling human gastric and small intestinal digestion. *Trends Biotechnol*. 30(11), 591-600.

He, P, Davis, S.S, Illum, L, 1999. Chitosan microspheres prepared by spray drying. *Int. J. Pharm*. 187, 53-65.

He, C, Chen, M, Liu, J, Yuan, Y, 2014. Host genetic factors respond to pathogenic step-specific virulence factors of *Helicobacter pylori* in gastric carcinogenesis. *Mut. Res*. 759, 14-26.

Hejazi, R, Amiji, M, 2002. Stomach-specific anti-*H. pylori* therapy. I: preparation and characterization of tetracyline-loaded chitosan microspheres. *Int. J. Pharm*. 235, 87-94.

Hejazi, R, Amiji, M, 2003. Stomach-specific anti-*H. pylori* therapy. II. Gastric residence studies of tetracycline-loaded chitosan microspheres in gerbils. *Pharm. Dev. Technol*. 8, 253-262.

Hejazi, R, Amiji, M, 2004. Stomach-specific anti-*H. pylori* therapy Part III: effect of chitosan microspheres crosslinking on the gastric residence and local tetracycline concentrations in fasted gerbils. *Int. J. Pharm*. 272, 99-108.

Hennig, E.E, Godlewski, M.M, Butruk, E, Ostrowski, J, 2005. *Helicobacter pylori* VacA cytotoxin interacts with fibronectin and alters HeLa cell adhesion and cytoskeletal organization *in vitro*. *FEMS Immunol. Med. Microbiol*. 44, 143-150.

Izzotti, A, Durando, P, Ansaldi, F, Gianiorio, F, Pulliero, A, 2009. Interaction between *Helicobacter pylori*, diet, and genetic polymorphisms as related to noncancer diseases. *Mut. Res*. 667(1), 142-157.

Janes, K.A, Calvo, P, Alonso, M.J, 2001. Polysaccharide colloidal particles as delivery systems for macromolecules. *Adv. Drug Deliv. Rev*. 47, 83-97.

Jing, Z.W, Jia, Y.Y, Wan, N, Luo, M, Huan, M.L, Kang, T.B, Zhou, S.Y, Zhang, B.L, 2016. Design and evaluation of novel pH-sensitive ureido-conjugated chitosan/TPP nanoparticles targeted to *Helicobacter pylori*. Biomater. Accepted Manuscript.

Joensuu, H, 2006. Gastrointestinal stromal tumor (GIST). *Ann. Oncol*. 17(10), 280-286.

Kalish, R.J, Clancy, P.E, Orringer, M.B, Appelman, H.D, 1984. Clinical, epidemiologic.

Kasper D.L., Braunwald, E., Hauser, S., Longo, D., Jameson, J.L., Fauci, A.S., 2005. *Harrison's principels of internal medicine*, 16th ed., McGraw-Hill medical publishing division, New York, pp. 1746-1762.

Kenny, D.T, Skoog, E.C, Linden, S.K, Struwe, W.B, Rudd, P.M, Karlsson, N.G, 2012. Presence of terminal N-acetylgalactosamine1-4N-acetylglucosamine residues on O-linked oligosaccharides from gastric MUC5AC: Involvement in *Helicobacter pylori* colonization? *Glycobiol*. 22(8), 1077-1085.

Ko, J.A, Lim, H.J, Park, H.J, 2011. Effect of microencapsulated precipitants of *Lactobacillus casei* ATCC 393 on *Helicobacter pylori* eradication. *Process Biochem*. 46, 631-635.

Kusters, J.G, van Vliet, A.H.M, Kuipers, E.J, 2006. Pathogenesis of *Helicobacter pylori* infection. *Clin. Microbiol. Rev*. 19(3), 449-490.

Lai, W.F, Lin, M.C, 2009. Nucleic acid delivery with chitosan and its derivatives. *J. Control. Rel.* 134, 158-168.

Lehane, M.J, 1997. Peritrophic matrix structure and function. *Annu. Rev. Entomol.* 42, 525-550.

Lin, Y.H, Mi, F.L, Chen, C.T, Chang, W.C, Peng, S.F, Liang, H.F, Sung, H.W, 2007. Preparation and characterization of nanoparticles shelled with chitosan for oral insulin delivery. *Biomacromol.* 8, 146-152.

Lin, Y.H, Chang C.H, Wu, Y.S, Hsu, Y.M, Chiou, S.F, Chen, Y.J, 2009. Development of pH-responsive chitosan/heparin nanoparticles for stomach-specific anti-*Helicobacter pylori* therapy. *Biomater.* 30, 3332-3342.

Lin, Y.H, Chiou, S.F, Lai, C.H, Tsai, S.C, Chou, C.W, Peng, S.F, 2012. Formulation and evaluation of water-in-oil amoxicillin-loaded nanoemulsions using for *Helicobacter pylori* eradication. *Proc. Biochem.* 47(10), 1469-1478.

Lin, Y.H, Tsai, S.C, Lai C.H, Lee, C.H, He, Z.S, Tseng, G.C, 2013. Genipin-cross-linked fucosechitosan/heparin nanoparticles for the eradication of *Helicobacter pylori. Biomater.* 34, 4466-4479.

Luo, D, Guo, J, Wang, F, Sun, J, Li, G, Cheng, X, Chang, M, Yan, X, 2009. Preparation and evaluation of anti-*Helicobacter pylori* efficacy of chitosan nanoparticles *in vitro* and *in vivo*. *J. Biomater. Sci.* 20, 1587-1596.

Lutay, N, Nilsson, I, Wadström, T, Ljungh, A, 2011. Effect of heparin, fucoidan and other polysaccharides on adhesion of enterohepatic helicobacter species to murine macrophages. *Appl. Biochem. Biotechnol.* 164(1), 1-9.

Martien, R, Loretz, B, Schnurch, A.B, 2006. Oral gene delivery: design of polymeric carrier systems shielding toward intestinal enzymatic attack. *Biopolym.* 83, 327-336.

Martien, R, Loretz, B, Thaler, M, Majzoob, S, Bernkop-Schnurch, A, 2007. Chitosanthioglycolic acid conjugate: an alternative carrier for oral nonviral gene delivery? *J. Biomed. Mater. Res.* A 82, 1-9.

Nogueira, F, Goncalves, I.C, Martins, M.C, 2013. Effect of gastric environment on *Helicobacter pylori* adhesion to a mucoadhesive polymer. *Acta Biomater.* 9, 5208-5215.

Palacios-Espinosa, J.F, Arroyo-García, O, García-Valencia, G, Linares, E, Bye, R, Romero, I, 2014. Evidence of the anti-*Helicobacter pylori*, gastroprotective and anti-inflammatory activities of Cuphea aequipetala infusion. *J. Ethnopharmacol.*, 151(2), 990-998.

Park, J.W, Choi K.H, Park, K.P, 1983. Acid-base equilibria and related properties of chitosan. *Bull. Korean Chem.* Soc. 4(2), 68-72.

Patel, J.K, Patel, M.M, 2007. Stomach specific anti-*Helicobacter pylori* therapy: preparation and evaluation of amoxicillin-loaded chitosan mucoadhesive microspheres. *Curr. Drug Deliv.* 4, 41-50.

Pedersen, P.B, Vilmann, P, Bar-Shalom, D, Müllertz, A, Baldursdottir, S, 2013. Characterization of fasted human gastric fluid for relevant rheological parameters and gastric lipase activities. *Eur. J. Pharm. Biopharm.* 85(3), 958-965.

Portero, A, Remunan-Lopez, C, Criado, M.T, Alonso, M.J, 2002. Reacetylated chitosan microspheres for controlled delivery of anti-microbial agents to the gastric mucosa. *J. Microencapsul.* 19, 797-809.

Rezaei, M, Ghafarian-Shirazi, H.R, Karimi, Z, Parsa, M, 2009. The effect of Mentha longifolia on children acute nonbacterial diarrhea (a double blind randomized clinical trial). *J. Jahrom. Univ. Med. Sci.* 7, 7-14.

Shah, S, Qaqish, R, Patel, V, Amiji, M, 1999. Evaluation of the factors influencing stomachspecific delivery of antibacterial agents for *Helicobacter pylori* infection. *J. Pharm. Pharmacol.* 51, 667-672.

Siegel, R., Ma, J., Zou, Z., Jemal, A, 2014. Cancer statistics.

Siewert, J.R, Bottcher, K, Stein, H.J, 1998. Relevant prognostic factors in gastric cancer: ten-year results of the German Gastric Cancer Study. *Ann. Surg.* 228(4), 449-461.

Song, W, Wang, Y, Zhang, L, Fu, S, Zeng, Y, Hu, H, 2014. Preparation and evaluation of polysaccharide sulfates for inhibiting *Helicobacter pylori* adhesion. *Carbohyd. Polym.* 103, 398-404.

Vaz, M, Hogg, T, Couto, J.A, 2012. The antimicrobial effect of wine on *Bacillus cereus* in simulated gastro-intestinal conditions. *Food Cont.* 28(2), 230-236.

Vere, C.C, Cazacu, S, Comnescu, V, Mogoant, L, Rogoveanu, I, Ciurea, T, 2005. Endoscopical and histological features in bile reflux gastritis. *Rom. J. Morphol. Embryol.* 46, 269-274.

Wallis-Crespo, M.C, Crespo, A, 2004. *Helicobacter pylori* infection in pediatric population: epidemiology, pathophysiology and therapy. *Fetal Pediatr. Pathol.* 2004, 23, 11-28.

Xiang, J.Y, Wu, L.G, Huang, X.L, Zhang, M, Pen, L, Ouyan, Q, Gan, H.T, 2009. Amelioration of murine dextran sulfate sodium-induced colitis by nuclear factor-kappaB decoy oligonucleotides. *Am. J. Surg.* 197, 797-805.

Yan, X.L, Khor, E, Lim, L.Y, 2001. Chitosan–alginate films prepared with chitosans of different molecular weights. *J. Biomed. Mater. Res.* 58, 358-365.

Zhu, X, Zhou, D, Guan, S, Zhang, P, Zhang, Z, Huang, Y, 2012. Preparation and characterization of novel multi-core chitosan microspheres for stomach-specific delivery of hydrophilic antibiotics. *J. Mater. Sci. Mater. Med.* 23, 983-990.

Ziaei, N, Mozafari, N.A, Kouhsari, H, 2009. Prevalence of Campylobacter jejuni in diarrhea samples in Gorgan, East north of Iran. *Med. Lab. J.* 2, 36-42.

In: Disorders of Gastrointestinal Systems …
Editors: S. Rajagopal, S. Murugan and R. Saravanan
ISBN: 978-1-63485-366-8

Chapter 17

FLAVONOIDS IN GASTRO PROTECTION

R. M. Veerappan[1,*], PhD, and M. Rajadurai[2,#], PhD
[1]Department of Biochemistry, Enathi Rajappa College of Arts and Science, Pattukkottai. TN, India
[2]Sri Venkateswara College, Dharmapuri, TN, India

ABSTRACT

Peptic ulcer is the most common gastrointestinal tract (GIT) disorder in clinical practice. Oxygen-derived free radicals play an important role in the pathogenesis of digestive system. The major underlying factor of ulcer formation is the generation of free radicals. Peptic ulcers causes due to an imbalance between aggressive factors (acid, pepsin, bile salts) and defensive factors (mucus, bicarbonate, blood flow, eptithelial cell restoration, and prostaglandins) mucosal blood flow, cell renewal and migration, nonenzymatic and enzymatic antioxidants and some growth factors. Flavonoids are having wide range of biological effects, including anti-ulcer activity. In recent years flavonoids have attracted the interest of researchers because they have promising powerful antioxidant properties that protect the human body from free radicals by their hydrogen donating abilities. Flavonoids can prevent injury caused by free radicals by Activation of antioxidant enzymes, Metal chelating activity, Inhibition of oxidative stress, and Increase in antioxidant properties of low molecular antioxidants. One of the most studied flavonoids is quercetin protects the gastrointestinal mucosa from acute lesions induced by various experimental models and against different necrotic agents. **Conclusion:** consumption of flavonoids, play a significant role in the prevention and treatment of peptic ulcer under oxidative stress conditions.

Keywords: gastrointestinal tract, peptic ulcer, pediatrics, antioxidants

* Corresponding author: Dr. R. M. Veerappan, PhD., Assistant Professor, Dept. of Biochemistry, Enathi Rajappa College of Arts and Science, Pattukottai, Tamilnadu, India, Email: drrmveera@gmail.com, Mo: 9965618963.
≠ M. Rajadurai, PhD., Research and Development Director.

INTRODUCTION

Peptic ulcer is a disease of chronic development, characterized by an imbalance between the factors that damages the mucosa and those for its protection, resulting in a lesion of the lining of the upper digestive tract (Nieto 2022). It has been one of the most prevalent diseases in the world, and some of its complications have been the major causes of morbidity and mortality (Sung et al., 2012).

Ulcers in the gastrointestinal tract could be divided into two common types according to location; ulcerative colitis (lower) and peptic ulcer (upper). Ulcerative colitis (UC) is an inflammatory bowel disease that primarily affects the colonic mucosa. In its most limited form it may be restricted to the distal rectum, while in its most extended form, the entire colon is involved (DiPiro et al., 2002).

Peptic ulcer disease (PUD) is an illness that affects a considerable number of people worldwide. It develops when there is an imbalance between the "aggressive" and "protective" factors at the luminal surface of the epithelial cells. Aggressive factors include Helicobacter pylori, HCl, pepsins, nonsteroidal anti-inflammatory drugs (NSAIDs), bile acids, ischemia, hypoxia, smoking and alcohol. While defensive factors include bicarbonate, mucus layer, mucosal blood flow, PGs and growth factors (Harold et al., 2007).

Peptic ulcer disease is a group of disorders characterized by the presence of ulcers in any portion of gastrointestinal tract (GIT) exposed to acid in sufficient concentration and duration. Although these ulcerations most commonly occur in the stomach (gastric ulcer), or small intestine (duodenal ulcer), this disease also includes Barrett ulcer of the esophagus (Barrett's esophagus or Barrett's metaplasia) and other upper GI ulcers (Helms et al., 2006). An ulcer is a crater like lesion in a membrane; ulcers that develop in areas of the GIT exposed to acidic gastric juice are called peptic ulcers (Tortora and Derrickson 2006). Word 'peptic' derives from the Greek term 'peptikos,' meaning related to digestion (Boston 2009).

1. EPIDEMIOLOGY

Indigestion and heartburn have been described for thousands of years, but it was only in the 16th century that the disease peptic ulcer was established by autopsy. One of the first autopsies - proven pyloric peptic ulcers was studied in 1586 by Donatus of Mantua. Bauhin, in 1679, concluded that inflammation of the stomach led to a gastric ulcer which then ruptured. The first known gastric hemorrhage was reported in 1704 (Baron 2000). First classification of stomach diseases came in 1793 from Matthew Baillie, with clear descriptions of acute inflammation (arsenic), trichobezoar, ulcer, perforation, and pyloric stenosis, scirrhous and ulcerated cancer. In 1817, patients with perforated gastric ulcer were reported in Dublin by Crampton and patients with perforated duodenal ulcer were reported in London by Travers, who also noted bleeding, stenosing and penetrating gastric ulcers (Crampton 1817). The first epidemiological study on peptic ulcer in North India was conducted in 1963 (Sharma and Ahuja 2003).

Approximately 5, 00,000 new cases and 4 million recurrences of peptic ulcer are reported each year, contributing to the approximately 10% of Americans developing peptic ulcer disease during their lifetime (Sonnenberg 1997). Complications of peptic ulcer disease, including perforation, bleeding, and obstruction, occur in up to 20% of cases; overall, gastric outlet obstruction may affect 5% - 12% of peptic ulcer patients (Barksdale and Schwartz 2002).

Peptic ulcer has a multifactor etiology. Environmental elements such as alcohol and nicotine can inhibit or reduce secretion of mucus and bicarbonate, increasing acid secretion. Genetic factors can influence, and children of parents with duodenal ulcer are three times more likely to have ulcer than the population (Lafortuna et al., 2004).

Peptic ulcers are defects in the GI mucosa that extend throughout the muscularis mucosa, and which are often associated with Helicobacter pylori (H. pylori) infection or with consumption of NSAIDs. As the prevalence of H. pylori infection has declined in Western countries, gastric ulcers have increasingly been linked to NSAID use, with acetylsalicylic acid (Yuan et al., 2006) being an important cause of morbidity and rising health care costs related to work loss, hospitalization, and outpatient care (Ramakrishnan and Salinas, 2007).

A systematic review of the worldwide literature estimated that the annual incidence of peptic ulcer disease ranged from 0.1 to 0.19 percent for physician-diagnosed and 0.01 to 0.17 percent when based upon hospitalized patients (Sung et al., 2009). Upper GI symptoms, such as dyspepsia, occur in 15% to 60% of NSAID users, twice as often as in individuals not taking NSAIDs. The prevalence of gastric or duodenal ulcers in patients taking NSAIDs regularly is approximately 15% to 30%. The annual incidence of NSAID-related clinical upper GI events (complicated and symptomatic ulcers) is approximately 2.5% to 4.5%, with the annual incidence of serious complications (severe bleeding, perforation, and obstruction) running about 1% to 1.5% (Laine, 2002).

2. Life Style Risk Factors

Several studies implied that modulating life style factors as dietary factors, controlling stress, reducing smoking and alcohol intake may directly prevent the initiation of gastric ulcers, especially in predisposed people. Some even suggested certain physical exercises to reduce the risk of ulcer formation or recurrence. Such exercises were seen to directly improve psychological and cardiovascular conditions and thus may be indirectly related to decreasing gastric ulcer development.

2.1. Diet

Diet rich in fibers may decrease the risk of developing gastric ulcers by about 50%. Fiber found in fruits and vegetables is particularly protective, as vitamin A contained in many of these foods may increase the benefit. Milk, previously thought to aid in decreasing ulcer symptoms, actually encourages the production of acid in the stomach, although moderate amounts (2-3 cups/day) appear to do no harm. However, yogurt may protect against gastric ulcer, as it contains probiotics. Coffee (caffeinated and decaffeinated), soft drinks and fruit juices with citric acid increase stomach acid production. Although no studies have proven that any of these drinks contribute to ulcers, consuming more than 3 cups of coffee per day may increase susceptibility to Helicobacter pylori infection (University of Maryland Medical Center website). Studies conducted on spices and peppers have yielded conflicting results.

In general, these substances should be used moderately, and should be avoided if they irritate the stomach. Some studies suggest that high amounts of garlic may have some protective properties against stomach cancer, although a recent study concluded that garlic offered no benefits against Helicobacter pylori and, in large amounts, can cause considerable gastrointestinal distress. Studies have shown that phenolic compounds in virgin olive oil may be effective against Helicobacter pylori infection. Although no vitamins have been shown to protect against Helicobacter pylori-induced ulcers, Helicobacter pylori appears to impair the absorption of vitamin C, which may play a role in the higher risk of stomach cancer.

Table 1. Recommended daily diet for peptic ulcer

Characteristics	Recommendations	
Daily energy needs (DEN)	Sufficient to maintain or recover the nutritional status 20-25 Kcal/Kg: weight loss 25-30 Kcal/Kg: maintenance 30-35 Kcal/Kg: weight gain31	
	Acute phase	Recovery phase
Carbohydrate (%)[29]	50-60	50-60
Protein (g/Kg/weight)	1.2	1.5
Lipid (%)	25-30	25-30
Zinc (mg)[13]	11	40
Selenium (μg)20	55	400
Vitamin A (μg)1	900	3000
Vitamin C (mg)	75	500
Vitamin B^{12} (μg)	2.4	2.4
Folic acid (μg)	400	400
Iron (mg)	45	45
Fibers (g)	20-30	20-30
Probiotics (UFC/day)	10^9 to 10^{11} lactic acid bacteria	$10^9$to 10^{11} lactic acid bacteria

Sources: Marrota& Floch (1991); Reis (2003); DRI'S (UL) and DRI'S (RDA) Mentz (1989).

2.2. Psychological Factors: Stress

As a body response to stress, many diseases may develop. There is debate as to whether psychological stress can influence the development of gastric ulcers. Some studies still suggest that stress may predispose a person to ulcers or prevent existing ulcers from healing. Some even believe that the relationship between stress and ulcers is so strong that people with ulcers should be treated for psychological conditions. Stress causes the digestive tract to slow down and more gastric acid is allowed to accumulate in the stomach. Increased stomach acidity may predispose to or aggravate an already present ulcer. Stress can also cause change in appetite, leading to over-eating or lack of appetite. Overeating causes the stomach to produce more acid while lack of appetite will subject the stomach mucosa to the acid produced in an empty stomach. Although psychological stress is no longer considered a direct cause of ulcers, it surely can delay the healing and aggravate already existing gastric ulcers. Physical stress, however, is definitely a risk factor for developing gastric ulcers, as in patients with injuries such as severe burns or patients undergoing major surgeries.

2.3. Smoking

Cigarette smoking appears to be a risk factor for the development and recurrence of gastric ulcer. The incidence of gastric ulcer is higher among smokers than non-smokers. Compared with non-smokers, people who smoke cigarettes are twice as likely to develop gastric ulcer. Smoking may lead to initiation of ulceration, slow ulcer healing and an increased risk of gastric ulcer recurrence. Smoking may have an inconsistent effect on gastric acid secretion; however it reduces prostaglandin and bicarbonate production, reduces mucosal blood flow, interferes with the action of histamine H2 receptor antagonists and accelerates gastric emptying of liquids. Cessation of smoking or reducing it is usually associated with the prompt relief of already existing gastric ulcer symptoms.

2.4. Excess Alcohol Intake

Alcohol increases the production of acid in the stomach, which may irritate an existing ulcer. Alcohol also relaxes the lower esophageal sphincter, allowing stomach contents to reflux back up into the esophagus, increasing the discomfort associated with gastric ulcer. Patients suffering of gastric ulcer should, thus, avoid taking alcohol. People predisposed to gastric ulcer may dilute alcoholic beverages to reduce their concentration, restrict the number of drinks to one or two a day, replace red wine with white wine of less toxic content, or better, have drinks which are non-alcoholic.

2.5. Helicobacter Pylori

Helicobacter pylori can survive in the highly acidic medium of the stomach by producing urease, an enzyme that generates ammonia to neutralize the acid. These bacteria then produce a number of toxins causing inflammation and damage to the stomach, leading to ulcers especially in predisposed individuals. The bacteria also alter certain immune factors that allow them to evade detection by the immune system and cause persistent inflammation. Even if ulcers do not develop, the bacterium is considered to be a major cause of active chronic inflammation in the stomach (gastritis). Helicobacter pylori together with unavoidable risk factors as genetics and concomitant diseases may contribute in gastric ulcer formation and the subsequent metaplasia and dysplasia leading to gastric cancer. Avoidance of risk factors, therapeutic intervention and some protective herbs can be employed to prevent the initiation of this sequence. Less than 15% of people infected with Helicobacter pylori develop gastric ulcer. Factors that trigger gastric ulcers in Helicobacter pylori carriers include genetic factors, which explain the higher incidence of development of ulcers in certain ethnicity. Another factor is abnormal immune response, which allows the bacteria to injure the stomach lining.

Frequent interruption of sleep is thought to weaken the immune system's ability to protect against harmful bacterial substances. Using certain medications as non-steroidal anti-inflammatory drugs or corticosteroids may contribute to higher infection rates of Helicobacter pylori. Patients with prior gastric ulcer, Zollinger-Ellison syndrome, congenital stomach malformations, malignant diseases such as mastocytosis and basophilic leukemia, head trauma, severe traumatic injuries, burns, radiation, or recently had major surgery are also more prone to Helicobacter pylori infection. Increased risk of Helicobacter pylori infection is seen among people who live in crowded places with unsanitary conditions. Some genetic predispositions for Helicobacter pylori infection cure rate may exist. One example is cytochrome P450-2C19 polymorphism that seems to predict the cure of Helicobacter pylori infection and predisposition to gastric ulcer (Lay and Lin, 2010). Therapeutic interventions to eradicate Helicobacter pylori are needed to prevent ulcer formation and its transformation to gastric cancer, one of the major complications of chronic gastric ulcer. Helicobacter pylori eradication therapy comprises a combination of two or more drugs including antimicrobials, proton pump inhibitors and gastro-protective agents. Several eradication methods were suggested. Dual eradication therapy using proton pump inhibitor with amoxicillin was tried (Graham et al., 2010).

2.6. Effects of NSAIDs on Gastric Mucosa

The pathophysiology of gastric injury associated with NSAID administration depends partly on cyclooxygenase inhibition and partly on cyclooxygenase-independent mechanisms, which result mainly from local direct actions (Scarpignato and Hunt, 2010). Cyclooxygenase blockade has been shown to increase the susceptibility of gastric mucosa to NSAID-induced injury by suppression of a number of prostaglandin-mediated protective functions. For instance, prostaglandins reduce the activation of neutrophils and the local release of reactive oxygen species (ROS). The production of prostacyclin by the endothelium of mucosal microcirculation is also highly relevant in ensuring a tonic inhibition of neutrophil adhesion. Therefore, NSAIDs can shift the mucosal balance toward the recruitment and endothelial adhesion of circulating neutrophils through the inhibition of prostaglandin biosynthesis (Whittle, 2002). Once adhered, neutrophils clog the microvasculature causing a local decrease in mucosal blood flow and a marked release of tissue damaging factors, including proteolytic enzymes and leukotrienes, which enhance the vascular tone, exacerbate tissue ischaemia, stimulate the production of ROS, and promote the destruction of intestinal matrix, leading to a severe degree of focal tissue necrosis, particularly in the presence of a low luminal pH (Whittle, 2002; Jimenez et al., 2004).

As anticipated above, cyclooxygenase-dependent inhibition of bicarbonate secretion contributes also to the gastric mucosal injury elicited by NSAIDs. Indeed, the secretion of bicarbonate ions in the mucus gel layer generates a pH gradient on the mucosal surface, thus providing a first line defense against luminal acid (Allen and Flemstrom, 2005). A number of studies have demonstrated the expression of bicarbonate/chloride ion exchangers in the apical membranes of gastric surface epithelial cells, and shown that cyclooxygenase-derived prostaglandins stimulate bicarbonate secretion via activation of EP1 receptors (Rossmann et al., 1999). Most NSAIDs are weakly acidic in nature and this property accounts for their local cyclooxygenase-independent injuring actions on the gastric mucosa. In the presence of gastric acidity, the undissociated lipophilic form of acidic NSAIDs can impair the hydrophobic surface barrier of the stomach. This transformation of the gastric mucosal surface from a non-wettable to a wettable state appears to be linked with the ability of acidic NSAIDs to destabilize the extracellular lining of zwitterionic phospholipids, particularly phosphatidylcholine, which are present within and on surface of the mucus gel layer (Lichtenberger et al., 2007). Previous studies have demonstrated that such an effect contributes significantly to NSAID-induced gastric injury in experimental models, and that it can persist for prolonged periods after discontinuation of NSAID administration (Lichtenberger, 2001). There is also consistent evidence that the protonophore actions of aspirin and other acidic NSAIDs take a significant part in the topical damage to gastric mucosa.

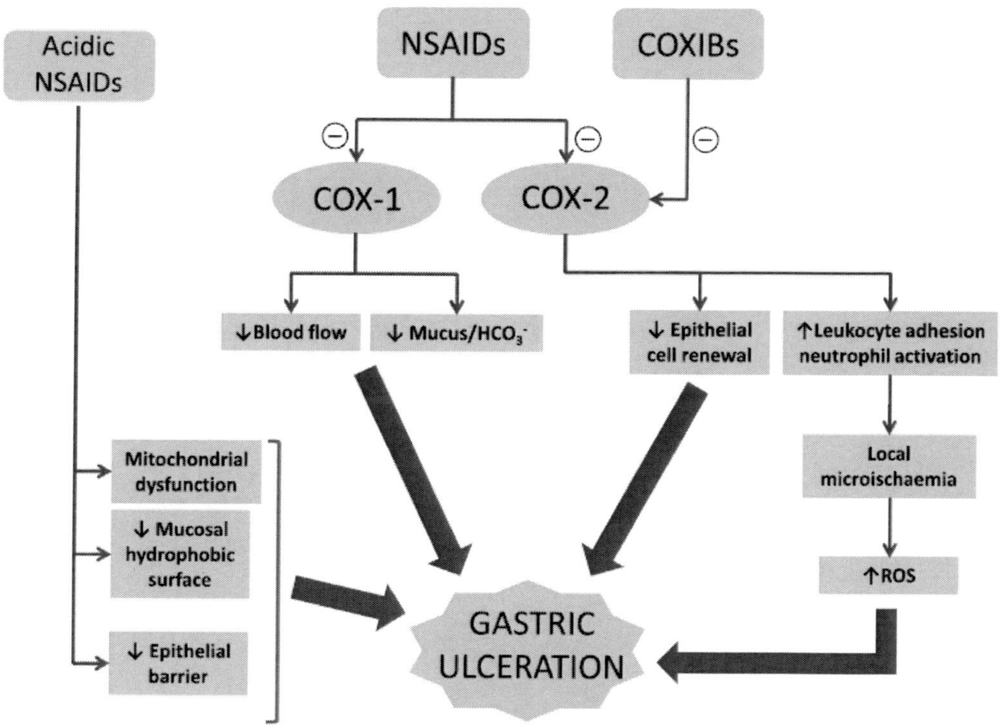

Figure 1. Pathophysiology of gastric injury induced by non-selective NSAIDs.

These anti-inflammatory drugs exert their detrimental effects on the gastric mucosa through two key mechanisms: simultaneous inhibition of COX-1 and COX-2, and direct topic cytotoxic effects. The topic injuring actions depend on the acidic chemical structure of NSAIDs. Coxibs do not harm the gastric mucosa owing to their ability to selectively inhibit COX-2, while not affecting the protective functions of COX-1. ROS: reactive oxygen species.

An additional mechanism, involved in the injurious effects of NSAIDs on gastrointestinal mucosa, is related to the detrimental actions of these drugs on the integrity of epithelial tight junctions, which are known to segregate the apical from basolateral cell surface domains, in order to establish cell polarity and provide a barrier function against the back diffusion of acid and other solutes through the paracellular space (Schneeberger and Lynch, 2004). It has been suggested that cyclooxygenase inhibition may be implicated in NSAID-induced alterations of intercellular epithelial permeability (Joh et al., 2003). However, recent evidence indicates that aspirin can elicit gastric epithelial barrier dysfunction through downregulation of claudin-7, a member of the claudin protein family, which plays important roles in the formation of tight junctions (Oshima et al., 2008).

Coxibs do not alter the integrity of normal gastric mucosa in preclinical models, and their clinical development was based on the assumption that COX-2 is not expressed in the gastric mucosa (Laine et al., 2008). However, this initial hypothesis has not been supported by subsequent observations, demonstrating the constitutive presence of both COX-1 and COX-2 in human and rodent gastric mucosa (Zimmermann et al., 1998). In addition, studies on COX-1-knockout mice have provided no evidence of spontaneous gastric injury and demonstrated the ability of NSAIDs to damage the gastric mucosa via COX-2-dependent mechanisms (Langenbach et al., 1995). Wallace et al. (2000) investigated further the functional roles of COX isoforms in the gastric mucosa, showing that COX-1-dependent prostaglandins are involved in the maintenance of mucus/bicarbonate secretion and blood flow, while COX-2 protects the mucosa from leucocyte endothelial adhesion and supports epithelial renewal. In addition, these Authors observed that selective COX-1 or COX-2 inhibitors did not damage the stomach when tested alone, while NSAIDs or the combined administration of COX-1 plus COX-2 selective inhibitors resulted in gastric erosions (Wallace et al., 2000). A schematic diagram illustrating the mechanisms of gastric mucosal injury exerted by cyclooxygenase inhibitors is provided in Figure. Overall, it is currently acknowledged that NSAIDs can impair gastric protection via a concomitant blockade of COX-1 and COX-2, while coxibs lack damaging actions on gastric mucosa by preserving COX-1-dependent prostaglandin production (Wallace, 2006).

3. Symptoms

Small ulcers may not cause any symptoms however some big ulcers can cause serious bleeding. Although there are common shared symptoms (Malagelada et al., 2007) which include:

- Feeling of fullness, unable to drink as much fluid.
- Hunger and an empty feeling in the stomach, often 1–3 h after a meal.
- Mild nausea (vomiting may relieve symptom).
- Pain or discomfort in the upper abdomen.
- Upper abdominal pain that wakes you up at night.

In addition to some symptoms in some cases:

- Bloody or dark stools
- Chest pain
- Fatigue
- Vomiting
- Weight loss.

4. TYPES OF PEPTIC ULCER

Ulceration of the gastrointestinal mucosa is caused by disruption of normal balance of the corrosive effect of gastric juice and the protective effect of mucus on gastric epithelial cells. On the basis of location, peptic ulcers are categorized as follows - Gastric ulcer: means occurrence of ulcer in stomach. These ulcers occur more generally in the older age group.

Duodenal ulcer: Occurrence of ulcer in the duodenum is referred as duodenal ulcer. These ulcers are more common than gastric ulcers. They occur commonly in younger individuals and are evenly distributed among various socio-economic groups. Duodenal ulcer patients have higher than normal levels of acid secretion rates (Marieb 2007). Depending on severity, peptic ulcers are also classified as: Acute peptic ulcers: These ulcers involve tissues to the depth of the sub mucosa. They may arise in the form of single or multiple lesions. They are found in many sites of stomach and in the first few centimeters of duodenum. Chronic peptic ulcers: These ulcers penetrate through the epithelial and muscle layers of stomach wall and may include the adjacent pancreas or liver. In majority of cases, they occur singly in the pyloric antrum of the stomach and in duodenum (Waugh A, Grant 2001).

5. REGULATION OF GASTRIC ACID SECRETION

Stomach secretes about 2.5 liters of gastric juice daily. The primary exocrine secretions are pepsinogens, from the chief or peptic cells, and hydrochloric acid and intrinsic factor from the parietal or oxyntic cells (Rang et al., 2003). Men secrete more acid than women. This can be explained partially by differences in body size (Richardson 1990). Gastric acid secretion is regulated by intricate central and peripheral mechanisms. Parietal cells have receptors for several stimulants of acid secretion and these cells possess a specific Hydrogen Potassium-ATPase enzyme (proton pump), which is responsible for the exchange of H+ for K+ ions across the apical surface of the parietal cells. The final process of acid transport per se rests with this enzyme. Three distinct but interdependent pathways deliver chemical messengers that stimulate acid secretion as shown in Figure 2 and are summarized in the following text.

- The neurocrine pathway, that acts through the transmitters such as acetylcholine.
- The paracrine pathway delivers tissue factors, such as histamine from enterochromaffin like cells.
- The endocrine pathway delivers hormones such as gastrin from antral G cells (Satoskar).

The receptors on the surface of parietal cell include H2 receptors responding to histamine released from specialized mast cells, receptors that are sensitive to the muscarinic effects of acetylcholine released from the vagus nerve and probably receptors responsive to endogenous circulating gastrin. A stimulated receptor modifies the activity of other receptors and at the same time releases an intracellular second messenger. Calcium ions and cyclic AMP are the principal second messengers, and these in turn activate the gastric proton pump situated near the luminal apex of the parietal cell (Tasman-Jones 1987).

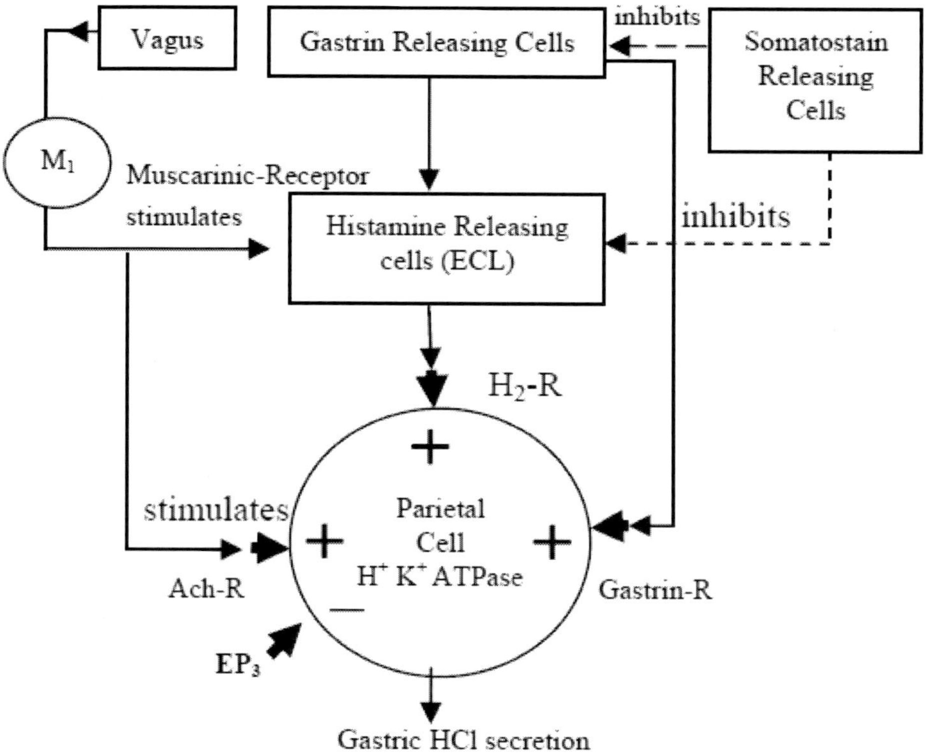

Figure 2. Mechanism involved in regulation of gastric acid secretion by the parietal cells R= Receptors, EP3= PG receptor for PGE2, M1= Muscarinic receptor, ECL= Enterochromaffin like cells, Ach = Acetylcholine, H2 = Histamine.

More data are also available on the role of GI hormones in the regulation of aggressive factors, especially gastric acid. In fact, the antral hormone gastrin was detected by its property to stimulate gastric acid secretion (Lamers 1988). In 1971, McGuigan and Trudeau observed that patients with duodenal ulcer had an exaggerated gastrin release in response to meals and suggested that the trophic effect of gastrin might be responsible for the increase in parietal cell mass characteristic of duodenal ulcer disease (McGuigan and Trudeau 1973). In the late 1980s, several investigators also examined meal-stimulated gastrin release in relation to H. pylori infection (Dore and Graham 2000).

6. Diagnostic Tests

Until early 20th century, the diagnosis of peptic ulcer was made on clinical grounds. In 1950's various flexible endoscopies revolutionized the direct visualization of ulcer disease (Nawaz 2008). Various diagnostic tests which are frequently employed by gastroenterologists depending upon patient's symptoms are summarized in the following text.

6.1. Esophagogastroduodenoscopy

This is a special test performed by gastroenterologists in whom a thin tube with a camera on the end is inserted through mouth into the GI tract to see stomach and small intestine. During this examination, the doctor may take a biopsy from the wall of stomach for detection of H. pylori (Rakesh Pahwa et al., 2009).

6.2. X-Ray

In this, patient is made to swallow a white chalky substance called barium that is visible on X-ray and then patient is made to lie down on a tilted examining table. The tilting distributes the barium evenly around upper digestive tract and X-ray can capture images at different angles. This allows the doctor to locate the ulcer and determine its type and severity (Nawaz 2008).

6.3. Computed Tomography

It is a rapid way to confirm an uncertain diagnosis of perforation and penetration associated with peptic ulcer disease. This study is carried out retrospectively to review the abdominal computed tomography findings in patients with peptic ulcer disease and correlated them with the clinical history, endoscopic and upper GIT series findings, and surgery when it is performed (Moller 2009).

7. Basal Acid Secretion

The normal human stomach secretes 2 to 5 mEq of HCI per hour in the fasting state. Since vagotomy decreases this basal secretion by some 85%, it has been presumed that vagal tone is important in determining the rate of basal acid production. However, Hz-receptor blockers have also been demonstrated to inhibit basal acid secretion by about 80%. One might conclude, therefore, that ambient histamine concentration in the interstitial fluid bathing the parietal cell as well as vagal tone are important in sustaining basal acid secretion.

Gastrin does not appear to play an important role in basal acid secretion in normal individuals. Patients with the Zollinger-Ellison syndrome, however, may secrete in excess of 10 mEq of acid per hour in the fasting state and, in this pathological condition, basal acid secretion is stimulated by gastrin. Critically ill patients, particularly those who are septic or have increased intracranial pressure, will also have increased "basal" acid secretion.

7.1. Stimulated Acid Secretion

Phasic vagal discharge in response to the thought, sight, or smell of food stimulates acid secretion directly by a cholinergic mechanism. Vagal discharge also inhibits gastric somatostatin release. Since somatostatin inhibits parietal cell secretion, inhibition of somatostatin release may be an additional mechanism by which the vagus stimulates acid secretion. The direct cholinergic action of the parietal cell has the more important role, however. The cephalic phase component of acid secretion, as determined by sham-feeding of normal individuals, is about 10 mEq/hr. This vagally controlled component of acid secretion represents approximately 40% of the maximal acid response to gastrin infusion. When food enters the stomach, distention triggers neural reflexes and gastrin release is activated. A technique of continuous intragastric titration can be used to estimate the amount of acid the stomach secretes in response to a meal. These estimates range from 15 to 25 mEq/hr, or approximately 75% of maximal response to exogenous gastrin or histamine. The reason that the maximal response to a meal is somewhat lower than the response to exogenous stimulants may be the concomitant release of somatostatin by food.

Gastrin is the most important mediator of the gastric phase of acid secretion. It is of interest that women secrete twice as much gastrin as men in response to food. Since their meal-stimulated acid response is equal to or less than that of men, the parietal cells in women may be less sensitive to gastrin. The reason for these differences is unknown. When food enters the small intestine, an additional mechanism for acid secretion is activated. The "intestinal phase hormone" OI "enterooxyntin" is released. Purification and chemical characterization of this putative hormone has not been accomplished. Physiological studies suggest that although enterooxyntin is a weak stimulant of acid secretion, it is capable of markedly augmenting the acid response to both submaximal and maximal doses of gastrin and histamine.

8. Diagnosis of Peptic Ulcer Disease

The diagnosis of peptic ulcer disease is usually based on clinical features and specific testing, although it is important to be aware that individual signs and symptoms are relatively unreliable.

8.1. Clinical Features

Typical symptoms of peptic ulcer disease include episodic gnawing or burning epigastric pain; pain occurring two to five hours after meals or on an empty stomach; and nocturnal pain relieved by food intake, antacids, or antisecretory agents. A history of episodic or epigastric pain, relief of pain after food intake, and nighttime awakening because of pain with relief following food intake are the most specific findings for peptic ulcer and help rule in the diagnosis.14 Less common features include indigestion, vomiting, loss of appetite, intolerance of fatty foods, heartburn, and a positive family history. The physical examination is unreliable in one study; tenderness to deep palpation reduced the likelihood of ulcer (Spiegelhalter 1987).

9. FREE RADICALS AND ANTIOXIDANT DEFENCES

Gastroduodenal disease is associated with a variety of risk factors, including tobacco smoke, hereditary influences, sex, diet, stress and the actions of drugs (NSAIDs) (Wallace, 1992). There is evidence that free radicals and antioxidants may be important components in the pathophysiology of gastroduodenal disease caused by many of these factors, implicating H. pylori. Free radicals have been involved in a wide spectrum of human diseases including other digestive disorders such as inflammatory bowel, toxic liver injury or pancreatic disease (Phull et al., 1995).

Table 2. Peptic Ulcer Disease in Different Populations

Population	Features
Children	Incidence: Rare; most ulcers occur between eight and 17 years of age; duodenal ulcer up to 30 times more common than gastric ulcer Cause: Helicobacter pylori infection contributory Presentation: Patients may present with poorly localized abdominal pain Testing: EGD should be performed if ulcer suspected; test and- treat strategy not recommended; H. pylori testing and treatment recommended only if ulcer is documented by EGD or contrast studies Treatment: Antisecretory agents Complications: 25 percent of bleeding duodenal ulcers may be silent; perforation and penetration rare
Older patients	Presentation: More likely to have painless ulcers; 50 percent present acutely (e.g., with perforation); may present with nonspecific complaints (e.g., confusion, restlessness, abdominal distention, fall) Complications: Perforations associated with mortality three times higher than in younger patients; hemorrhagic complications more likely (20 percent from silent ulcers); more likely to have continued bleeding and to need transfusions and surger
Patients with stress ulcers	Cause: Breakdown of mucosal protectants as a result of stress leads to splanchnic hypoperfusion and ulcer; risk factors include mechanical ventilation longer than 48 hours, burns, coagulopathy, moderate to severe trauma, head or spinal cord injury, liver failure, and organ transplantation Presentation: Patients may be asymptomatic or may develop bleeding or perforation Treatment: Early institution of PPI prophylaxis with oral or intravenous pantoprazole (Protonix) minimizes ulcer risk; histamine H2 blockers and sucralfate (Carafate) are other options for prophylaxis
Pregnant Women	Presentation: Ulcer symptoms milder and may improve during pregnancy; vomiting is nocturnal or postprandial and worse in third trimester Testing: Ultrasonography and EGD are safe diagnostic tests Treatment: Early, aggressive treatment with PPI recommended; misoprostol (Cytotec) contraindicated; H. pylori infection treated as usual; avoid tetracyclines throughout pregnancy and metronidazole (Flagyl) during first trimester Complications: Infrequent; hypotension treated vigorously to minimize placental risk of miscarriage, abruption, and preterm labor if complications ensue

EGD = esophagogastroduodenoscopy; PPI = proton pump inhibitor.

Table 3. Tests Used in the Diagnosis of Peptic Ulcer

EGD	Indicated in patients with evidence of bleeding, weight loss, chronicity, or persistent vomiting; those whose symptoms do not respond to medications; and those older than 55 years More than 90 percent sensitivity and specificity in diagnosing gastric and duodenal ulcers and cancers
Barium or diatrizoate meglumine and diatrizoate sodium (Gastrografin) contrast radiography (double-contrast hypotonic duodenography)	Indicated when endoscopy is unsuitable or not feasible, or if complications such as gastric outlet obstruction suspected Diagnostic accuracy increases with extent of disease; 80 to 90 percent sensitivity in detecting duodenal ulcers
Helicobacter pylori testing Serologic ELISA	Useful only for initial testing (sensitivity, 85 percent; specificity, 79 percent); cannot be used to confirm eradication
Urea breath test	More expensive Sensitivity, 95 to 100 percent; specificity, 91 to 98 percent; can be used to confirm eradication PPI therapy should be stopped for two weeks before test
Stool antigen test	Inconvenient but accurate (sensitivity, 91 to 98 percent; specificity, 94 to 99 percent) Can be used to confirm eradication
Urine-based ELISA and rapid urine test	Sensitivity, 70 to 96 percent; specificity, 77 to 85 percent Cannot be used to confirm eradication
Endoscopic biopsy	Culture (sensitivity, 70 to 80 percent; specificity, 100 percent), histology (sensitivity,> 95 percent; specificity, 100 percent), rapid urease (CLO) test (sensitivity, 93 to 97 percent; specificity, 100 percent)

EGD = esophagogastroduodenoscopy; ELISA= enzyme-linked immunosorbent assay; PPI= proton pump inhibitor; CLO= Campylobacter-like organism.**p1005.**

ROS can be defined as any chemical species capable of independent existence that contain one or more unpaired electrons in their outer orbital. Considering that the most stable molecular species have the electrons within their outer orbital arranged in pairs, free radicals tend to be unstable and highly reactive. Oxygen is the most abundant radical in biological systems. The seemingly paradoxical consequences of the beneficial and harmful effects of oxygen (O_2) have been shown for several decades. While more than 95% of the O_2 consumed by the aerobic organisms is fully reduced to water during the process of mitochondrial respiration, a small percentage (<5%) is converted to semireduced species such as superoxide anion radical (O2.-), hydrogen peroxide (H_2O_2) and hydroxyl radical (OH.). These species are collectively named "Reactive Oxygen Species or ROS." ROS are formed continuously as normal byproducts of cellular metabolism and several of their sources are mitochondrial oxidative phosphorylation, prostaglandin synthesis, non-mitochondrial respiratory burst of neutrophils, and possibly the inhibition of mitochondrial electron transport.

9.1. Antioxidant Defences

Free radicals play a number of physiological roles, but due to their high reactivity tend to attack the first biochemical component that they encounter inside cells, including macromolecules such as lipids, proteins or nucleic acids and bring about oxidative damage (Reilly et al., 1991). To avoid the oxidative damage, cells have development defense mechanisms to limit or prevent the toxicity caused by an excessive ROS activity. These defenses include non-enzymatic compounds such as vitamin (Vit) A, E and C, and enzymatic substances such as superoxide dismutase, catalase, glutathione peroxidase, and glutathione S-transferase; the latter two enzymes using glutathione (GSH) as a cofactor. Tissue damage may result from excessive ROS activity, from any deficiency in the defense mechanisms or from both of them. It is well known that low/moderate concentrations of ROS affect a great number of physiological functions. However, when ROS concentration exceeds the antioxidative capacity of an organism, cells enter a state termed oxidative stress, in which the excess ROS induces oxidative damage on cellular components. So, ROS have been implicated in the pathogenesis of many human sufferings like Parkinson's, Alzheimer, Huntington's diseases and many other neurodegenerative conditions (Halliwell B, 1989). There is sample evidence that free radicals and antioxidants may be important components in the pathophysiology of gastroduodenal disease, in fact, as noted above, an exacerbated synthesis of free radicals has been implicated in inflammatory bowel disease, toxic liver injury or pancreatic disorders.

9.2. Free Radicals, Antioxidant Defenses and Gastro Duodenal Diseases

A growing body of experimental and clinical evidence suggests that gastric mucosal damage by ethanol, NSAIDs and by H. pylori (Davies et al., 1994) is mediated through ROS (Phull et al., 1995). The cause could be the excessive synthesis, the deficiency of antioxidants defenses or the coexistence of both reasons. Most of the studies in this area have focused on the link between low intakes of fresh fruit and/or vegetables and gastric cancer. Several data show that exist an increased risk of gastric cancer specifically related to low intakes of Vit C and β-carotene or that β-carotene and Vit E levels were significantly lower in subjects with gastric dysplasia, a precursor of gastric cancer (Haenszel et al., 1985). Lower plasma levels of Vit A, C and E in subjects with chronic atrophic gastritis (Jaskiewicz et al., 1990) has been detected in a cross-sectional and prospective studies showing that an increased risk of gastric cancer is associated with low plasma β-tocoferol (Knekt et al., 1991), Vit C, β -carotene (Stahelin et al., 1991), retinal levels and with low selenium levels (van den Brandt et al., 1993). Respect to the selenium, some evidence suggests that the diet of dyspeptic patients is deficient in the micronutrient selenium, which is an important constituent of the antioxidant enzyme glutathione peroxidase (GSH-Px).

Involvement of ROS in the pathogenesis of gastric ulceration was first evident from the studies of ischemia-reoxygenation-induced gastric mucosal injury. Many of the works in this area have been performed by Davies et al. using a chemiluminiscence assay (Davies et al., 1994). They have shown significantly greater free radical production in duodenal mucosal biopsies from patients with duodenal ulceration and severe duodenitis that in patients with mild duodenitis or controls. This increased free radical activity in duodenal ulcer patients is accompanied by reduced levels of plasma glutathione (GSH). Recent studies show the same conclusions: there is an increased ROS production in gastric ulceration compared with gastric antral mucosa (Peng et al., 2008). Gastric ulceration also appears to be associated with increased plasma free radical activity and lower levels of Vit C and E, but not with superoxide dismutase (SOD) or catalase. ROS also decrease the level of endogenous antioxidants such as GSH, α-tocopherol and ascorbate, and make the mucosa more prone to oxidative damage.

Moreover, ROS may play an important role in gastric ulceration induced by several kinds of stress. The pathogenesis of gastric mucosal lesions by water immersion restraint stress and burn shock in rat is associated with increased lipid peroxidation. Furthermore, cold restraint stress has been shown to alter the level of various damaging and cytoprotective factors of rat gastric mucosa to cause gastric ulceration (Das et al., 1997). It was reported (Yoshikawa et al., 1989) that the gastric mucosal injury induced by ischemia-reperfusion is avoided after administration of SOD and catalase, indicating the role of lipid peroxidation and ROS in the origin of the lesion. Similarly, astaxanthin has been shown to provide protection against naproxen-induced and stress-induced gastric ulceration by reducing the level of lipid peroxides and free radicals indicating again the role of ROS in gastric damage (Oh et al., 2005). The inhibitory effect of diacerein on indomethacin-induced gastric ulceration by inhibition of neutrophil activation (Tamura et al., 2001), and consequently the suppression of ROS production by these cells, leads to similar conclusions.

Furthermore, Davies et al. (Davies et al., 1994) also detected higher levels of ROS in antral mucosa infected with H. pylori and they affirmed that there is no evidence for ROS participation in gastric mucosal injury in cases not related to H. pylori infection. Other works show that ROS levels are directly correlated with the infective load of H. pylori (Zhang et al., 2007) and lipid peroxidation has been also shown to be increased in H. pylori-positive gastric mucosa. But although it has been established a clear association between bacterial infection and impaired synthesis of ROS, many other clinical data suggest that other factors inherent to host conditions (stress, diet, tobacco, hygiene, genetics...) contribute to the pathogenesis of this infection (Oh et al., 2005). It should be noted that some of these factors, including ingested food and tobacco smoke, directly influence in mucosal oxidative status, since they expose the gastric epithelium to the ROS that they generate within the gastric lumen in a sustained manner.

10. Treatment with Synthetic Drugs

Management of peptic ulcer disease continues to evolve because of the emergence of various novel therapeutic agents, advancements in several operative techniques and pharmacological oriented strategies. With the development of various therapies, as well as recognition and understanding of H. pylori infection along with mechanism, the medical management of ulcer has been largely successful (Barksdale AR, Schwartz 2000). Several drugs are extensively used for the reduction of acidity in peptic ulcer, gastro esophageal reflux disease and in many form of gastritis. Enormous drugs are also employed in the regimens for treating H. pylori infection. Various therapeutic agents utilized in management of ulcer and in the regimens for treating H. pylori infection includes H2 blockers, proton pump inhibitors, antacids, prostaglandins etc.

Several classes of pharmacological agents have proved to be effective in the management of the acid peptic disorders. These groups include: antacids (aluminum hydroxide, magnesium trisilicate), acid suppressive agents (Antisecretory drugs) which include proton pump H+/K+ ATPase inhibitors (omeprazole, lanzoprazole), histamine H2 receptor antagonist (cimetidine, ranitidine) and anticholinergic (M1) (pirenzepine), cytoprotective agents (sucralfate and prostaglandin analogs (misoprostol), antimicrobials for eradication of H. pylori (amoxicillin, clarithromycin) and Triple therapy (one week triple therapy consisting of a proton pump inhibitor such as Omeprazole and the antibiotics Clarithromycin and Amoxicillin) (Waller et al., 2005; Katzung, 2004).

A widespread search has been launched to identify new anti-ulcer therapies from natural sources to replace currently used drugs of doubtful efficacy and safety. Herbs, medicinal plants, spices, vegetables and crude drug substances are considered to be a potential source to control various diseases including gastric ulcer and ulcerative colitis. In the scientific literature, a large number of medicinal plants and their secondary metabolites with anti-ulcer potential have been reported.

Despite the remarkable achievements in various management strategies, few issues associated with this disease still remain unaddressed or partially defined. Exciting opportunities along with advanced pharmacotherapeutic approaches must be developed, and the mechanism involved in regulation of gastric acid secretion and H. pylori pathogenicity should be elucidated more evidently which holds great potential for the treatment in the future. Furthermore, innovative research should also attempt to solve the enigma related with various factors and causes on the prevalence of this disease. Extensive experiments must be carried out to establish the mechanisms and for development of new and safe drugs with advanced therapeutic interventions. Moreover, explorations in this field have to address the different etiologies of gastric and duodenal ulcer and other acid-peptic conditions as well as attempting to cure the disease rather than simply heal the ulcer. Advanced research on various novel gastroretentive dosage forms with several new antimicrobial agents for eradication of H. pylori infection would lead to management of complicated ulcer cases; thereby creating an exciting revolution in treatment strategies. Understanding and further study of complete genome of the bacterium should also aid in the development of most effective genetically engineered therapeutic regimens in times to come. Such knowledge might facilitate the design of specific vaccination regimens, allowing exclusive tissue-specific targeting drug delivery. New medical and pharmaceutical developments should also be conducted in close collaboration with gastroenterologist surgeons utilizing innovative surgical approaches.

Peptic ulcers result from an imbalance between factors that maintain mucosal integrity with high concentration of acid and the proteolytic enzyme pepsin. Patients with peptic ulcer frequently have symptoms of indigestion and bowel dysfunction or acid related symptoms of pain and dyspepsia. *H. pylori* colonization of gastric mucosa is also recognized to be strongly associated with both chronic active gastritis and peptic ulcer disease. Enormous potential benefits of *H. pylori* eradication in the management of peptic ulcer disease will provide the necessary stimulus for continued research into the treatment of this infection. It is emphasized that suitable management and treatment strategies along with proper diagnosis of peptic ulcer are imperative considerations in decreasing patient morbidity and efficient eradication of the bacterium.

References

Allen, A. and Flemström, G. Gastroduodenal mucus bicarbonate barrier: protection against acid and pepsin. *Am J Physiol Cell Physiol.* 2005 Jan;288(1):C1-19.

Barksdale AR, Schwartz RW. Current management of perforated peptic ulcer. *Curr. Surg.* 2000; 57(6): 594-599.

Barksdale AR, Schwartz RW. The evolving management of gastric outlet obstruction from peptic ulcer disease. *Curr Surg.* 2002; 59(4): 404-409.

Baron JH. Peptic ulcer. *MT Sinai J Med.* 2000; 67 (1): 58-62.

Boston MA. Peptic ulcer disease. http://knol.google.com/k/peptic-ulcer-disease online publication 7 July 2008. Accessed 15 Oct 2009.

Crampton J. Rupture of the stomach and escape of its contents into the cavity of the abdomen. *Med Chir Trans.* 1817; 8: 228- 231.

Das D, Bandyopadhyay D, Bhattacharjee M, Banerjee RK. Hydroxyl radical is the major causative factor in stress-induced gastric ulceration. Free Radic Biol Med. 1997;23(1):8-18.

Davies GR, Simmonds NJ, Stevens TR, Sheaff MT, Banatvala N, Laurenson IF, Blake DR, Rampton DS. Helicobacter pylori stimulate antral mucosal reactive oxygen metabolite production *in vivo*. *Gut.* 1994 Feb; 35(2): 179–185.

DiPiro J.T., Talbert R.L., Yee G.C., Matzke G.R., Wells B.G., Posey L.M., 2002. In: *Pharmacotherapy: A Pathophysiologic Approach.* Fifth eds. The McGraw-Hill companies, pp. 625–669 (Chapter 34).

Dore MP, Graham DY. Pathogenesis of duodenal ulcer disease: The rest of the story. Bailliere's *Clin Gastroenterol.* 2000; 14(1): 97-107.

Graham DY; Javed SU, Keihanian S, Abudayyeh S, Opekun, AR. Dual proton pump inhibitor plus amoxicillin as an empiric anti-H. pylori therapy: studies from the United States. *J. Gastroenterol.* 2010 Aug;45(8):816-20.

Haenszel W, Correa P, Lopez A, Cuello C, Zarama G, Zavala D, Fontham E. Serum micronutrient levels in relation to gastric pathology. *Int J Cancer.* 1985 Jul 15;36(1):43-8.

Halliwell B, G. J. (1989). Free radicals in biology and Medicine. 2nd eds. Clarendon Press,

Harold, Kalant, Grant, Denis M., Mitchel, Jane, 2007. In: Principles of Medical Pharmacology, seventh eds. Elsevier Canada Ltd., pp.557- 559.

Helms RA, Herfindal ET, Quan DJ, Gourley DR. Peptic Ulcer Disease and Gastroesophageal Reflux Disease. In: Text Book of Therapeutics Drug and Disease Management. 8th eds, Lippincott Williams and Wilkins Publication, Philadelphia, 2006, pp. 1227-1256.

Institute of Medicine. DRIs – Dietary Reference Intakes: Applications in Dietary Planning. National Academy Press. Washington, D.C. 2003. [*Acesso em* 2012 out 30]. Disponível em: URL: http://www. nap.edu/.

Jaskiewicz K, Van Helden PD, Wiid IJ, Steenkamp HJ, Van Wyk MJ. Chronic atrophic gastritis, gastric pH, nitrites and micronutrient levels in a population at risk for gastric carcinoma. *Anticancer Res.* 1990 May-Jun;10(3):833-6.

Jimènez, M.D., Martin MJ, Alarcon de la Lastra C, Bruseghini L, Esteras A, Herrerias JM, and Motilva V. Role of L-arginine in ibuprofen-induced oxidative stress and neutrophil infiltration in gastric mucosa. *Free Radic Res.* 2004 Sep;38(9):903-11.

Joh, T, Takezono, Y, Oshima, T, Sasaki, M, Seno, K, Yokoyama, Y, Ohara, H, Nomura, T. Alexander, JS and Itoh, M. The protective effect of rebamipide on paracellular permeability of rat gastric epithelial cells. *Aliment Pharmacol Ther.* 2003 Jul;18 Suppl 1:133-8.

Katzung BG, (2004). Basic and clinical pharmacology, ninth eds. Mc Graw-Hill Companies, p. 1009.

Knekt P, Aromaa A, Maatela J, Aaran RK, Nikkari T, Hakama M, Hakulinen T, Peto R, Teppo L. Vitamin E and cancer prevention. *Am J Clin Nutr.* 1991;53(1) 283S-286S.

Kurata JH, Nogawa AN. Meta analysis of risk factors for peptic ulcers: Nonsteroidal anti-inflammatory drugs, Helicobacter pylori and smoking. *J Clin Gastroenterol.* 1997; 24: 2-17

Lafortuna CL, Agosti F, Marinone PG, Marazzi N, Sartorio A. The relationship between body composition and muscle power output in men and women with obesity. *J Endocrinol Invest.* 2004;27:854-861.

Laine L, Takeuchi K, Tarnawski A. Gastric mucosal defense and cytoprotection: bench to bedside. *Gastroenterology.* 2008 Jul;135(1):41-60.

Laine L. The gastrointestinal effects of nonselective NSAIDs and COX-2-selective inhibitors. *Semin Arthritis Rheum.* 2002 Dec;32(3 Suppl 1):25-32.

Lamers CBHW. Hormonal regulation of gastric acid in peptic ulcer disease. *Scand J Gastroenterol.* 1988; 23(1): 5-10.

Langenbach, R, Morham SG, Tiano HF, Loftin CD, Ghanayem BI, Chulada PC, Mahler JF, Lee CA, Goulding EH, Kluckman KD, Kim HS, Smithies O. Prostaglandin synthase 1 gene disruption in mice reduces arachidonic acid-induced inflammation and indomethacin-induced gastric ulceration. *Cell.* 1995 Nov 3;83(3):483-92.

Lay CS, Lin CJ. Correlation of CYP2C19 genetic polymorphisms with helicobacter pylori eradication in patients with cirrhosis and peptic ulcer. *J. Chin Med. Assoc.* 2010 Apr;73(4):188-93.

Lichtenberger LM, Romero JJ, Dial EJ. Surface phospholipids in gastric injury and protection when a selective cyclooxygenase-2 inhibitor (Coxib) is used in combination with aspirin. *Br J Pharmacol.* 2007 Apr;150(7):913-9.

Lichtenberger, L.M. Romero JJ and Dial EJ. Where is the evidence that cyclooxygenase inhibition is the primary cause of nonsteroidal anti-inflammatory drug (NSAID)-induced gastrointestinal injury? Topical injury revisited. *Biochem Pharmacol.* 2001 Mar 15;61(6):631-7.

Malagelada, J.R., Kuipers, E.J., Blaser, M.J., 2007. Acid peptic disease: clinical manifestations, diagnosis, treatment, and prognosis. In: Goldman, L., Ausiello, D., (Eds.), *Cecil Medicine.* 23rd eds. Philadelphia, PA: Saunders Elsevier (chap. 142).

Marieb EN. Peptic Ulcers. In: Anatomy and Physiology. 8th eds. South Asia, 2007, pp. 472-474.

Marotta K, Floch MH. Diet and nutrition in ulcer disease. Med Clin North Am. 1991 Jul;75(4):967-79.

McGuigan JE, Trudeau WL. Differences in rates of gastrin release in normal persons and patients with duodenal ulcer disease. *N Engl J Med.* 1973; 288: 64-66.

Mentz LA, Schekel EP. Medicinal Plants: Coherence and Confidence of Therapeutic Indications. Caderno de farmácia. 1989;5:93-119.

Moller MH, Adamsen S, Wojdemann M, Moller AN. Perforated peptic ulcer: How to improve outcome? *Scand J Gastroenterol.* 2009; 44(1): 15-22.

Nawaz M, Jehanzaib M, Khan K, Zari M. Role of barium meal examination in diagnosis of peptic ulcer. *J Ayub Med Coll.* 2008; 20(4): 59-61.

Nieto Y.B. Therapeutic protocol of peptic ulcer. *Medicine.* 2012;11:179-82.

Oh TY, Yeo M, Han SU, Cho YK, Kim YB, Chung MH, Kim YS, Cho SW, Hahm KB. Synergism of Helicobacter pylori infection and stress on the augmentation of gastric mucosal damage and its prevention with alpha-tocopherol. *Free Radic Biol Med.* 2005 Jun 1;38(11):1447-57.

Oshima T, Miwa H, Joh T. Aspirin induces gastric epithelial barrier dysfunction by activating p38 MAPK via claudin-7. *Am J Physiol Cell Physiol.* 2008 Sep;295(3):C800-6 Oxford, pp. 416.

Peng YC, Hsu CL, Tung CF, Chou WK, Huang LR, Hung DZ, Hu WH, Yang DY. Chemiluminescence assay of mucosal reactive oxygen species in gastric cancer, ulcer and antral mucosa. *Hepatogastroenterology*, 2008 Mar-Apr;55(82-83):770-3.3,

Phull PS, Green CJ, Jacyna MR. A radical view of the stomach: the role of oxygen-derived free radicals and anti-oxidants in gastroduodenal disease. *Eur J Gastroenterol Hepatol.* 1995 Mar;7(3):265-74.

Rakesh Pahwa, Neeta, Vipin Kumar, Kanchan Kohli. Clinical Manifestations, Causes and Management Strategies of Peptic Ulcer Disease. *Int. J. Pharm. Sci. Drug Res.* 2010; 2(2): 99-106,

Ramakrishnan K, Salinas RC. Peptic ulcer disease. *Am Fam Physician.* 2007 Oct 1;76(7):1005-1012.

Rang HP, Dale MM, Ritter JM, Moore PK. Diseases of the Stomach and Duodenum. In: Pharmacology. 5th eds, Churchill Livingstone Publication, Philadelphia, 2003, pp. 368-372.

Reilly PM, Schiller HJ, Bulkley GB. Pharmacologic approach to tissue injury mediated by free radicals and other reactive oxygen metabolites. *Am J Surg, Vol.* 1991 Apr;161(4):488-503.

Reis NT. clinical nutrition: digestive system. 1 ed. Rio de Janeiro: Rubio; 2003.

Richardson CT. Role of aggressive factors in the pathogenesis of peptic ulcer disease. *Scand J Gastroenterol.* 1990; 25(1): 37- 43.

Rossmann, H, Bachmann O, Vieillard-Baron D, Gregor M, Seidler U. Na+/HCO3 cotransport and expression of NBC1 and NBC2 in rabbit gastric parietal and mucous cells. *Gastroenterology.* 1999 Jun;116(6):1389-98.

Satoskar RS, Bhandarkar SD, Ainapure SS. Pharmacotherapy of Peptic Ulcer Disease. In: Pharmacology and Pharmacotherapeutics. 18th eds, Popular Prakashan, Mumbai. pp. 601 - 616.

Scarpignato C, Hunt, RH. Nonsteroidal antiinflammatory drug-related injury to the gastrointestinal tract: clinical picture, pathogenesis, and prevention. *Gastroenterol Clin North Am.* 2010 Sep;39(3):433-64.

Schneeberger, E.E. and Lynch, R.D. The tight junction: a multifunctional complex. *Am J Physiol Cell Physiol.* 2004 Jun;286(6):C1213-28.

Sharma MP, Ahuja V. Current management of acid peptic disorders. *J Indian Acad Clin Med.* 2003; 4(3): 228-233.

Sonnenberg A, Everhart JE. Health impact of peptic ulcer in the United States. *Am J Gastroenterol*. 1997; 92: 614-620.

Spiegelhalter DJ, Crean GP, Holden R, Knill-Jones RP. Taking a calculated risk: predictive scoring systems in dyspepsia. *Scand J Gastroenterol Suppl*. 1987;128:152-60.

Stähelin HB, Gey KF, Eichholzer M, Lüdin E.. Beta-carotene and cancer prevention: the Basel Study. *Am J Clin Nutr*. 1991;53(1) 265S-269S.

Sung JJ, Kuipers EJ, El-Serag HB. Systematic review: the global incidence and prevalence of peptic ulcer disease. *Aliment Pharmacol Ther*. 2009 May 1;29(9):938-46.

Sung JJ, Tsoi KK, Ma TK, Yung MY, Lau JY, Chiu PW. Causes of mortality in patients with peptic ulcer bleeding: a prospective cohort study of 10,428 cases. *Journal Gastroenterol*. 2012;105:84-89.

Tamura T, Yokoyama T, Ohmori K. Effects of diacerein on indomethacin induced gastric ulceration. *Pharmacology*. 2001;63(4):228-33.

Tasman-Jones C. Pathogenesis of peptic ulcer disease and gastritis: Importance of aggressive and cytoprotective factors. *Scand J Gastroenterol*. 1986; 21(1): 1-5.

Tortora GJ, Derrickson B. Peptic Ulcer Disease. In: *Principles of Anatomy and Physiology*. 11th eds, Wiley Publication, USA, 2006, pp. 942-943.

van den Brandt PA, Goldbohm RA, van 't Veer P, Bode P, Dorant E, Hermus RJ, Sturmans F. A prospective cohort study on toenail selenium levels and risk of gastrointestinal cancer. *J Natl Cancer Inst*.1993;85 (3) 224-229.

Wallace JL. COX-2: a pivotal enzyme in mucosal protection and resolution of inflammation. *Scientific World J*. 2006 May 25;6:577-88.

Wallace JL. Non-steroidal anti-inflammatory drug gastropathy and cytoprotection: pathogenesis and mechanisms re-examined. *Scand J Gastroenterol Suppl*. 1992; 192:3-8.

Wallace, J.L, McKnight W, Reuter BK, Vergnolle N. NSAID-induced gastric damage in rats: requirement for inhibition of both cyclooxygenase 1 and 2. *Gastroenterology*. 2000 Sep;119(3):706-14.

Waller DG, Renwick AG, Hillier K, (2005). Medical Pharmacology and Therapeutics, second eds. El Sevier Limited, pp. 347–401.

Waugh A, Grant A. Diseases of the Stomach. In: Ross and Wilson Anatomy and Physiology in Health and Illness. 9th eds, Churchill Livingstone Publication, Spain, 2001, pp. 321-324.

Whittle, BJ. Gastrointestinal effects of nonsteroidal anti-inflammatory drugs. *Fundam Clin Pharmacol*. 2003 Jun;17(3):301-13.

Yoshikawa, T, Ueda S, Naito Y, Takahashi S, Oyamada H, Morita Y, Yoneta T, Kondo M. Role of oxygen-derived free radicals in gastric mucosal injury induced by ischemia or ischemia-reperfusion in rats. *Free Radic Res Commun*. 1989;7(3-6):285-91.

Zhang H, Fang DC, Lan CH, Luo YH. Helicobacter pylori infection induces apoptosis in gastric cancer cells through the mitochondrial pathway. *J Gastroenterol Hepatol*. 2007 Jul;22(7):1051-6.

Zimmermann, K.C, Sarbia M, Schrör K, Weber AA. Constitutive cyclooxygenase-2 expression in healthy human and rabbit gastric mucosa. *Mol Pharmacol*. 1998 Sep;54(3):536-40.

INDEX

B

C

D

E

F

G

H

I

J

K

L

M

N

O

P

Q

R

S

T

U

V

W

X

Y

Z